Beyond One Health

Beyond One Health

From Recognition to Results

Edited by John A. Herrmann and Yvette J. Johnson-Walker

University of Illinois, IL, USA

WILEY Blackwell

Registered Office(s)
John Wiley & Sons, Inc., 111 River Street, Hoboken, NJ 07030, USA

Editorial Office
111 River Street, Hoboken, NJ 07030, USA

For details of our global editorial offices, customer services, and more information about Wiley products visit us at www.wiley.com.

Wiley also publishes its books in a variety of electronic formats and by print-on-demand. Some content that appears in standard print versions of this book may not be available in other formats.

Library of Congress Cataloging-in-Publication Data

9781119194491 [paperback]

Cover design: Wiley
Cover image: Courtesy of John Herrmann

Set in 10/12pt Warnock by SPi Global, Pondicherry, India

Printed in the United States of America

10 9 8 7 6 5 4 3 2 1

For Wanda, who always knew the way; and for Anne and Kate, who are my guideposts.

J.A. Herrmann

For Mom, Lauren, and Lamar – my shelter from the storm; and for Ikenna, Ndidi, and Amaya – my windows of hope.

Y.J. Johnson-Walker

Contents

List of Contributors

Jonathan D. Alpern, MD
Infectious Disease Fellow
Department of Medicine, Division of
Infectious Diseases & International
Medicine
School of Medicine
University of Minnesota
Minneapolis, Minnesota, USA

**Casey Barton Behravesh, MS, DVM, DrPH,
DACVPM**
Captain, US Public Health Service
Director, One Health Office
National Center for Emerging and Zoonotic
Infectious Diseases
Centers for Disease Control and Prevention
Atlanta, Georgia, USA

Val R. Beasley, DVM, PhD, Diplomate ABVT
Professor of Veterinary, Wildlife, and
Ecological Toxicology
Department of Veterinary and Biomedical
Sciences
College of Agricultural Sciences
The Pennsylvania State University
University Park, Pennsylvania, USA

Matteo Convertino, PhD, PE
Assistant Professor
Division of Environmental Health Sciences
& PH Informatics
School of Public Health
University of Minnesota
Minneapolis, Minnesota, USA

Meggan Craft, PhD
Assistant Professor of Disease Ecology
Department of Veterinary Population
Medicine
College of Veterinary Medicine
University of Minnesota
Minneapolis, Minnesota, USA

William J. Craven, JD
Chief Consultant
California State Senate
Sacramento, California, USA

Timur Durrani, MD, MPH, MBA
Co-Director of the Western States Pediatric
Environmental Health Specialty Unit
Assistant Clinical Professor
University of California at San Francisco
School of Medicine
San Francisco, California, USA

Robert V. Ellis, MD, FAAFP
Associate Professor
University of Cincinnati College of
Medicine
Cincinnati, Ohio, USA

Thomas R. Gillespie, PhD
Associate Professor
Departments of Environmental Sciences &
Environmental Health
Emory University & Rollins School of Public
Health
Math and Science Center
Georgia, USA

Marja-Liisa Hänninen, DVM
Professor Emeritus
Department of Food Hygiene and
Environmental Health
University of Helsinki
Helsinki, Finland

John A. Herrmann, DVM, MPH, DACT
Clinical Associate Professor
Director, DVM/MPH Joint Degree Program
Center for One Health Illinois
College of Veterinary Medicine
University of Illinois at Urbana-Champaign
Urbana, Illinois, USA;
Division Affiliate
Epidemiology and Biostatistics
School of Public Health
University of Illinois at Chicago
Chicago, Illinois, USA

Ronald C. Hershow, MD
Director, Division of Epidemiology and
Biostatistics
School of Public Health
University of Illinois at Chicago
Chicago, Illinois, USA

Ari Hörman, DVM, PhD, MPH
Department of Food Hygiene and
Environmental Health
University of Helsinki
Helsinki, Finland

Daniel Hryhorczuk, MD, MPH, FACMT
Clinical Professor of Medical Toxicology
Director, Environmental Health, Center for
Global Health
College of Medicine
University of Illinois at Chicago
Chicago, Illinois, USA;
Professor Emeritus
Environmental and Occupational Health
Sciences and Epidemiology
School of Public Health
University of Illinois at Chicago
Chicago, Illinois, USA

**William D. Hueston, DVM, PhD, Diplomate
ACVPM, Epidemiology Specialty**
Professor Emeritus
College of Veterinary Medicine and
School of Public Health

Global Leadership Programs
Center for Animal Health and Food Safety
University of Minnesota
Minneapolis, Minnesota, USA

Yvette J. Johnson-Walker DVM, MS, PhD
Clinical Epidemiologist
Center for One Health Illinois
University of Illinois Urbana-Champaign
College of Veterinary Medicine
Urbana, Illinois, USA

Laura H. Kahn, MD, MPH, MPP
Research Scholar
Program on Science and Global Security
Woodrow Wilson School of Public and
International Affairs Princeton University
Princeton, New Jersey, USA;
Co-Founder, One Health Initiative

John B. Kaneene DVM, MPH, PhD, FAES, FAVES
University Distinguished Professor of
Epidemiology and Public Health
Director, Center for Comparative
Epidemiology
Michigan State University
East Lansing, Michigan, USA

Shaun Kennedy, PhD
President and CEO
Food Systems Institute
St Paul, Minnesota;
Adjunct Associate Professor
College of Veterinary Medicine, University
of Minnesota
Minneapolis, Minnesota, USA

**Sandra L. Lefebvre, BA, BSc (Hons
Neuroscience), DVM, PhD**
Assistant Editor, JAVMA and AJVR
American Veterinary Medical Association
Schaumburg, Illinois, USA

Jeffrey M. Levengood, PhD
Illinois Natural History Survey, Prairie
Research Institute
University of Illinois at Urbana-Champaign
Urbana, Illinois, USA

Thomas P. Meehan, DVM
Vice-President of Veterinary Services
Chicago Zoological Society
Adjunct Clinical Assistant Professor
Veterinary Clinical Medicine
College of Veterinary Medicine
Brookfield Zoo
University of Illinois at Urbana-Champaign
Brookfield, Illinois, USA

Yvonne Nadler, DVM, MPH
Program Manager
Zoo and Aquarium All Hazards
Preparedness, Response, and Recovery
Fusion Center
Silver Spring, Maryland, USA

Megin Nichols, DVM, MPH, DACVPM
Lead, Enteric Zoonoses Activity
Division of Foodborne, Waterborne, and
Environmental Diseases
National Center for Emerging and Zoonotic
Infectious Diseases (NCEZID)
Centers for Disease Control and Prevention
Atlanta, Georgia, USA

Kenneth E. Nusbaum, DVM, PhD
Professor Emeritus
College of Veterinary Medicine
Auburn University
Auburn, Alabama, USA

Kevin O'Brien, PhD
Director
Illinois Sustainable Technology Center
Prairie Research Institute
University of Illinois at Urbana-Champaign
Urbana, Illinois, USA

Robert H. Poppenga, DVM, PhD, DABVT
Professor
CAHFS Toxicology Laboratory
School of Veterinary Medicine
University of California
West Health Sciences Drive
Davis, California, USA

Cheryl Robertson, PhD, MPH, RN, FAAN
Associate Professor
Chair, Population Health and Systems
Cooperative Unit
School of Nursing

University of Minnesota
Minneapolis, Minnesota, USA

Innocent B. Rwego, BVM, MSc, PhD
Assistant Professor
Department of Veterinary Population
Medicine
College of Veterinary Medicine
University of Minnesota
Minneapolis, Minnesota, USA;
Senior Technical Lead for Africa
USAID One Health Workforce Project
University of Minnesota-Makerere
University Uganda Hub
Kampala, Uganda

Christopher A. Shaffer, PhD
Assistant Professor
Department of Anthropology
Grand Valley State University
Allendale, Michigan, USA

William Stauffer, MD, MSPH, FASTMH
Professor
Department of Medicine, Division of
Infectious Diseases & International
Medicine
Department of Pediatrics, Infectious
Diseases
School of Medicine and Public Health
University of Minnesota
Minneapolis, Minnesota, USA

Lauren Stevenson, MHS
Assessment Epidemiologist
Division of Foodborne, Waterborne, and
Environmental Diseases
National Center for Emerging and Zoonotic
Infectious Diseases
Centers for Disease Control and Prevention,
Atlanta, Georgia, USA

Robert V. Tauxe, MD, MPH
Director
Division of Foodborne, Waterborne, and
Environmental Diseases
National Center for Emerging and Zoonotic
Infectious Diseases
Centers for Disease Control and Prevention
Atlanta, Georgia, USA

Dominic A. Travis, DVM, MS
Associate Professor
Division of Ecosystem Health
Department of Veterinary Population
Medicine
College of Veterinary Medicine
University of Minnesota
Minneapolis, Minnesota, USA

Ed G.M. van Klink, DVM, PhD, Dipl. ECVPH, MRCVS
Senior Lecturer in Veterinary Public Health
School of Veterinary Science
University of Bristol
Lower Langford
Bristol, United Kingdom;
Wageningen Bioveterinary Research
Lelystad, The Netherlands

Donald J. Wuebbles, PhD
Harry E. Preble Endowed Professor
of Atmospheric Sciences
Department of Atmospheric Sciences
University of Illinois
Urbana, Illinois, USA

Foreword

We encourage you to set aside time to read *Beyond One Health: From Recognition to Results.* We hope that you will be as inspired by its contents as we are.

One Health is one of the great innovations of our time. It is an idea, a concept, a way of thinking and working, and a means to organize action. One Health starts from a recognition that 75% of the new infections affecting humans come from animals. The risks of animal diseases can be decreased through proper attention to livestock health in livestock production: the One Health approach guides efforts to intensify production. It recognizes the benefits of food systems that are sensitive to nutrition and the threats posed by infections that are resistant to antimicrobial therapies.

The One Health idea came to life in 2004 as scientists considered how best to tackle diseases that move between human, domestic animal, and wildlife populations. It reflected experiences with the Ebola virus disease, avian influenza, and chronic wasting disease. It is set out as the Manhattan principles (https://www.cdc.gov/onehealth/pdfs/manhattan/twelve_manhattan_principles.pdf) for *One World, One Health.*[1] It is an international, interdisciplinary approach for tackling threats to the health of life on Earth. It has practical application for reducing risks of unsafe foods and diseases that move from animals to humans.

One Health connects science and systems to the needs of society. It has matured into a new way of thinking and working and contributes to the health of both humans and animals. It links several disciplines that focus on health. It helps professionals to see their work differently and to do it with new purpose. It stimulates integration when remaining separate is less effective. One Health frames how we speak and act: it encourages us to focus on the interfaces between human, animal, and environmental systems. It helps us make sense of multiple interacting determinants of illness. It helps us to better reduce risk and prepare for threats.

Many of us with coordination responsibilities have found that One Health makes our joint working more effective and efficient. It makes sense on the farm, in the factory, and at home, encouraging us to prevent costly outbreaks.

More recently, One Health has helped with restructuring institutions and transforming education. It helped drive collaboration between the World Health Organization (WHO), the World Organisation for Animal Health (OIE), and the Food and Agriculture Organization of the United Nations (FAO). It stimulated new academic departments and degree programmes. It provided a basis for local and national governments to combine animal, human, and environmental health programs, and to reap economic benefits.

Beyond One Health: from Recognition to Results offers us an update on One Health topics from the perspectives of different professional and academic disciplines. It includes

---

1 Organized by the Wildlife Conservation Society and hosted by The Rockefeller University (http://www.oneworldonehealth.org).

an analysis of different threats to people and planet (including zoonoses and climate change), the epidemiology that underlies One Health, as well as the evidence base for different One Health policies and their benefits. It shows how One Health is best approached from a systems perspective and explains the importance of good leadership in making One Health a reality.

If we want to learn how One Health can best be applied in practice, we should study its use in different situations. In this book, we can see how One Health approaches help when analyzing risk and devising prevention, preparedness, and response strategies; when monitoring the evolution of threats and establishing early warning systems; or when prioritizing actions and coordinating actors during implementation. We can understand how One Health has been used in responses to avian influenza, yellow fever, Zika, Middle East respiratory syndrome (MERS), and Ebola.

When combining animal and environmental health practice, we must be sensitive to variations in motivations, responsibilities, and accountability of practitioners in these disciplines. In our experience, the One Health approach is especially useful when coalitions of actors are being established and a consensus is being built. It should be applied in ways that are sensitive to context, adapted to capabilities of systems (for public, veterinary, and environmental health), and adjusted to ecosystem, economic, and societal realities of interfaces between humans, animals, and nature.

We are starting to see One Health approaches being used to frame analyses of costs, benefits, acceptability, and scalability of different interventions. Academic groups are often asked to provide the evidence base for One Health policies and interventions. Their inputs are most helpful when interdisciplinary research methods are used. This is especially necessary when exploring links among environmental dynamics, disease vectors, pathogens, and human susceptibility.

Enlightened approaches like One Health – which focus on prevention and response from the perspectives of multiple disciplines – are vital to success in achieving the 2030 Agenda for Sustainable Development and in building a common future for all. This book will help you move along that path.

Chadia Wannous
David Nabarro

Chadia Wannous, PhD, is a Public Health professional and expert in prevention, emergency preparedness, and risk reduction for health threats. She previously served in several senior policy advisory positions with the UN.

David Nabarro, MD, is a medical doctor and Adviser on Sustainable Development. He previously served as Special Adviser to the United Nations Secretary-General.

Foreword

The naturalist and conservationist, John Muir, once stated, "When one tugs at a single thing in nature, he finds that it is attached to the rest of the world." The interconnectedness that Muir described in the early twentieth century is much more profound today, and much more consequential, regarding our health. The globalization of trade, travel, information, and investments, integrated and consolidated global food systems, urbanization, and a group of anthropogenic drivers that negatively impact our ecosystems, have created a new dynamic and an unprecedented interdependence among the health and well-being of people, animals, and our environment. The complex construct that describes these three domains of health is termed "One Health" and, indeed, tugging on any one of these domains demonstrates their significant attachments to one another. As a corollary to this axiom, we can no longer focus on health through a single lens or discipline.

Our new twenty-first century interdependence, including social, economic, political, and biological factors, has created new threats and risks to our health and has produced ecological changes that have fractured our planet. Several decades ago, the concept of One Health re-emerged from past medical thinking and gained important traction and acceptance. Recently, there have been many articles and books published focusing on One Health but, fortunately and very timely, this book has added special insights and brought together diverse disciplines and thinking to give us a better understanding of One Health in our contemporary lives, with an important and unique emphasis on operationalizing the concept. The book's authors have substantially improved our understanding of the key themes of One Health, added to our knowledge base, and stressed that new skills and competencies need to be acquired to successfully address the threats to human, animal, and ecosystem health.

The factors and drivers of our interdependent world, and increasingly risky lives, show no signs of abating; rather, they are accelerating. These drivers are leading to the intensification of the human-animal-ecosystem interface and causing further ecological damage. One consequence of this reality has been the dramatic increase in zoonotic diseases worldwide over the last few decades, which is thoroughly detailed in several chapters. This book also discusses the serious consequences of the degradation of our water resources and ecosystems, as well as threats to biodiversity and food security, all underpinned by climate change. The authors present evidence that our complex and interconnected world has generated a group of "wicked problems" that demand our attention and resources to resolve. A key feature of "wicked problems" is the recognition that past solutions and practices are not likely to be relevant or effective when applied to today's unparalleled challenges. A One Health mindset and an ability to work holistically across disciplines need to become the new norm to address complex problems and to take appropriate actions. In addition, we must champion new partnerships and innovations, and learn to effectively lead and manage change.

However, our medical fields continue to become progressively more specialized and, at the same time, progressively more isolated and siloed. While we appreciate the impressive advances in medicine, our health systems are increasingly disease-oriented and reactive. One Health, on the other hand, stresses disease prevention, shifting interventions closer to the origins of the problem, often in our animals and environment. *Beyond One Health:From Recognition to Results* argues that improving animal and environmental health can be a very effective and cost-beneficial public health strategy. As this text points out so well, maintaining and improving health must go beyond a strictly disease-oriented approach to consider the impact of the environment, social-economic status, genetics and human behavior, and other social determinants of health, which is truly a One Health perspective. This timely book makes the case that we need to normalize good health through this larger and more comprehensive context.

In differentiating *Beyond One Health: From Recognition to Results* from past One Health books, this book emphasizes the need to translate new knowledge into practice. We know that this transformation is a difficult and dynamic process that involves synthesis, dissemination, exchange, and finally application of One Health knowledge to the maintenance and improvement of health in all of its domains and dimensions. The book's authors acknowledge and present compelling evidence that critical gaps exist today between the promise of good health and actual results. The book reiterates that developing and implementing new strategies and polices represent the tactics necessary to support a One Health framework and plan of action. In addition, the authors argue in favor of the growing evidence that One Health thinking can offer a favorable value proposition, demonstrating that maintaining the status quo for our current healthcare delivery and disease response system is no longer acceptable, cost-effective, or scientifically valid.

While we remember John Muir as an outstanding ecological thinker, we also recognize that he was a very effective political spokesperson who understood the importance of translating science and knowledge into policies in support of conservation. Likewise, we need to move One Health from an abstract concept to a catalyst for new policies and interventions that can change the existing dynamic and improve health outcomes across all the domains of health. We understand that there are three stages of translating knowledge into practice, and this book discusses all three throughout its chapters. Awareness, acceptance, and adoption comprise the sectors of translation and all are integrated throughout the text. The authors also stress an important lesson: as we develop and adopt new strategies and policies, we also must design and carry out processes for outcome measurement and evaluation and continuous improvement for them to remain relevant and effective.

We are indebted to the editors and authors who have successfully built momentum toward a more universal acceptance of One Health and, perhaps even more importantly, have been especially instructive in helping us appreciate the need to enact new policies and shift One Health from theory to effective field implementation. They have reminded us, throughout this text, that One Health is likely just to be relegated to an academic exercise if it is not accompanied by a new value proposition, new policies, and more efficient interventions in the rapidly changing human, animal, and environmental health dynamic. Finally, we are grateful for both the intellectual and practical contributions of the book's editors and authors and are well advised to use their ideas and examples to better address the threats to our health, in all its dimensions.

Lonnie King, DVM, MS, MPA, DACVPM
Professor and Dean Emeritus
College of Veterinary Medicine
Ohio State University

Preface

"One Health" has caught on, some 140 years after Virchow coined the term "zoonoses" and said, "between animal and human medicine there are no dividing lines – nor should there be" (Schultz, 2008). The principles of One Health are often assigned singular ownership of that conceptual triad. However, other models, such as the Ecological Model in public health, eco-social theory, EcoHealth, conservation medicine, ecological medicine, and others, also take the holistic view that individual or population health outcomes are the result of many interrelated exposures, determinants, and contributing factors, and that an understanding of them, and their relatedness to each other, is required to formulate effective public policy designed to improve health.

Much has been written about One Health, its history and importance, especially in the context of emerging infectious diseases. One cannot minimize previous essays and textbooks focused on the need for viewing modern challenges to population health through a One Health lens, or the many peer reviewed journal articles that framed their research findings as examples of the demand for One Health thinking. We also must appreciate the excellent efforts of various national and international groups devoted to promoting One Health concepts and spreading awareness of their importance. However, we are at an inflection point in world events at which it has never been more critical that policy-makers set aside their ideologies and prejudices and promote science and technology policies that affect health, broadly defined. Those policies must be based on scientific consensus drawn from independent, well-constructed, repeatable research that is published for all to read and analyzed in well-respected, peer reviewed journals. We need to get beyond the abstract and actually do. Centuries ago, the German writer and statesman, Johann Wolfgang von Goethe, counseled that knowing and willing to do something is all well and good but eventually we must actually do it.

When we received a request from our publisher to edit a textbook about One Health, we initially declined. There were already four or five excellent books that describe One Health thinking and the challenges associated with it. It was only after we discussed our interest in public policy, and our experiences in the policy formation process, that we came up with the idea to edit a One Health book that is directed at policy solutions. The title of this textbook should be instructive. Our book is intended to serve as a reference for students and professionals in many disciplines, from architecture through urban planning, and not just for those working in traditional healthcare and health-related fields. The concept of One Health, that human, animal, and ecosystem health are inextricably linked, is an idea that is, at its core, about prevention. One Health may be easy to describe but it is a challenge to operationalize as policy. One Health thinking recognizes the interrelatedness of determinants of health and uses the scientific method to discover how strongly exposures are related to outcomes. Data are tested until they are accepted as fact; those facts can, gradually, after the iterative process of the scientific method, be translated into policy that should be designed to prevent the adverse effects of natural and human-derived phenomena on an ecosystem and to improve health.

Population growth, climate change, environmental degradation, inconsistent food production and distribution, water resource management, nonparticipatory governance, lack of civil society – all of the many determinants of global health – indicate that we are at a critical point in world history. To make significant improvements in global health, to improve the lives of global societies, we must engage thinkers from virtually all academic and professional fields and develop solutions, in public policy and in individual behaviors, that are effective, efficient, and sustainable. This is true One Health.

So, it is in this context that we offer this collection of critical population health topics, written by an international group of experts, that addresses not only the technical aspects of their topics but also offers potential policy solutions to help mitigate current threats and to prevent additional threats from occurring. Too often, public policy is based on the short-term benefit for the few at the long-term cost to the many. Too often, short-sighted policies defer current costs to future generations.

Reference

Schultz, M. (2008). Rudolf Virchow. *Emerging Infectious Diseases* 14(9), 1480–1481.

John A. Herrmann
Yvette J. Johnson-Walker

Section 1

The Science of One Health

1

Epidemiology: Science as a Tool to Inform One Health Policy

Yvette J. Johnson-Walker[1] and John B. Kaneene[2]

[1] *University of Illinois Urbana-Champaign, Urbana, IL, USA*
[2] *Michigan State University, East Lansing, MI, USA*

1.1 Introduction

Epidemiology is the study of disease dynamics in populations. It seeks to understand patterns of disease as a means of identifying potential prevention and control measures. It has been described as "an interesting and unique example of cross-fertilization between social and natural sciences" (Vineis, 2003). The basic principle of epidemiology is that disease is not a random event. Each individual in a population has a unique set of characteristics and exposures (risk factors) that determine his or her probability of disease. Clinical medicine is focused on the health of the individual while epidemiology and public health seek to apply assessment of risk factors at the community level. Understanding how those risk factors impact a community provides public health officials with the tools to develop policies and interventions for disease control and prevention in the community as a whole.

The One Health concept is coherent with the principles of epidemiology because risk factors for many diseases occur at the interface between humans, animals, and the environment. Failure to consider the interactions between them may result in public health policies that fail to effectively control disease and protect the environment. The One Health triad (Figure 1.1) of humans, animals, and the environment is analogous with the other triads that epidemiologists use to describe disease dynamics within a population:

- The host, agent, environment triad (Figure 1.2) is used to describe the interplay between these three key components of infectious disease transmission. Changes in any of these components alters the probability of disease.
- The three states of infectious disease status are illustrated by the susceptible, infected, removed (SIR) triad (Figure 1.3).
- Outbreaks of disease are characterized in terms of person or animal, place, and time as the first step of identifying the population at risk.
- Risk factors for disease causation are categorized as: necessary, sufficient, and component causes (Figure 1.4).

The goal of public health policy is to prevent transmission of disease agents to the susceptible segment of the population by controlling and treating disease among the infected and increasing the segment of the population that is removed (recovered or resistant). Identification and isolation of cases, quarantine of the exposed, and vaccination of the

Beyond One Health: From Recognition to Results, First Edition.
Edited by John A. Herrmann and Yvette J. Johnson-Walker.
© 2018 John Wiley & Sons, Inc. Published 2018 by John Wiley & Sons, Inc.

The one health triad

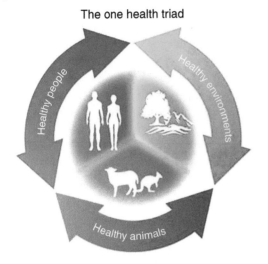

Figure 1.1 The One Health triad. *Source:* Thompson, 2013. Reproduced with permission of Elsevier.

susceptible are the primary tools employed by public health practitioners for infectious disease control. Development of effective programs to accomplish these goals requires an understanding of the:

1) Causes of disease (etiologic agent, pathophysiology, and risk factors.
2) Impact of the disease on the population (number of cases, ease of transmission, economic and social impact).
3) Natural course of the disease (reservoirs for the agents of disease, means of introduction of the agent into the population, period of infectivity, severity of disability, length of immunity, and potential for long-term sequelae) (Figure 1.5).

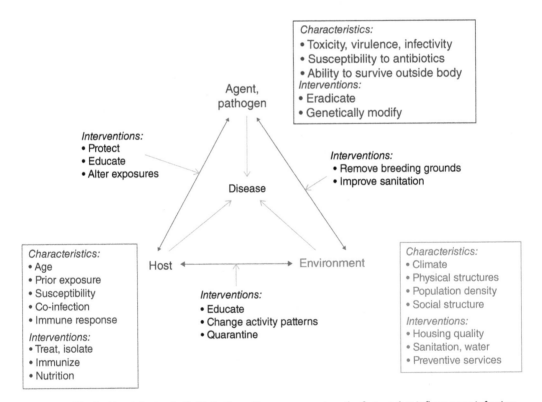

Figure 1.2 The "epidemiologic triad" of infectious disease summarizes the factors that influence an infection, and the measures you might take to combat the infection. *Source:* Used with permission from Ian McDowell (http://www.med.uottawa.ca/SIM/data/Pub_Infectious_e.htm#epi_triad).

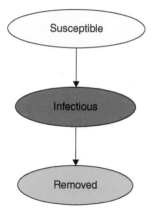

Figure 1.3 Infection modeling: the SIR model. **Susceptible** nodes – have not been infected yet and are therefore available for infection. They do not infect other nodes. **Infectious** nodes – have been infected and infect other nodes with a certain probability. **Removed** (recovered) nodes – have gone through an infectious period and cannot take part in further infection (neither actively nor passively). *Source:* Used with permission from Michael Jaros (http://mj1.at/articles/infection-modelling-the-sir-model/).

The goals of this chapter are to elucidate how epidemiology can 1) provide a tool for understanding the causes, impacts, and course of disease in human and animal populations within various ecosystems, and 2) form the basis for evidence-based health and environmental policy development.

1.2 Enhancing Our Understanding of Health and Disease

1.2.1 Causes of Disease

Epidemiology is unique among biomedical investigative approaches because of the observational nature of many of the study designs. Unlike laboratory studies, the epidemiologist often studies a naturally

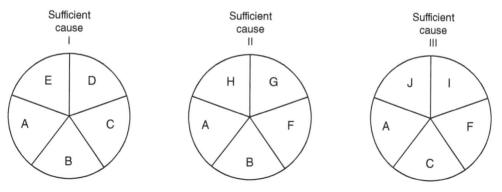

Figure 1.4 Necessary, sufficient, and component causes. The individual factors are called component causes. The complete pie (or causal pathway) is called a sufficient cause. A disease may have more than one sufficient cause. A component that appears in every pie or pathway is called a necessary cause, because without it, disease does not occur. *Source:* Rothman, 1976. Reproduced with permission of Oxford University Press.

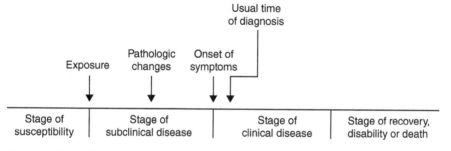

Figure 1.5 Natural history of disease timeline. *Source:* CDC, 1992.

occurring disease within a free-living population in which study subjects are not assigned to intervention groups (except in the case of clinical trials). Individuals may have a variety of independent exposures during the study period. Whether studying human or animal populations, the epidemiologist seeks to identify exposures that are associated with the probability of disease using statistical analysis of data from carefully documented exposures and outcomes. However, even if a statistically significant association between an exposure and disease outcome has been identified, that does not necessarily mean that a cause and effect relationship has been established. Much more rigorous standards have been set for establishing a causal relationship between a risk factor and the probability of disease.

1.2.1.1 Deterministic Models of Disease

Criteria for establishing causation for infectious disease have been described since the nineteenth century. Research by Robert Koch, Friedrich Loeffler, and Jakob Henle resulted in the Koch–Henle postulates published in 1882 (Sakula, 1983; Gradmann, 2014) (Figure 1.6). While this approach is useful when seeking to identify the etiologic agent responsible for an infectious disease, it has many limitations. The simplistic approach of a deterministic model for establishing disease causation is insufficient for identifying risk factors for chronic noninfectious diseases (such as type II diabetes) or even infectious diseases with a multifactorial etiology (such as new variant Creutzfeldt–Jakob disease, or CJD). In more recent years more complex

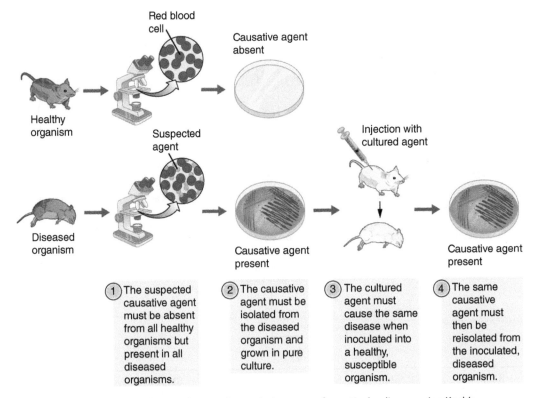

Figure 1.6 The steps for confirming that a pathogen is the cause of a particular disease using Koch's postulates.

models have been used to establish a causal relationship between a putative risk factor and disease.

1.2.1.2 Hill's Causal Criteria

Austin Bradford Hill published "The environment and disease: association or causation?" in 1965 (Hill, 1965). The manuscript describes nine criteria necessary for establishing a causal relationship between a risk factor and a disease:

1) *Strength of association:* the greater the magnitude of the association between the risk factor and the outcome, the more likely the relationship is to be causal.
2) *Temporality:* the risk factor must precede the onset of the disease.
3) *Consistency:* the same association should be observed in multiple studies with different populations.
4) *Theoretical plausibility:* the association should be biologically plausible and consistent with the pathophysiology of the disease.
5) *Coherence:* the association should be consistent with what is known about the disease.
6) *Specificity in the causes:* a risk factor should be associated with a single disease or outcome.
7) *Dose-response relationship:* as the dose of the risk factor is increased the probability and severity of the disease should increase in a linear fashion.
8) *Experimental evidence:* data from *in vitro* studies and animal models should support the causal association between the risk factor and the disease.
9) *Analogy:* similar causal relationships should be known.

The nature of these criteria makes it impossible for a single observational study to establish a causal relationship between an exposure and a disease outcome. The criterion of consistency requires that multiple studies, in different populations, show the same association. The criterion of temporality also requires that the association

be demonstrated in prospective studies. Prospective study designs monitor the study population prior to the onset of disease and follow their exposures over time until the disease of interest occurs. However, as we learn more about the complexity of the interactions between hosts and their exposures, limitations of the Bradford Hill Causal Criteria have also been described (Rothman, 2012). Some of Hill's Causal Criteria have been challenged by known causal associations that are contradictory. Specificity of effect, dose-response gradient, and coherence are all criteria whose validity has been challenged.

The criterion of specificity fails to acknowledge the potential for a single exposure to cause a multiplicity of pathologic effects. One well-known example of this is seen with exposure to tobacco smoke, which is associated with lung cancer, chronic obstructive pulmonary disease, heart disease, stroke, asthma, impaired fertility, diabetes, premature/low birthweight babies, blindness, cataracts, age-related macular degeneration, and cancers of the colon, cervix, liver, stomach, and pancreas (American Lung Association, 2017).

Many disease-causing exposures fail to produce a linear dose-response gradient. Goldsmith and Kordysh (1993) reviewed the literature for examples of nonlinear dose-response relationships and concluded that nonlinear causal relationships are equally as common as linear associations. Their analysis of the literature concluded that dose-response relationships are often nonlinear when countervailing outcomes are likely. They cautioned against linear extrapolation of dose-response data to develop policies and regulations for the protection of human populations. Exposures such as ionizing radiation and vitamin toxicity have been reported to produce U- or J-shaped dose-response curves (May and Bigelow, 2005). Inadequate sample size in the research study, insufficient range in the exposure dosages, and variability in individual susceptibility are all factors that impede the identification of these nonlinear dose-response causal relationships.

The criterion of coherence doesn't allow for paradigm shifts in models of disease causation. Identification of new mechanisms of disease pathogenesis may require elucidation of relationships that are not coherent with the current body of knowledge about the disease process. This is illustrated by the work of Marshall and Warren (1984) and their discovery of the role of *Helicobacter pylori* in the etiology of gastritis and peptic ulcers. Prior to their research, acid production was believed to be the key risk factor for the development of gastritis and peptic ulcers. Gastritis was thought to be a chronic inflammatory disease; the concept that it was actually due to a bacterial infection, was not coherent with the theory of the disease at the time of the findings by Marshall and Warren.

1.2.1.3 Multifactorial Models of Disease Causation

Krieger (1994) describes the transition in epidemiology from a focus on acute and infectious diseases to research focused on chronic disease. These more complex disease etiologies were first described as a "web of causation" in 1960. Multifactorial causes of disease have been framed as host-agent-environment models and social determinants of health. The public health application of these models is manifested as identification of the necessary component causes of disease and directing policies and interventions at those causes that are most amenable to alteration (see Figure 1.4).

In summary, epidemiology has evolved from a monocausal (deterministic) model to the multicausal concept of the "web of causation" (Vineis, 2003). The models that seek to describe disease causation continue to evolve. More recently, an "ecosocial framework" has been proposed as a more holistic, comprehensive approach to describing the how and why of disease occurrence (Krieger, 1994) (Figure 1.7). Unlike the web of causation, this model takes a One Health approach

to understanding disease in human populations. Krieger concludes that "encouraging a social and ecologic point of view, this image also serves as a reminder that people are but one of the species that populates our planet; thus implies that the health of all organisms is interconnected."

1.2.1.4 Breaking the Chain of Transmission

The goal of epidemiology is to enhance the health of populations. The rationale for researching risk factors for disease is to identify policies and interventions that can be employed to prevent disease. One of the most important lessons of epidemiology is that disease can be controlled even when there is incomplete knowledge of the etiologic agent responsible for the disease. Louis Pasteur conducted research that led to the germ theory of disease between 1860 and 1864. Prior to this discovery, John Snow's classic work on the epidemiology of the 1854 cholera epidemic in London demonstrated that an infectious disease outbreak can be controlled by understanding risk factors for disease, even if the etiologic agent is unknown. In the 1854 outbreak, new cases of cholera were prevented by removing the handle from the Broad Street pump once the water source was identified as being the important exposure associated with cholera deaths in that part of London.

More recently, the first case of acquired immune deficiency syndrome (AIDS) was reported in 1981 and it wasn't until 1984 that the etiologic agent, human immunodeficiency virus (HIV), was discovered. However, in 1982, it was known that the disease was caused by a blood-borne or sexually transmitted virus and high-risk segments of the population had been identified. Even before the etiologic agent had been discovered, measures to prevent disease transmission were identified, including condom use and avoidance of needle-sharing among IV drug users (https://history.nih.gov/nihinownwords/docs/page_02.html) (Poundstone et al., 2004).

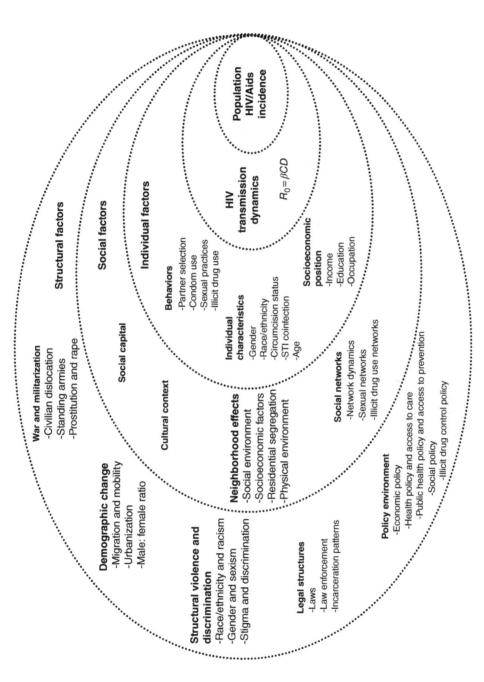

Figure 1.7 Ecosocial framework. An heuristic framework for the social epidemiology of human immunodeficiency virus (HIV)/acquired immunodeficiency syndrome (AIDS). The dotted lines separating the levels illustrate the porous nature of the distinctions made between levels of analysis. In reality, there are extensive linkages between factors at all levels that give rise to observed epidemic patterns. STI, sexually transmitted infection. *Source:* Poundstone et al., 2004. Reproduced with permission of Oxford University Press.

1.2.2 Assessing the Impact of Disease

The foundation of assessing a population health problem is determining the impact of the disease on the population. How big is the problem? Answering this question requires establishing the:

- number of individuals in the population with the disease (prevalence);
- number of new cases of disease that will occur in a given period of time (incidence);
- ease with which the disease spreads within the population (infectiousness);
- severity of the illness (agent virulence); and
- cost of the disease to society.

The *prevalence* of disease is a measure of the number of cases of disease at a given point in time. Prevalence of disease includes both recently diagnosed cases and chronic cases that have lived with the disease for some time. Knowing the prevalence of a disease in a community allows public health personnel to determine the resources necessary to manage the disease in the community. The *incidence* of disease is focused only on those new cases of disease identified within a given time period. Incidence tells how frequently new cases of the disease are occurring.

Infectiousness is a description of how easily an agent is transmitted from one host to another. Some agents are inherently very infectious and can spread quickly and easily to multiple susceptible hosts. The basic reproduction number, or R_0, is a measure of infectiousness of an agent in a totally susceptible population. The R_0 is the number of new cases of disease a single case will generate during its infectious period. Examples of highly infectious pathogens include measles virus in humans and foot-and-mouth disease (FMD) virus in livestock. Measles has an R_0 of 12–18 (CDC and WHO, 2014) meaning that in an unvaccinated population, each case of measles can be expected to infect an additional 12 to 18 people. A recent study of FMD transmission in dairy cattle reported an R_0 of infinity for nonvaccinated dairy cattle

in the same pen. In contrast, other agents are inherently less infectious. Estimates of infectiousness of the seasonal influenza virus report an R_0 of approximately 1.3 (Biggerstaff et al., 2014). R_0 is an inherent characteristic of an infectious agent. However, it is the interaction between the population, the environment, and the agent that best describes the spread of disease within a population. This is expressed by the effective reproduction number (R). "R" is the average number of new cases generated by a single case in a population that consists of both immune and nonimmune individuals. If R is less than 1.0, sustained transmission within a population cannot occur. As long as the R is greater than 1.0, meaning each case spreads the disease to more than one new case, the disease will continue to spread in the population. Without intervention the entire population will eventually get the disease.

The basic reproduction number (R_0) not only provides information about how likely an agent is to cause an epidemic, it also indicates the percentage of the susceptible population that must be vaccinated or be immune through natural infection to prevent disease transmission. This is referred to as *herd immunity* – a state in which enough members of the population are immune to the disease to prevent spread, thus protecting those who are not immune. So, for measles, 83–94% of the population must be vaccinated to achieve herd immunity (CDC and WHO, 2014), while for influenza it has been reported that only 13–40% (depending on the influenza strain) of the population needs to be vaccinated to establish herd immunity (Plans-Rubio, 2012).

The practical application of this information is that it can be used to direct public health interventions that have the potential to stop transmission. Vaccination programs reduce the number of individuals in the population who are susceptible to the disease, and the population can achieve a state of herd immunity if a sufficient percentage is vaccinated. Case finding efforts, combined with treatment and isolation of infectious individuals, and education programs, such as hand washing and social distancing campaigns, can reduce the number of individuals in the population who are exposed to the agent, thereby preventing spread of the agent to new susceptible hosts.

The *virulence* of an agent is an indication of the severity of the illness it causes. Some pathogens cause mild, self-limited illnesses with few clinical signs, while more virulent agents result in debilitating disease or even death. Agent virulence is assessed using the *case-fatality rate* (CFR). The CFR is simply the rate of death due to a disease among all cases of the disease. The CFR for chickenpox in children (varicella) is 0.001% or 1 in 100 000 (Heymann, 2008). In comparison the CFR for rabies is 100% (WHO, 2017). Thus, the virus causing rabies in humans is much more virulent than that causing chickenpox.

In addition to considering the number of sick individuals, the rate of disease spread, and the severity of the illness, assessing the impact of a disease must also take into consideration the burden of the disease on society (Figure 1.8). Direct economic costs of disease include the cost to diagnose, treat, or prevent the disease. Indirect economic costs

may include lost productivity due to absenteeism from work or losses due to declines in trade and tourism caused by fear of the disease, and so forth. Lastly the social disruption caused by the disease, or fear of the disease, can be more costly than the actual cases of disease. Remnants of this disruption may last years beyond the disease event.

It is easy to see how an outbreak of a high-incidence, rapidly spreading disease, caused by a very virulent agent, can have a huge economic and social impact on a community. This was apparent during the 2014–2016 West African Ebola virus disease outbreak in which there were an estimated 28 652 human cases and 11 325 deaths in 10 countries (CDC, 2016). The 2015 United Nations Development Group (UNDG) report on the socioeconomic impact of Ebola virus disease in West African countries indicates that the impact of the 2014–2015 Ebola outbreak was pervasive in the affected countries: labor markets shrank; access to food and the quality and quantity of food consumed was decreased; access to education declined for children, due both to mortalities among educators and school staff and to school closures; access to health services declined substantially; and there was an erosion of

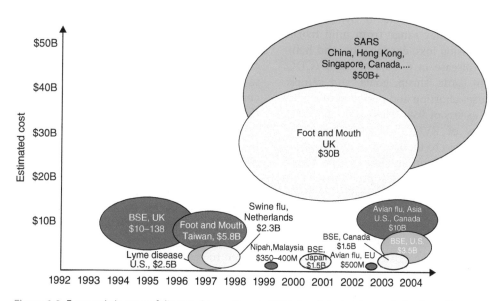

Figure 1.8 Economic impact of disease. *Source:* Karesh, 2007. Reprinted with permission from Bio-era.

communal cooperative behaviors and relationships (UNDG, 2015). Declines in gross domestic product (GDP) for the most severely impacted countries were estimated to range from 3.4% for Guinea to 13.7% for Liberia (UNDG, 2015). As a result, prior trends in poverty reduction are expected to slow or reverse in Guinea, Liberia, and Sierra Leone. In fact, the economic impact will be felt throughout the entire region. West Africa is expected to incur losses of approximately 3.6 billion US dollars per year for the period 2014–2017 (UNDG, 2015).

In some cases, the devastating socioeconomic impact of a disease outbreak is caused by a combination of illness and death in both human and domestic animal populations. Rift Valley fever (RVF) is a mosquito-borne emerging viral disease that causes severe disease in human and animal populations. First reported in Kenya in 1930, outbreaks have been documented in several countries in sub-Saharan Africa. However, in the year 2000 a large outbreak of human cases was reported in Saudi Arabia and Yemen. A total of 516 human cases of severe RVF, with 87 deaths, were documented between August and November of 2000 (CDC, 2000). A 2007 outbreak of RVF in the Sudan was reported to have caused an estimated 75 000 human cases (Anyamba et al., 2010). Symptoms in human cases may range from mild febrile illness to vision loss, encephalitis, and hemorrhagic disease in 8–10% of cases (CDC, 2013). In cattle, sheep, goats, and camels, RVF causes abortion and perinatal mortality rates in excess of 95% (Hassan et al., 2011). Outbreaks of RVF in livestock result in reduced access to food, loss of income from livestock production, and loss of export markets due to trade bans, in addition to costs to the government for disease control, surveillance, and assistance to producers (Hassan et al., 2011). A 2007 RVF outbreak in Kenya was reported to cause US$32 million in losses (Rich and Wanyoike, 2010).

However, a relatively rare disease with few cases in any community can still place a huge burden on society in terms of the direct and indirect economic and social costs of the disease. The economic and social impact of diseases like severe acute respiratory syndrome (SARS) and bovine spongiform encephalopathy (BSE, or mad cow disease) illustrate that a limited number of human cases of disease can have huge social and economic consequences on the affected community and beyond (Figure 1.8). The SARS pandemic occurred from November 2002 through July 2003. During that period there were 8098 total cases of SARS with 774 deaths across 29 countries with an estimated economic impact of US$30–50 billion. Human exposure to the prion that causes BSE in cattle is a cause of variant Creutzfeldt–Jakob disease (vCJD) in humans. There were 178 human cases of vCJD in the UK between 1995 and 2016 (CDC, 2017), while concern that BSE may pose a human health risk resulted in losses of 740–980 million GBP in 1992 in the UK (Atkinson, 2014).

Even a disease outbreak in which only domestic animal health is at risk can have a substantial economic impact. From December of 2014 through June of 2015, the USA experienced its largest foreign animal disease outbreak in history. Only avian species were affected in this outbreak of highly pathogenic avian influenza, which spread across three migratory bird flyways and resulted in the death or euthanasia of more than 50 million birds on 232 premises (https://www.aphis. usda.gov/aphis/ourfocus/animalhealth/animal-disease-information/avian-influenza-disease/sa_detections_by_states/hpai-2014-2015-confirmed-detections). Laying hens and turkeys were the predominant agricultural species impacted by the outbreak. Total economic losses associated with the outbreak were estimated to be US$3.3 billion (https://www.aphis.usda.gov/aphis/ourfocus/animalhealth/animal-disease-information/avian-influenza-disease/sa_detections_by_states/hpai-2014-2015-confirmed-detections). In the UK, the 2001 outbreak of FMD was estimated to causes losses of 3.1 billion GBP to the food and agricultural segment alone, with additional losses to tourism that were similar in magnitude (Thompson et al., 2002). Over 10 million cows and sheep were euthanized to get the outbreak under control. Although human health was not directly impacted by FMD, the outbreak response activities, which included the mass depopulation of livestock, restrictions in human movement, social isolation, and resultant job losses, took a heavy psychological toll on affected communities. As a result, increased rates of psychological morbidity were reported in affected areas, with morbidity rates in farmers correlated with the level of livestock culling and movement restrictions (Peck, 2005). These events highlight the inextricable connections between human, animal, and ecosystem health – demonstrating that events effecting one segment of the triad inevitably impact the others even if indirectly.

1.2.3 Natural Course of Disease

Each case of a disease in a population follows a progression from susceptible to recovery or death (see Figure 1.5). Interactions between the host, the agent, and the environment influence the rate of progression and the end result. *Susceptible* individuals are those at risk for becoming a case of the disease. Exposure to risk factors for the disease or to the infectious agent increases the probability of becoming a case only for those members of the population who are susceptible. Once a susceptible population member is exposed, the disease process may begin. This early phase of the disease often poses the greatest risk to the rest of the susceptible population because clinical signs of illness have not developed and the disease is difficult, if not impossible, to detect. For infectious diseases, this means that infected humans or animals may infect others in the population without showing clinical signs. The length of time from exposure to a disease-causing agent to the onset of clinical signs is referred to as the *incubation period*. Agents have different incubation periods, with some as short as a few minutes, while others may take decades before clinical signs develop (Table 1.1).

Once clinical signs appear, there is the possibility that the disease can be detected and steps taken to intervene and prevent

transmission to other susceptible population members. Even if control measures or treatments are not implemented, the simple onset of signs can reduce contacts with noninfected susceptible population members. Animals that are clinically ill often distance themselves from the rest of the herd or flock (Lopes et al., 2016). In human populations, public health policies focused on social distancing have been shown to effectively reduce transmission of infectious disease (Glass et al., 2006).

The final stage of disease is also influenced by host and agent factors. As discussed earlier in this chapter, virulence of the agent influences severity of the illness, degree of disability, and the rate of death among cases. Agent *immunogenicity* reflects the host's ability to develop immunity to the disease upon recovery and the duration of this immunity. These agent characteristics also impact the ease with which effective vaccines can be developed to reduce the number of susceptible individuals in the population. The duration of the period of time from onset of clinical signs to the resolution of any secondary sequelae or long-term disability has a large potential impact on the economic and social costs of the disease.

1.2.3.1 Reservoirs of Disease

So far in this chapter, host factors and agent factors have been the focus of discussion. Where does the environment fit into this triad? Where does the infectious disease agent "live" when it is not infecting a host? In addition to understanding the agent and the susceptible hosts that it infects, breaking the chain of transmission requires understanding where that agent can be found in nature and how the host becomes exposed to it. The *reservoir* of a disease is the habitat in which the agent normally lives, grows, and multiplies (http://www.cdc.gov/ophss/csels/dsepd/ss1978/lesson1/section10.html). Humans, animals, and the environment are potential reservoirs for infectious disease agents and, in some cases, insects serve as vectors transmitting infectious disease agents to new hosts (Table 1.2). Identifying the reservoir and finding measures to control or eradicate

Table 1.1 Incubation periods of selected exposures and diseases.

Exposure	Clinical effect	Incubation/latency period
Saxitoxin and similar toxins from shellfish	Paralytic shellfish poisoning (tingling, numbness around lips and fingertips, giddiness, incoherent speech, respiratory paralysis, sometimes death)	Few minutes to 30 minutes
Organophosphorus ingestion	Nausea, vomiting, cramps, headache, nervousness, blurred vision, chest pain, confusion, twitching, convulsions	Few minutes to a few hours
Salmonella	Diarrhea, often with fever and cramps	Usually 6–48 hours
SARS-associated corona virus	Severe acute respiratory syndrome (SARS)	3–10 days, usually 4–6 days
Varicella-zoster virus	Chickenpox	10–21 days, usually 14–16 days
Treponema pallidum	Syphilis	10–90 days, usually 3 weeks
Hepatitis A virus	Hepatitis	14–50 days, average 4 weeks
Hepatitis B virus	Hepatitis	50–180 days, usually 2–3 months
Human immunodeficiency virus	AIDS	<1 to 15+ years
Atomic bomb radiation (Japan)	Leukemia	2–12 years
Radiation (Japan, Chernobyl)	Thyroid cancer	3–20+ years
Radium (watch dial painters)	Bone cancer	8–40 years

Source: Centers for Disease Control and Prevention (http://www.cdc.gov/OPHSS/CSELS/DSEPD/SS1978/Lesson1/Section9.html#_ref44).

the agent from that reservoir is a goal of epidemiology that often proves to be elusive.

1.2.3.2 Humans as a Reservoir

The best hope for disease eradication is found in those diseases in which humans are the only reservoir. In 1980 the world was declared free of smallpox. Stuart-Harris (1984) identified features of smallpox that facilitated eradication, including: characteristic rash, identifiability of virus location, lack of subclinical cases, absence of an animal reservoir, no vector, seasonality, no latency, only one serotype, and a stable vaccine. Poliomyelitis is considered by many to be the next disease in line for global eradication in part because it also lacks an animal reservoir or insect vector (Stuart-Harris, 1984; Kew et al., 2005). When an infectious disease is only transmitted from person to person and has an effective vaccine, there is the potential to achieve a global vaccination rate that induces herd immunity. As the number of susceptible individuals in the population declines over time, that disease may cease to exist.

1.2.3.3 Domestic Animal Reservoirs

Unfortunately, most emerging and re-emerging infectious diseases are *zoonotic*. That means they can be transmitted under natural conditions between animals and humans. Diseases with an animal reservoir are inherently more difficult to control effectively because control efforts must target both the animal and human susceptible populations. Although it is more challenging

Table 1.2 Important anthroponoses, zoonoses, and sapronoses.

Category	Diseases
Anthroponoses	Measles*; rubella; mumps; influenza; common cold; viral hepatitis; poliomyelitis; AIDS*; infectious mononucleosis; herpes simplex; smallpox; trachoma; chlamydial pneumonia and cardiovascular disease*; mycoplasmal infections*; typhoid fever; cholera; peptic ulcer disease*; pneumococcal pneumonia; invasive group A streptococcal infections; vancomycin-resistant enterococcal disease*; meningococcal disease*; whooping cough*; diphtheria*; *Haemophilus* infections* (including Brazilian purpuric fever*); syphilis; gonorrhea; tuberculosis* (multidrug-resistant strains); candidiasis*; ringworm (*Trichophyton rubrum*); *Pneumocystis* pneumonia* (human genotype); microsporidial infections*; cryptosporidiosis* (human genotype); giardiasis* (human genotype); amebiasis; and trichomoniasis
Zoonoses transmitted by direct contact, alimentary (foodborne and waterborne), or aerogenic (airborne) routes	Rabies; hemorrhagic fever with renal syndrome*; hantavirus pulmonary syndrome*; Venezuelan*, Brazilian*, Argentinian, and Bolivian hemorrhagic fevers; Lassa, Marburg, and Ebola hemorrhagic fevers*; Hendra and Nipah hemorrhagic bronchopneumonia*; hepatitis E*; herpesvirus simiae B infection; human monkeypox*;Q fever; sennetsu fever; cat-scratch disease; psittacosis; mammalian chlamydiosis*; leptospirosis; zoonotic streptococcosis; listeriosis; erysipeloid; campylobacterosis*; salmonellosis*; hemorrhagic colitis*; hemolytic uremic syndrome*; yersiniosis; pseudotuberculosis; sodoku; Haverhill fever; brucellosis*; tularemia*; glanders; bovine and avian tuberculosis*; zoonotic ringworm; toxoplasmosis; and cryptosporidiosis* (calf genotype 2)
Zoonoses transmitted by hematophagous arthropods Hard ticks (*Ixodidae*)	Russian spring-summer encephalitis; Central European encephalitis; louping ill; Kyasanur Forest disease; Powassan; Crimean-Congo hemorrhagic fever*; Colorado tick fever; Rocky Mountain spotted fever; boutonneuse fever; African tick typhus*; other rickettsial fevers*; human granulocytic ehrlichiosis*; Lyme disease*; tularemia; and babesiosis
Soft ticks (Argasidae)	Tickborne relapsing fever
Mites (Trombiculidae, Dermanyssidae)	Scrub typhus; rickettsialpox
Lice (*Anoplura*)	Epidemic typhus; trench fever*; and epidemic relapsing fever
Triatomine bugs (Triatominae)	Chagas disease
Sandflies (Phlebotominae)	Sandfly fever; vesicular stomatitis; Oroya fever; and leishmaniasis
Mosquitoes (Culicidae)	Eastern, Western, and Venezuelan equine encephalomyelitides; Sindbis fever; Chikungunya and O'nyong nyong fevers*; Ross River epidemic polyarthritis*; Japanese encephalitis*; West Nile fever*; St Louis encephalitis; yellow fever; dengue/dengue hemorrhagic fever*; Murray Valley encephalitis; California encephalitis; Rift Valley fever*; and malaria*
Biting midges (Ceratopogonidae)	Oropouche fever; vesicular stomatitis
Tsetse flies (Glossinidae)	African trypanosomiasis
Fleas (Siphonaptera)	Murine typhus*; cat-scratch fever*; plague

(Continued)

Table 1.2 (Continued)

Category	Diseases
Sapronoses	Chlamydia-like pneumonia* (amoebic endosymbionts *Parachlamydia acanthamoebae* and other Parachlamydiaceae); tetanus; gas gangrene (*Clostridium perfringens, C. septicum, C. novyi*); intestinal clostridiosis* (*C. difficile, C. perfringens*); botulism; food poisoning* (*Bacillus cereus*); anthrax; vibrio gastroenteritis* or dermatitis (*Vibrio parahaemolyticus, V. vulnificus*); nosocomial *Klebsiella pneumoniae* and *Pseudomonas aeruginosa* bacteremia* (including antibiotic-resistant strains); bacterial infections associated with cystic fibrosis* (*Burkholderia cepacia; Ralstonia* spp.); melioidosis* (*B. pseudomallei*); legionellosis* and Pontiac fever* (*Legionella pneumophila, L. micdadei,* and other spp.); atypical bacterial meningitis and sepsis* (*Chryseobacterium meningosepticum*); acinetobacter bacteremia* (*Acinetobacter calcoaceticus, A. baumannii, A. radioresistens*); corynebacterial endocarditis* (*Corynebacterium serosis, C. amycolatum,* and other nondiphtheriae corynebacteria); rhodococcosis* (*Rhodococcus equi*); possibly leprosy (some strains of *Mycobacterium leprae* were detected as living saprophytically in wet moss habitats); Buruli ulcer disease* (*Mycobacterium ulcerans*); mycobacterial diseases other than tuberculosis* (*M. kansasii, M. xenopi, M. marinum, M. haemophilum, M. fortuitum, M. scrofulaceum, M. abscessus,* and other spp.); nocardiosis (*Nocardia asteroides, N. brasiliensis*); actinomycetoma (*Actinomadura madurae, A. pelletieri, Streptomyces somaliensis*); dermatophytosis (*Microsporum gypseum*); histoplasmosis* (*Histoplasma capsulatum, H. duboisii*); blastomycosis (*Blastomyces dermatitidis*); emmonsiosis (*Emmonsia crescens, E. parva*); paracoccidioidomycosis (*Paracoccidioides brasiliensis*); coccidioidomycosis* (*Coccidioides immitis*); sporotrichosis (*Sporothrix schenckii*); cryptococcosis* (*Cryptococcus neoformans*); aspergillosis (*Aspergillus fumigatus*); mucormycosis (*Absidia corymbifera* and some other Mucorales); entomophthoromycosis (*Basidiobolus, Conidiobolus,* and *Entomophthora* spp.); maduromycetoma (*Madurella mycetomatis, M. grisea, Pseudoallescheria boydii, Leptosphaeria senegalensis, Neotestudina rosatii*); chromoblastomycosis (*Phialophora verrucosa, Exophiala jeanselmei, Fonsecaea compacta, F. pedrosoi, Cladosporium carioni, Rhinocladiella aquaspersa*); phaeohyphomycosis (*Wangiella dermatitidis, Dactylaria gallopava, Exophiala spinifera*); fusariosis* (*Fusarium oxysporum, F. solani*); primary amoebic meningoencephalitis* (*Naegleria fowleri*); and amoebic keratitis or chronic granulomatous amoebic meningoencephalitis* (*Acanthamoeba castellanii, A. polyphaga*)

Source: Centers for Disease Control and Prevention (https://wwwnc.cdc.gov/eid/article/9/3/02-0208-techapp1.pdf).
* Denotes emerging and re-emerging diseases.

than controlling a disease that is only present in human populations, it can be accomplished, especially if the susceptible animal population is a domestic animal species. Regulations requiring vaccination of pets or livestock, mandatory tests and slaughter programs for livestock, animal travel and trade restrictions, and requirements for health certifications can be enacted as public health policies to control zoonotic disease in animal populations and thereby enhance both animal and human health. The impact on human health of public health policies directed at animals can be seen in the effects of US control efforts targeting rabies in dogs, and brucellosis and tuberculosis in cattle, on the rates of those diseases in the human population in the USA.

1.2.3.4 Wildlife Reservoirs

More challenging for disease control efforts is when the reservoir of disease is found in free-living wildlife. A variety of risk factors have been identified that may explain the emergence of new zoonotic infectious diseases into human populations in recent years. These phenomena are global in scope and not just an issue for developing countries. Population growth, civil unrest, population displacement, and urban/suburban sprawl contribute to humans now residing in previously pristine natural habitats where direct and indirect contact with wildlife is more likely to occur. Climate change and alteration of geographic home ranges of reservoir animals and insect vectors may result in the exposure of susceptible populations to new agents of infectious disease. Expansion of livestock and other agricultural production systems into new habitats can also result in increased exposure of domestic livestock and farm workers to wildlife reservoirs of disease. Global trade and travel also mean that a spillover event in one corner of the globe has the potential to move novel disease agents to any other area of the world in a matter of a few days. After its discovery in 1975, Lyme disease spread from deer, ticks, and humans in Connecticut to, in 2015, being the most commonly reported vector-borne illness in the USA (CDC, 2015). SARS traveled from Guangdong Province in southeast China to 29 countries in less than seven months, from November 2002 to July 2003. Nipah virus initially appeared in swine and swine farm workers in 1999 in Malaysia. There were 300 human cases of encephalitis associated with this outbreak, which resulted in 100 deaths. Over one million pigs were euthanized as a result. The reservoir was later determined to be fruit bats (*Pteropus* spp.) commonly known as flying foxes (http://www.searo.who.int/entity/emerging_diseases/links/nipah_virus_outbreaks_sear/en/). Since

2001, repeated outbreaks have been reported in Bangladesh and India resulting in a total of 280 cases and 211 deaths between 2001 and 2012. Person-to-person transmission in healthcare settings (*nosocomial infection*) has been a predominant feature in the outbreaks in India (Chadha et al., 2006). Cases in Bangladesh have been linked to the consumption of raw date palm sap contaminated by fruit bats (Islam et al., 2016).

One of the greatest challenges is identifying the wildlife reservoir of a new disease. When SARS appeared in 2002, the search began to find the wildlife reservoir that was the source of the spillover event. In 2003, it was reported that a SARS-like virus had been isolated from palm civets (Guan et al., 2003), triggering a province-wide effort to cull 10 000 palm civets in Guangdong Province.

1.2.3.5 Environmental Reservoirs

Lastly, the very environment itself can serve as a reservoir for infectious disease agents, with the potential to impact the health of humans, domestic animals, and wildlife. Air, water, and soil may be the site for disease agents to live, grow, and multiply.

Airborne transmission of infectious disease is illustrated by *Coxiella burnetii*, the agent that causes Q fever in several species, including humans. *C. burnetii* is a hardy agent that can travel long distances on dust particles and remain infectious for years outside of a living host. Infection of humans usually occurs by inhalation of these organisms from air that contains airborne barnyard dust contaminated by dried placental material, birth fluids, and excreta of infected animals (https://www.cdc.gov/qfever/stats/index.html). The acute phase of the disease causes flu-like signs. Sequelae associated with Q fever may include pneumonia, inflammation of the heart and liver, and central nervous system complications. Pregnant women are at increased risk for pre-term delivery or miscarriage. In 1983 a large outbreak of Q fever was reported in Switzerland in which there were 415 confirmed human cases (Dupuis et al., 1987). Epidemiologic

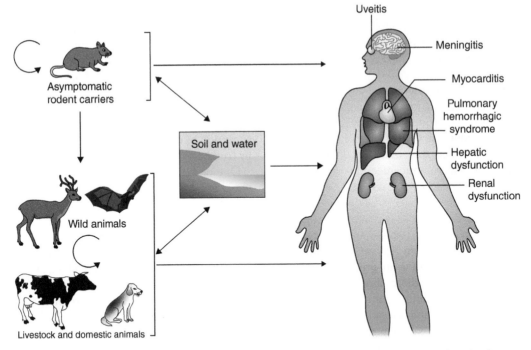

Figure 1.9 Leptospirosis reservoirs and transmission to humans. *Source*: Ko et al., 2009. Reproduced with permission of Nature Publishing Group.

investigation revealed that the outbreak was associated with 12 flocks of sheep returning to the valley from Alpine pastures. Those who resided near roads traveled by the sheep were at increased risk of becoming ill. The agent was also isolated from sheep on several facilities in the region. The authors concluded that better collaborations between physicians and veterinarians could prevent such outbreaks in the future (Dupuis et al., 1987).

Leptospirosis is one of the most common bacterial zoonotic diseases globally (Pappas et al., 2008). In humans, leptospirosis may begin with flu-like symptoms, vomiting, and diarrhea. A second phase of the disease may then occur, manifested by meningitis or liver and kidney failure. It is treatable with antibiotics (https://www.cdc.gov/leptospirosis/symptoms/index.html) but must be diagnosed correctly. Water contaminated with urine from infected animals is the most frequent means of human exposure (Figure 1.9). It has

been classified as a re-emerging infectious disease since outbreaks are occurring with increasing frequency in several parts of the world. Extreme weather events, such as flooding, typhoons, and hurricanes, associated with the ecological effects of climate change, have been associated with an increase in human cases of leptospirosis (Lau et al., 2010). Studies have reported that the Caribbean, Latin America, India, Southeast Asia, Oceania, and eastern sub-Saharan Africa are regions with the highest morbidity and mortality due to leptospirosis (Pappas et al., 2008, Costa et al., 2015). This is consistent with reports of an outbreak of leptospirosis in Mumbai, India, in the summer of 2015 with 54 cases and an unusually high case-fatality rate of one-third (Herriman, 2015). In addition, studies have documented a substantial increase in the number of leptospirosis-positive dogs in the USA (Moore et al., 2006; Alton et al., 2009).

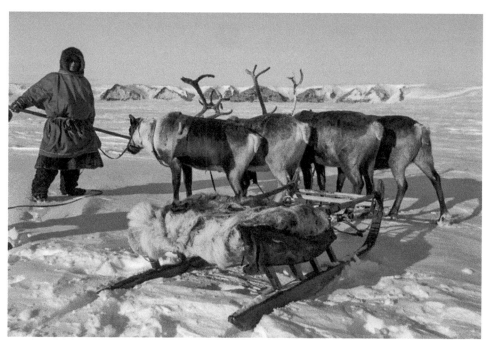

Figure 1.10 A Nenets herder in a malitsa with his reindeer-drawn sledge on the Yamal Peninsula in the Siberian Arctic in winter. Yamal Peninsula, Yamalo-Nenets, Russia (2014). *Source:* Image by Nick Mayo/ RemoteAsiaPhoto.

Soil has been identified as the reservoir for three outbreaks of anthrax reported in Siberia during the summer of 2016. These outbreaks offer additional illustrations of the interdependent relationships between humans, animals, and the environment. Record high temperatures in the region, attributed to climate change, have resulted in the thawing of deep layers of permafrost. Underneath that permafrost was soil harboring the bacterium that causes anthrax (*Bacillus anthracis*), believed to be from a reindeer carcass of a previous anthrax outbreak in the region. As a result, 1500 reindeer died from the disease, thousands were euthanized, and 100 human cases, including one death, have been reported (Guarino, 2016). To control the spread of the disease, Russian officials are reported to have planned to euthanize 250 000 deer by the end of 2016 (Doucleff, 2016). Concerns have been raised that the disease and the control efforts may threaten the future of the Nenets, pastoralists who herd and raise the reindeer in

the traditional nomadic manner (Doucleff, 2016) (Figure 1.10).

1.3 From Understanding Epidemiology to Public Policy

The previous sections of this chapter have discussed how epidemiology provides the tools for understanding the causes, impacts, and course of disease in human and animal populations within various ecosystems. Figure 1.11 illustrates the role of epidemiology research in prevention and control of infectious disease. Epidemiology is routinely used to inform health policies and standards of care at both the individual patient and the population levels. Here are examples of the application of the principles of epidemiology for use in clinical and public health decision making. Many of these concepts introduced in this chapter form the basis of the discussions in the subsequent chapters of this text.

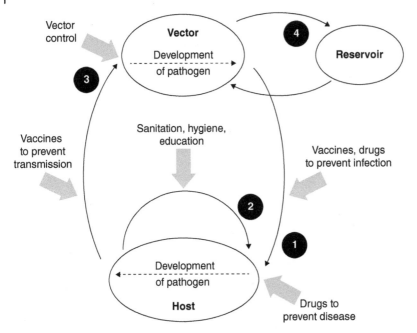

Figure 1.11 Role of epidemiology research in prevention and control of infectious disease. The black arrows illustrate a generalized infectious cycle; the shaded arrows indicate points where infectious diseases can be prevented. (1) A host is infected by the reservoir or a vector for the pathogen. This individual may infect (2) other hosts in a population or (3) new vectors. (4) The pathogen also may cycle between the vector and a reservoir. *Source:* Reproduced with permission of the National Institute of Medical Science.

1.3.1 Assessments of Diagnostic Test Reliability

When a physician or veterinarian conducts a diagnostic test on a patient, how certain are we that the results are valid? Epidemiologists assess the validity of diagnostic tests by determining their sensitivity and specificity. *Sensitivity* is defined as the ability of the test to correctly identify those who have the disease, and *specificity* is defined as the ability of the test to correctly identify those who do not have the disease (Gordis, 2014). These characteristics, which are inherent to the particular diagnostic test, are important especially when screening a population for a disease. However, at the level of the individual patient, predictive value is more informative. The *positive predictive value* is the probability of disease in an individual patient with a positive test result. It answers the question, "What are my chances of having the disease when my test result is positive?" Conversely, *negative predictive value* is the probability of being free of the disease given a negative test result. Predictive value incorporates the sensitivity and specificity of the test and the prevalence of the disease in the population from which the patient originates. Interpreting a diagnostic test in an individual patient requires epidemiologic data on the prevalence of the disease in the patient population. A diagnostic test that is very sensitive and specific may still have a low positive predictive value in an individual patient if he or she is from a population with a very low prevalence of the disease in question.

1.3.2 Determination of Safety and Effectiveness of New Treatments and Vaccines

The clinical trial is the primary method employed by epidemiologists to assess the safety and effectiveness of new treatments and vaccines. It is a research study conducted in the population for which the intervention is intended, as opposed to a laboratory study in a model animal species. Humans or animals at risk of a disease may participate in a clinical trial to assess the safety and effectiveness of a new vaccine intended to prevent the disease in that population. Patients with a disease may participate in a clinical trial to determine the safety and effectiveness of a new treatment for the disease. Clinical trials produce the best data available for healthcare decision making (https://www.nhlbi.nih.gov/studies/clinicaltrials). By standardizing the treatment approach and the subjects participating in the clinical trial, researchers are able to make unbiased assessments of how well the intervention performed, which types of patients were best suited for the intervention, and if there were negative side effects attributable to the intervention.

1.3.3 Assessing Health at the Level of the Individual, Community, or Ecosystem and Establishing Standards of Care for Prevention and Treatment Protocols/Programs

In addition to clinical trials for assessing the safety and effectiveness of vaccine and treatments, epidemiologists use three observational study designs to identify both risk factors for disease and preventive measures: the *cross-sectional, case-control,* and *cohort* studies. Due to the observational nature of these studies, conducted within the population of interest, data generated can be used by health policy makers to establish real world standards of care for prevention and treatment protocols, assess the effectiveness of public health programs, recommend vaccination schedules, and even assess environmental and ecosystem health.

The *cross-sectional* study uses a representative sample of the population to determine the approximate prevalence of disease and to identify behaviors and characteristics that are associated with having the disease.

Individuals are sampled at a single point in time to determine whether or not they have the disease in question and to determine their exposure status to risk factors believed to be associated with disease occurrence. The odds of exposure among cases is compared with the odds of exposure among non-cases. The cross-sectional study is useful for determining the scope of the problem for a common disease in a population and provides data for making a rapid assessment of potentially important exposures. However, no attribution of causality can be applied since there is no way to determine if a potential risk factor occurred prior to an outcome of interest. When the disease is rare or it is not feasible to get a representative sample of the population, the case-control study design is often employed.

The *case-control* study begins with a set of cases (subjects with the disease of interest) identified by the researchers and a set of controls (similar subjects who do not have the disease of interest). Since the participants are not part of a representative sample of the population, disease prevalence is not determined. However, this approach does allow for assessment of associated exposures in rare diseases. As with the cross-sectional study design, case and control subjects are assessed for exposure to potential risk factors and the odds of exposure among cases and controls are compared.

The *cohort* design is the third observational study design. A cohort is simply a group of individuals with something in common. The cohort study sets inclusion and exclusion criteria for the group of individuals and then observes that group over time, recording exposures and occurrence of disease. The key to the cohort study is the criterion that cohort members must be free of the disease of interest at the start of the observation period. Subjects are monitored over time and the risk of disease in the exposed is compared to the risk of disease in the unexposed.

The cross-sectional and case-control study designs are limited by the retrospective nature of exposure assessment inherent in their design. In both approaches the onset of disease begins prior to the onset of data collection. Thus, it is not always possible to clearly establish whether exposure preceded onset of disease. The criterion of temporality is essential in the establishment of a causal association. The cohort study design is unique for its potential to demonstrate a temporal association between the exposure and the disease of interest.

1.3.4 Establishing Disease Response Regulations and Control Standards

In addition to providing data for intervention recommendations, epidemiology provides a tool for directed action in the face of an epidemic. Several types of exposures may contribute to disease outbreaks including exposure to infected humans, domestic animals, and wildlife; consumption of contaminated food or water; and contact with contaminated surfaces. The case-control study design and retrospective cohort design are used to investigate outbreaks of disease with the goal of determining the source. An outbreak of a disease is defined as more cases than anticipated in a given time and place. Establishing that an outbreak is occurring requires some knowledge of the anticipated baseline disease level (incidence or prevalence). Once it has been determined that there is a true increase in disease, epidemiologists use case-control and retrospective cohort studies to identify exposures associated with cases of the disease.

Applying the multifactorial web of causation approach may lead to several types of risk factors identified as associated with cases of the disease. They may be factors intrinsic to the host, such as age, sex, or physiological state; or extrinsic, such as dietary, lifestyle, or occupational risk factors. They may be characteristics inherent to the agent, as in mutations altering infectiousness or virulence, or environmental influences, such as temperature, relative humidity, or UV radiation. When the outbreak is caused by the introduction of a disease into a new geographic region or host, the outbreak investigation can result in the identification of human or animal movements associated with disease introduction.

In response to the identification of risk factors for disease, health and regulatory agencies can implement interventions to break the chain of transmission, stop the current outbreak, and prevent future outbreaks. Control measures such as isolation, quarantine, and movement restrictions for humans and animals that are known or suspected cases of infectious disease can be effective outbreak response measures when epidemiologic evidence supports that such activities are associated with disease spread.

The primary goal of food safety regulations is to prevent future outbreaks of food-borne disease. When food handling and processing procedures are identified as risk factors in a food-borne disease outbreak, evidence-based food safety regulations can be developed to improve the safety of the food supply. Similarly, if wildlife species are identified as disease reservoirs, epidemiologic data about the magnitude and distribution of disease in the wildlife population is vital for the establishment of policies for wildlife disease surveillance and control policies. Wildlife disease surveillance and ecosystem health data are also crucial for setting guidelines and monitoring safety standards in environmental health policy.

Knowledge attained through outbreak investigations provides the data to support disease control initiatives such as: vaccine development or modification; public education programs for behavioral changes to enhance personal hygiene, food handling, and social distancing; and introduction of new occupational and food safety standards to prevent disease transmission.

The next section details real world examples of public health challenges posed by zoonotic infectious diseases and the application of epidemiologic data to develop a One Health approach to policy measures undertaken to address those challenges.

1.4   Examples of the Benefits of Using a One Health Approach

One Health is generally viewed as incorporating: 1) animal health (including domestic and wildlife), 2) human health, and 3) environment/ecosystem health. Interwoven within these three is a fourth pillar: 4) food and water security (Katz et al., 2013). Cross-cutting these four pillars are communication and policy considerations. Epidemiology serves as a critical tool in connecting the four pillars and in providing opportunity to generate results that can be used to design intervention strategies and policy actions. Two real life examples will illustrate benefits of applying a One Health approach in two major zoonotic diseases, brucellosis (Box 1.1) and tuberculosis (Box 1.2).

Box 1.1   A One Health approach to conduct brucellosis outbreak investigations in Uganda, East Africa

Brucellosis is a zoonotic disease that affects humans and many animal species. While there are more than eight species of *Brucella*, five species of brucellosis (*B. abortus, B. melitensis, B. suis, B. ovis,* and *B. canis*) cause abortions, arthritis, and orchitis in animals. In humans, the disease causes undulating fever, neurological disease, endocarditis, and arthritis. It is commonly misdiagnosed as malaria in developing countries. Brucellosis is both a public health and economic concern in many countries of the world. We will illustrate One Health approaches used in conducting outbreak investigations and research in Uganda.

Outbreak investigation in Western Uganda – 2013

An apparent increase in the number of human cases of brucellosis was reported in two health centers within two districts (Figure 1.12). Medical officers interviewed reported that the normal incidence was two to three cases per month. During the same period, increased abortions in cattle were reported in the districts. The District Veterinary Office (DVO) indicated that, in the district, usually 10–15 abortions were reported per month. However, they were now receiving 30–50 cases per month. Therefore, it was decided to conduct a One Health-based outbreak investigation to get at the root of the problem using the following phases.

Planning
At the university level, the College of Veterinary Medicine and the School of Public Health at Makerere University were involved. At the governmental level, the Ministry of Agriculture, Animal Industry, Fisheries and Wildlife and the Ministry of Health were involved. From the aforementioned institutions and governmental agencies, an interdisciplinary Outbreak Investigation Team (OIT) was formed. The team consisted of epidemiologists, microbiologists, veterinary pathologists, wildlife ecologists, physicians, veterinarians, laboratory technologists, and media specialists. A communication strategy was determined ahead of time, and a single person was to be in charge of communication within the outbreak investigation team. Communication to the media was to be done jointly by animal health and public health authorities, and laboratory protocols for sample collection, preservation, transport, and processing were jointly developed, well as data collection instruments, data analysis, and interpretation.

Training
Prior to starting the investigation, a short training session was held, which lasted 3 days. The first day covered the principles of outbreak investigation and ethical conduct of research. The second

(Continued)

Box 1.1 (Continued)

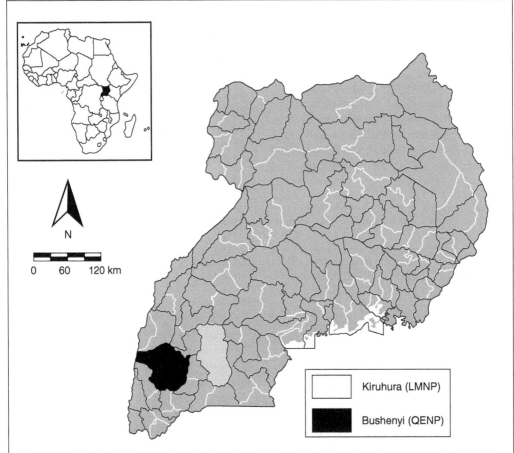

Figure 1.12 Districts in Western Uganda where brucellosis outbreak investigations were conducted 2013.

covered the type of questionnaires and different ways of administering them. The two questionnaires (one for human subjects and the other for livestock) that were going to be used were discussed, and because they were going to be administered in person, professional and cultural sensitivities were discussed in detail. The third day was devoted to how to assemble a team and preparation of the supplies needed. The individuals who were going to collect blood from humans were nurses and laboratory technologists familiar with blood collection. Individuals who were going to collect blood and milk from cattle and goats were veterinarians and veterinary technicians familiar with collection of the samples. A total of 24 individuals were trained.

Implementation
Fifteen livestock farms that reported abortions were identified, and the OIT visited them together and administered two simple questionnaires. The first questionnaire (human) was administered to 136 persons on the farms who came in contact with animals. The second questionnaire (animal) was administered to one person who was in charge of the livestock. From the available 168 cattle and 131 goats, blood and milk (where appropriate) were collected, and blood was collected from the 136 humans on the farms. The collected specimens were taken to a single regional laboratory for testing. The rose Bengal plate test (RBPT) with *B. abortus* and *B. melitensis* and the milk ring test were used to test for evidence of *Brucella* spp. exposure in cattle and goats. The Brucella micro-agglutination test (BMAT) and the lateral flow assay (LFA) for IgG and IgM were used on samples from humans. The outbreak investigation showed evidence of brucellosis in humans, cattle, goats, and milk. The seroprevalence was

Box 1.1 (Continued)

14% for cattle, 17% for goats, and 11% for humans from the outbreak investigation.

Communication of results
Communication of results to the public was accomplished jointly by representatives of the Ministry of Health and Ministry of Agriculture, Animal Industry, Fisheries and Wildlife.

Benefits of a One Health approach

The major benefits of a One Health approach that were realized in this example include: 1) shared facilities (lab) and activities, such as driving to the farms together to collect samples and needed data; 2) coordination of activities and responses, and communication to the public and policy makers; 3) education of farmers regarding how to reduce transmission of brucellosis within herds and between herds, transmission risk to humans through consumption of raw milk and dairy products, and handling livestock birth materials from infected animals; and 4) cost savings as a result of reduced time spent on the investigation, and sharing of resources (see Table 1.3 for illustration of monetary savings from applying a One Health approach). No follow-up data are available to assess whether this approach reduced human morbidity and mortality, but subjective information from the medical officers in the district suggests that there have been reduced cases of brucellosis in the district. Livestock and wildlife officials in the area have used the information in their outreach programs to the industry. In addition, there has been increased awareness of the disease in both the Ministry of Health and Ministry of Agriculture, and it has served as a catalyst for the use of a One Health approach in dealing with a zoonotic disease.

Table 1.3 Illustration of savings in US dollars as a result of applying a One Health approach to a brucellosis outbreak investigation and response in Western Uganda 2013.

	Supplies	Personnel	Others	Total
Animal health	600	2980	3005	6585
Public health	1098	3368	3877	8343
Animal and public health	1560	4295	3776	9631
Savings				5297

1.4.1 Overall Summary of Practical Experiences Applying a One Health Approach

The value of the One Health approach in dealing with zoonotic diseases, such as brucellosis and tuberculosis, would be:

1) Developing integrated approaches that will consider the role of humans, domesticated animals, wildlife, and the environment in the epidemiology of the disease.
2) Opportunities for shared resources; such as data and information, facilities, and personnel.
3) Increased efficiency and effectiveness.

Outbreak investigations and surveillance programs are often limited by funding in both resource-limited and high-income countries. Having public health, livestock, and wildlife agencies work together creates a strong voice to the policy makers of the need for continued funding. This is particularly true in Michigan, where the message to the policy makers has stressed both the economic and public health benefits of controlling and eradicating tuberculosis.

Box 1.2 A One Health approach for controlling *Mycobacterium bovis* **in cattle, deer, and humans in Michigan, USA**

In 1994, after a white-tailed deer (*Odocoileus virginianus*) with *M. bovis* was reported in the state of Michigan, surveillance programs were initiated in wildlife, livestock, captive cervid farms, and humans. Since 1994, cases of *M. bovis* have been reported in deer, followed by reports in cattle in 1998, and in humans in 2002 and 2004. To date, 52 beef herds, 15 dairy herds, four beef lots, four captive cervid herds, and one bison herd have been identified as infected with bovine tuberculosis (bTB) in Michigan (Figure 1.13), and the disease has cost millions of US dollars in surveillance and the testing and removal of infected animals. Bovine tuberculosis has a complex epidemiology with multiple, susceptible hosts and routes of transmission, and with ecosytems influencing host interaction and survival of the pathogen. Due to the complex epidemiology associated with this disease in the state of Michigan, multiple governmental agencies have had to use a One Health approach to work together to control the disease involving multiple disciplines. The One Health approach used in Michigan involves three pillars: 1) TB State Advisory Committee, 2) TB Interdisciplinary Technical Team, and 3) engagement of joint TB activities.

TB State Advisory Committee (TBAC)

A State Advisory Committee, whose responsibility was to advise the state on all matters relating to TB in livestock, wildlife, and humans, was formed in 1998. The committee is composed of individuals from all the relevant government departments in the state (Michigan Department of Agriculture & Rural Development, Michigan Department of Natural Resources, and Michigan Department of Community Health), federal agencies (USDA & CDC), Michigan State University (MSU), the livestock industries (dairy and beef), Michigan Farm Bureau, and deer hunting groups. The committee addresses policy issues, including surveillance strategies, outbreak investigation, and communication to the industries and the public at large.

TB Interdisciplinary Technical Team

An Interdisciplinary Technical Team was formed, composed of practicing veterinarians, TB epidemiologists, a TB program officer, deer ecologists, epidemiologists, pathologists, microbiologists, agricultural economists, sociologists, and extension specialists. The team addresses technical matters relating to strategies for control and eradication of TB, research, teaching, and communication of the problem and strategies for dealing with the disease.

Joint TB activities

Common TB activities handled in a One Health approach include: sharing of data between agencies, sharing of laboratory facilities, training of students, interdisciplinary research for new control strategies, and joint outbreak investigations of TB on a livestock farms. Examples of such investigations have been reported (Kaneene et al., 2002, 2014; Bruning-Fann et al., 2017).

Benefits

There are several benefits of applying a One Health approach in dealing with diseases. A specific example of such benefit in Michigan can be illustrated by the joint investigation of suspected bovine TB on a cattle farm. An earlier approach to investigating a suspected herd involved the different key government departments and the university going onto the farm separately. This approach was costly and caused a lot of stress and anxiety to the farmers affected. It was estimated (2015) that a single visit to each farm by a One Health team would cost US$3675, and would get just as much needed information. In contrast, multiple single visits by different agencies would cost US$5100. The other

Box 1.2 (Continued)

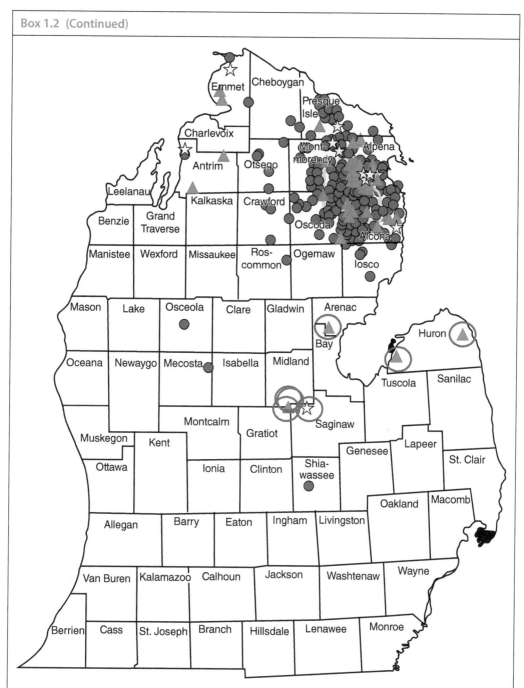

Figure 1.13 County map of the lower peninsula of Michigan depicting locations where *Mycobacterium bovis*-infected deer and *M. bovis*-affected beef and dairy herds have been identified between 1975 and 2016.

significant benefit is that, due to the One Health approach, the industries (livestock, wildlife, and captive cervid), as well as public health officials, jointly approach the state and federal authorities for increased funding relating to research and control programs in bTB.

References

Alton, G.D., Berke, O., Reid-Smith, R., Ojkic, D., and Prescott, J.F. (2009). Increase in seroprevalence of canine leptospirosis and its risk factors, Ontario 1998–2006. *Can J Vet Res* 73(3), 167–175.

American Lung Association (2017). 10 of the Worst Diseases Smoking Causes. Available at: http://www.lung.org/our-initiatives/tobacco/reports-resources/sotc/by-the-numbers/10-worst-diseases-smoking-causes.html (accessed November 14, 2017).

Anyamba, A., Linthicum, K.J., Small, J., Britch, S.C., and Pak, E. (2010). Prediction, assessment of the Rift Valley fever activity in East and Southern Africa 2006–2008 and possible vector control strategies. *Am J Trop Med Hyg* 83, 43–51.

Atkinson, N. (2014). The Impact of BSE on the UK Economy. Available at: http://www.veterinaria.org/revistas/vetenfinf/bse/14Atkinson.html (accessed November 14, 2017).

Biggerstaff, M., Cauchemez, S., Reed, C., Gambhir, M., and Finelli, L. (2014). Estimates of the reproduction number for seasonal, pandemic, and zoonotic influenza: a systematic review of the literature. BMC Infect Dis 14, 480.

Brunning-Fann, C.S., Robbe-Austerman, S., Kaneene, J.B., et al. (2017). The use of whole genome sequencing and evaluation of the apparent sensitivity and specificity of antemortem tuberculosis tests in the investigation of an unusual outbreak of Mycobacterium bovis in cattle herds in Michigan, USA, 2013. *Am J Vet Res* 251, 206–216.

CDC (Centers for Disease Control and Prevention) (1992). *Principles of Epidemiology*, 2nd edn. Atlanta: U.S. Department of Health and Human Services.

CDC (Centers for Disease Control and Prevention) (2000). *MMWR-Morbid Mortal W November 03*, 49(43), 982–985.

CDC (Centers for Disease Control and Prevention) (2013). Rift Valley Fever.

Available at: https://www.cdc.gov/vhf/rvf/symptoms/index.html (accessed November 14, 2017).

CDC (Centers for Disease Control and Prevention) (2015) Lyme Disease Fast Facts. Available at: https://www.cdc.gov/lyme/stats/index.html (accessed November 14, 2017).

CDC (Centers for Disease Control and Prevention) (2016). 2014 Ebola Outbreak in West Africa - Case Counts. Available at: https://www.cdc.gov/vhf/ebola/outbreaks/2014-west-africa/case-counts.html (accessed November 14, 2017).

CDC (Centers for Disease Control and Prevention) (2017). Variant Creutzfeldt-Jakob Disease (vCJD). Available at: https://www.cdc.gov/prions/vcjd/risk-travelers.html (accessed November 14, 2017).

CDC (Centers for Disease Control and Prevention) and WHO (World Health Organization) (2014). History and Epidemiology of Global Smallpox Eradication, slides 16 and 17. Available at: stacks.cdc.gov/view/cdc/27929/cdc_27929_DS1.pdf (accessed November 14, 2017).

Chadha, M.S., Comer, J.A., Lowe, L., et al. (2006) Nipah virus-associated encephalitis outbreak, Siliguri, India. *Emerg Infect Dis* 12, 235–240.

Costa, F., Hagan, J.E., Calcagno, J., et al. (2015). Global morbidity and mortality of leptospirosis: A systematic review. *PLoS Negl Trop Dis* 9(9), e0003898.

Doucleff, M. (2016). Killing reindeer to stop anthrax could snuff out a nomadic culture. National Public Radio (NPR). Available at: http://www.npr.org/sections/goatsandsoda/2016/10/12/496568291/killing-reindeer-to-stop-anthrax-could-snuff-out-a-nomadic-culture (accessed November 14, 2017).

Dupuis, G., Petite, J., Peter, O., and Vouilloz, M. (1987). An important outbreak of human Q fever in a Swiss Alpine Valley. *Int J Epidemiol* 16(2), 282–287.

Glass, R.J., Glass, L.M., Beyeler, W.E., and Min, H.J. (2006). Targeted social distancing design for pandemic influenza. *Emerg Infect Dis* 12(11). Available at: https://wwwnc.cdc.gov/eid/article/12/11/06-0255_article (accessed November 14, 2017).

Goldsmith, J.R. and Kordysh, E. (1993). Why dose-response relationships are often non-linear and some consequences. *J Expo Anal Environ Epidemiol* 3(3), 259–276.

Gordis, L. (2014). *Epidemiology*, 5th edn. Elsevier.

Gradmann, C. (2014). A spirit of scientific rigour: Koch's postulates in twentieth-century medicine. *Microbes Infect* 16(11), 885–892.

Guan, Y., Zheng, B.J., He, Y.Q., et al. (2003). Isolation and characterization of viruses related to the SARS coronavirus from animals in Southern China. *Science* 302(5643), 276–288.

Guarino, B. (2016). Anthrax sickens 13 in western Siberia, and a thawed-out reindeer corpse may be to blame. *Washington Post*, July 28. Available at: https://www.washingtonpost.com/news/morning-mix/wp/2016/07/28/anthrax-sickens-13-in-western-siberia-and-a-thawed-out-reindeer-corpse-may-be-to-blame/ (accessed November 14, 2017).

Hassan, O.A., Ahlm, C., Sang, R., and Evander, M. (2011). The 2007 Rift Valley fever outbreak in Sudan. *PLoS Negl Trop Dis* 5(9): e1229.

Herriman, R. (2015). Mumbai leptospirosis: High deaths linked to treatment delays. Outbreak News Today. Available at: http://outbreaknewstoday.com/mumbai-leptospirosis-high-deaths-linked-to-treatment-delays-55856/ (accessed November 14, 2017).

Heymann, D.L. (2008). *Control of Communicable Diseases Manual*, 19th edn. Washington, DC: American Public Health Association.

Hill, A.B. (1965). The environment and disease: association or causation? *Proc Roy Soc Med* 58, 295–300.

Islam, M.S., Sazzad, H.M.S., Satter, S.M., et al. (2016). Nipah virus transmission from bats to humans associated with drinking traditional liquor made from date palm sap, Bangladesh, 2011–2014. *Emerg Infect Dis* 22 (4).

Kaneene, J.B., Bruning-Fann, C.S., Granger, L.M., Miller, R., and Porter-Spalding, B.A. (2002). Environmental and farm management factors associated with tuberculosis on cattle farms in northeastern Michigan. *J Am Vet Med Assn* 221, 837–842.

Kaneene, J.B., Kaplan, B., Steele, J.H., and Thoen, C.O. (2014). Preventing and controlling zoonotic tuberculosis: a One Health approach. *Vet Ital* 50, 7–22.

Karesh, W.B. (2006). Animal disease surveillance. Presentation at the Institute of Medicine Forum on Microbial Threats, Washington, DC, December 12–13. Global Infectious Disease Surveillance and Detection: Assessing the Challenges—Finding Solutions, Workshop Summary. Washington, DC: National Academies Press.

Katz, D.J., Wild, D., and Elmore, J.G. (2013). *Jekel's Epidemiology, Biostatistics, Preventive Medicine, and Public Health*, 4th edn. Elsevier.

Kew, O.M., Sutter, R.W., de Gourville, E.M., Dowdle, W.R., and Pallansch, M.A. (2005). Vaccine-derived poliovirus and the endgame strategy for global polio eradication. *Ann Rev Microbiol* 59, 587–635.

Ko, A.I., Goarant, C., and Picardeau, M. (2009). Leptospira: the dawn of the molecular genetics era for an emerging zoonotic pathogen. *Nat Rev Microbiol* 7, 736–747.

Krieger, N. (1994). Epidemiology and the web of causation: has anyone seen the spider? *Soc Sci Med* 39(7), 887–903.

Lau, C.L., Smythe, L.D., Craig, S.B., and Weinstein, P. (2010). Climate change, flooding, urbanization and leptospirosis: fuelling the fire? *Trans R Soc Trop Med Hyg* 104(10), 631–638.

Lopes, P.C., Block, P., and König, B. (2016). Infection-induced behavioural changes reduce connectivity and the potential for disease spread in wild mice contact networks. *Sci Rep* 6, 31790.

Marshall, B.J. and Warren, J.R. (1984) Unidentified curved bacilli in the stomach of patients with gastritis and peptic ulceration. *Lancet* i, 1311–1315.

May, S. and Bigelow, C. (2005). Modeling nonlinear dose-response relationships in epidemiologic studies: statistical approaches and practical challenges. *Dose-Response* 3, 474–490.

Moore, G.E., Guptill, L.F., Glickman, N.W., Caldanaro, R.J., Aucoin, D., and Glickman, L.T. (2006). Canine leptospirosis, United States, 2002–2004. *Emerg Infect Dis* 12(6), 501–503.

Pappas, G., Papadimitriou, P., Siozopoulou, V., Leonidas Christou, S., and Akritidis, N. (2008). The globalization of leptospirosis: worldwide incidence trends. *Int J Infect Dis* 12, 351–357.

Peck, D.F. (2005). Foot and mouth outbreak: lessons for mental health services. *Adv Psychiatr Treat* 11, 270–276.

Plans-Rubió, P. (2012). The vaccination coverage required to establish herd immunity against influenza viruses. *Prev Med* 55(1), 72–77.

Poundstone, K.E., Strathdee, S.A., and Celentano,.D.D. (2004). The social epidemiology of human immunodeficiency virus/acquired immunodeficiency syndrome. *Epidemiol Rev* 26(1), 22–35.

Rich, K.M. and Wanyoike, F. (2010) An assessment of the regional and national socio-economic impacts of the 2007 Rift Valley fever outbreak in Kenya. *Am J Trop Med Hyg* 83, 52–57.

Rothman, K.J. (1976). Causes. *Am J Epidemiol* 104, 587–592.

Rothman, K.J. (2012). *Epidemiology: An Introduction*, 2nd edn. Oxford University Press.

Sakula, A. (1983). Robert Koch (1843-1910): founder of the science of bacteriology and discoverer of the tubercle bacillus. A study of his life and work. *Can Vet J* 24, 124–127.

Stuart-Harris, C. (1984) Prospects for the eradication of infectious diseases. *Rev Infect Dis* 6(3), 405–411.

Thompson, D., Muriel, P., Russell, D., et al. (2002). Economic costs of the foot and mouth disease outbreak in the United Kingdom in 2001. *Rev Sci Tech Off Int Epiz* 21(3), 675–687.

Thompson, R.C. (2013). Parasite zoonoses and wildlife: One health, spillover and human activity. *Int J Parasitol* 43, 1079–1088.

UNDG (United Nations Development Group)-Western and Central Africa (2015). Socio-economic impact of Ebola virus disease in West African countries: A call for national and regional containment, recovery and prevention. Available at: http://www.africa.undp.org/content/dam/rba/docs/Reports/ebola-west-africa.pdf (accessed November 14, 2017).

Vineis, P. (2003). Causality in epidemiology. *Soz Praventivmed* 48(2), 80–87.

WHO (World Health Organization) (2017). Rabies Fact Sheet. Available at: http://www.who.int/mediacentre/factsheets/fs099/en/ (accessed November 14, 2017).

2

Health Impacts in a Changing Climate
Donald J. Wuebbles

University of Illinois, Urbana, IL, USA

2.1 Introduction

The science is clear: the Earth's climate is changing, it is changing extremely rapidly, and the evidence shows it is happening primarily because of human activities (IPCC, 2013, 2014; Melillo et al., 2014; UKRS and NAS, 2014; and the thousands of papers referenced in these assessments). Climate change is happening now – it is not just a problem for the future – and it is happening throughout the world. There are many indicators of the changing climate. Surface temperature is just one of them. Trends in the severity of certain types of severe weather events are increasing. Sea levels are also rising because of the warming oceans and because of the melting land ice. Observations show that the climate is changing extremely rapidly, about ten times more rapidly than natural changes in climate based on paleoclimatic observations of the changes that occurred since the end of the last ice age. And the evidence clearly points to climate changes over the last half century as being primarily due to human activities, especially the burning of fossil fuels and also land use change, especially through deforestation. As a result, it is not surprising that many national and world leaders have concluded that climate

change, often referred to as global warming in the media, has become one of the most important issues facing humanity.

There is essentially no debate in the peer-reviewed scientific literature (or in the national and international assessments of the science prepared by hundreds of scientists) about the large changes occurring in the Earth's climate and the fact that these changes are occurring as a response to human activities. Natural factors such as changes in the energy output of the Sun have always affected our climate in the past and continue to do so today; but over the last century, human activities have become the dominant influence in producing many, if not most, of the observed changes occurring in our current climate.

People throughout the world are already feeling the effects from increasing intensity of certain types of extreme weather and from sea level rise that are fueled by the changing climate. Prolonged periods of heat and heavy downpours, and in some regions, floods, and in others, drought, are affecting our health, agriculture, water resources, energy and transportation infrastructure, and much more. The focus here is on human health, and although the discussion applies to what is happening worldwide, the examples given are aimed at the USA. Climate change, in combination with natural and other health stressors, is and will influence human health and disease in numerous ways, regardless of whether prevention and adaptation efforts are undertaken. Evidence indicates that, absent these other changes (prevention/adaptation activities, infrastructure improvements) and with increasing population susceptibilities (e.g., aging, limited economic resources), some existing health threats will intensify and new health threats will emerge. It is important to recognize that climate change is clearly a global public health problem, with serious health impacts predicted to manifest in varying ways in different parts of the world. Public health in the USA can be affected by disruptions of physical, biological, and ecological systems, both originating in the USA and elsewhere.

The harsh reality is that the present amount of climate change is already dangerous and will become far more dangerous in the coming decades. Climate change is itself likely to increase the risks for impacts on health, and the more intense extreme events associated with a changing climate pose a serious risk to human health.

The chapter begins with a discussion of the changes happening and projected to happen in the climate system and a summary of the underlying scientific basis for the human cause for these changes. Much more on each of these topics, and the projections of future changes in climate, can be found in the international (IPCC, 2013, 2014) and US National Climate (Melillo et al., 2014) assessments of the science mentioned earlier. The connections between health and the changing climate are then examined, with a special focus on health impacts in the USA. Much of this discussion is based on Chapter 9 (Human Health) in the third National Climate Assessment (NCA: Melillo et al., 2014) and also on a recently updated analysis of human health effects published as part of the sustained assessment process for the US Global Change Research Program (USGCRP, 2016).

2.2 Our Changing Climate

The fifth assessment report (AR5) of the Intergovernmental Panel on Climate Change (IPCC, 2013, 2014) is the most comprehensive analysis to date of the science of climate change and how it is affecting our planet. Over 800 scientists and other experts were involved in the four volumes of this assessment. Similarly, the third US National Climate Assessment (Melillo et al., 2014) is the most comprehensive analysis to date of how climate change is affecting the USA now and how it could affect it in the future. A team of more than 300 scientists and other experts (see complete list online at http://nca2014.globalchange.gov), guided by a 60-member National Climate Assessment and Development Advisory Committee, produced the assessment. Stakeholders involved in the development of the assessment included decision-makers from the public and private sectors, resource and environmental managers, researchers, representatives from businesses and nongovernmental organizations, and the general public. The resulting report went through extensive peer and public review before publication, including two sets of reviews by the National Academy of Sciences. The NCA collects, integrates, and assesses observations and research from around the country, helping us to see what is actually happening and understand what it means for our lives, our livelihoods, and our future. The report includes analyses of impacts on seven sectors – human health, water, energy, transportation, agriculture, forests, and ecosystems – and the interactions among sectors at the national level. The report also assesses key impacts on all parts of the USA and evaluated for specific regions: Northeast, Southeast and Caribbean, Midwest, Great Plains, Southwest, Northwest, Alaska, Hawaii and Pacific Islands, as well as the country's coastal areas, oceans, and marine resources. By being so comprehensive, the NCA's aim is to help inform Americans' choices and decisions about investments, where to build and where to live, how to create safer communities and secure our own and our children's future.

Climate is defined as long-term averages and variations in weather measured over multiple decades. The Earth's climate system includes the land surface, atmosphere, oceans, and ice. Scientists from around the world have compiled the evidence that the climate is changing, changing much more rapidly than tends to occur naturally (by a factor of 10 or more according to some studies), and that it is changing because of human activities; these conclusions are based on observations from satellites, weather balloons, thermometers at surface stations, ice cores, and many other types of observing systems that monitor the Earth's weather and climate. A wide variety of independent observations give a consistent picture of a warming world. There are many indicators of this change, not just atmospheric surface temperature. For example, ocean temperatures are also rising, sea level is rising, Arctic sea ice is decreasing, most glaciers are decreasing, Greenland and Antarctic land ice is decreasing, and atmospheric humidity is increasing.

2.2.1 Climate Change Effects on Temperature

Temperatures at the surface, in the troposphere – the active weather layer extending from the ground to about 8 to 16 km (5 to 10 miles) altitude – and in the oceans have all increased over recent decades. Consistent with our scientific understanding, the largest increases in temperature are occurring closer to the poles, especially in the Arctic (this is especially related to ice-albedo feedback, which, as snow and ice decrease, indicates that the exposed surface will absorb more solar radiation rather than reflect it back to space). Snow and ice cover have decreased in most areas on Earth. Atmospheric water vapor (H_2O) is increasing in the lower atmosphere, because a warmer atmosphere can hold more water (the basic physics is captured by the Clausius–Clapeyron equation,

which provides the relationship between temperature and available water vapor). Sea levels are also increasing. All of these findings are based on observations.

As seen in Figure 2.1, global annual average temperature (as measured over both land and oceans) has increased by more than 0.8 °C (1.5 °F) since 1880 (through 2012). Since then, 2014 was the warmest year on record, but this was greatly eclipsed by 2015, when a strong El Niño event (unusually warm water in the eastern portion of the Pacific Ocean) added to the effects of climate change. Then 2016 was even warmer, and 2017 will likely be either the second or third warmest year on record. While there is a clear long-term global warming trend, some years do not show a temperature increase relative to the previous year, and some years show greater changes than others. These year-to-year fluctuations in temperature are related to natural processes, such as the effects of ocean events like El Niños and La Niñas, and the cooling effects of atmospheric emissions from volcanic eruptions. At the local to regional scale, changes in climate can be influenced by natural variability for a few decades (Deser et al., 2012). Globally, natural variations can be as large as human-induced climate change over timescales of up to a decade (Karl et al., 2015). However, changes in climate at the global scale observed over the past 50 years are far larger than can be accounted for by natural variability (IPCC, 2013).

While there has been widespread warming over the past century, not every region has warmed at the same pace (Figure 2.2). A few regions, such as the North Atlantic Ocean and some parts of the US Southeast, have even experienced cooling over the last century as a whole, though the US Southeast has warmed over recent decades. This is due to the stronger influence of internal variability over smaller geographic regions and shorter timescales. Warming during the first half of the last century occurred mostly in the Northern Hemisphere. The last three decades have seen greater warming in response

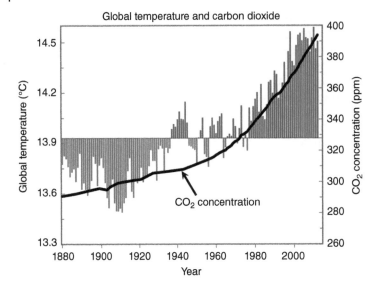

Figure 2.1 Changes in observed globally averaged temperature since 1880. Red bars show temperatures above the long-term average, and blue bars indicate temperatures below the long-term average. The black line shows the changes in atmospheric carbon dioxide (CO_2) concentration in parts per million (ppm) over the same time period (Melillo et al., 2014; temperature data from NOAA National Climate Data Center). *Source:* Adapted from Karl et al. (2009) in Melillo et al. (2014).

to accelerating increases in heat-trapping gas concentrations, particularly at high northern latitudes, and over land as compared to the oceans. These findings are not surprising given the larger heat capacity of the oceans leading to land-ocean differences in warming and the ice-albedo feedback leading to greater warming at higher latitudes. As a result, land areas can respond to the changes in climate much more rapidly than the ocean areas even though the forcing driving a change in climate occurs equally over land and the oceans.

Even if the surface temperature had never been measured, scientists could still conclude with high confidence that the global temperature has been increasing because multiple lines of evidence all support this conclusion. Figure 2.3 shows a number of examples of the indicators that show the climate on Earth has been changing very rapidly over the last century. Temperatures in the lower atmosphere and oceans have increased, as have sea level and near-surface humidity. Basic physics tells us that a warmer atmosphere can hold more water vapor; this

is exactly what is measured from the satellite data showing that humidity is increasing. Arctic sea ice, mountain glaciers, and Northern Hemisphere spring snow cover have all decreased. Over 90% of the glaciers in the world are decreasing at very significant rates. The amounts of ice on the largest masses of ice on our planet, on Greenland and Antarctica, are decreasing. As with temperature, many scientists and associated research groups have analyzed each of these indicators and come to the same conclusion: all of these changes paint a consistent and compelling picture of a warming planet.

2.2.2 Climate Change Effects on Precipitation

Precipitation is perhaps the most societally relevant aspect of the hydrological cycle and has been observed over global land areas for over a century. However, spatial scales of precipitation are small (e.g., it can rain several inches in Washington, DC, but not a drop in nearby Baltimore) and this makes interpretation of the point-measurements difficult.

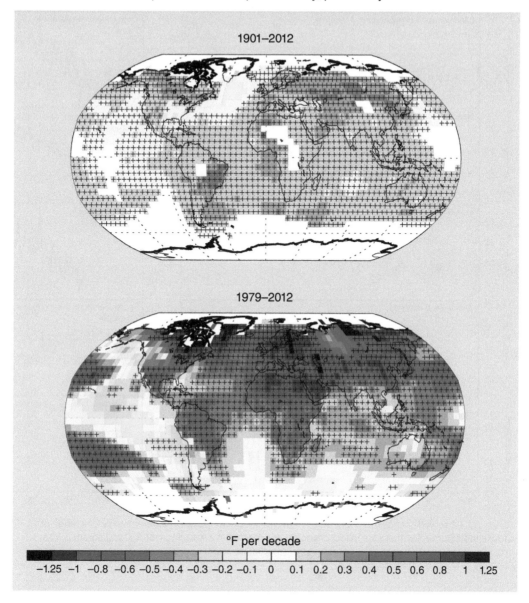

Figure 2.2 Surface temperature trends for the period 1901–2012 (top) and 1979–2012 (bottom) from NOAA National Climate Data Center's surface temperature product. Updated from Vose et al. (2012). *Source:* Adapted from Vose et al. (2012) in Melillo et al. (2014).

Based upon a range of efforts to create global averages, there does not appear to have been significant changes in globally averaged precipitation since 1900 (although, as we will discuss later, there has been a significant trend for an increase in precipitation coming as larger events). However, in looking at total precipitation there are strong geographic trends including a likely increase in precipitation in Northern Hemisphere mid-latitude regions taken as a whole (Figure 2.4). Stronger trends are generally found over the last four

Indicators of warming from multiple datasets

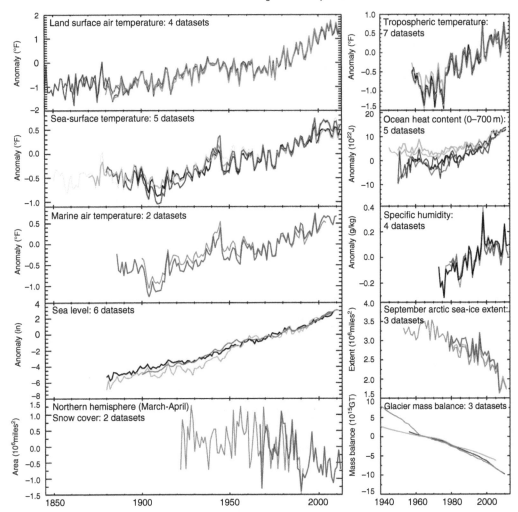

Figure 2.3 Observed changes, as analyzed by many independent groups in different ways, of a range of climate indicators. All of these are in fact changing as expected in a warming world. This diagram is from http://nca2014.globalchange.gov/report/appendices/climate-science-supplement. *Source:* Adapted from Kennedy et al. (2014) in Melillo et al. (2014).

decades. In general, the findings are that wet areas are getting wetter and dry areas are getting drier, consistent with an overall intensification of the hydrological cycle in response to the warming climate (IPCC, 2013).

As mentioned earlier, it is well known that warmer air can contain more water vapor than cooler air. Global analyses show that the amount of water vapor in the atmosphere has in fact increased over both land and oceans. Climate change also alters

dynamical characteristics of the atmosphere, which in turn affect weather patterns and storms. At mid-latitudes, there is an upward trend in extreme precipitation in the vicinity of fronts associated with mid-latitude storms. Locally, natural variations can also be important. In contrast, the subtropics are generally tending to have less overall rainfall and more droughts. Nonetheless, many areas show an increasing tendency for larger rainfall events when

Annual precipitation trends: past century, past 30+ years

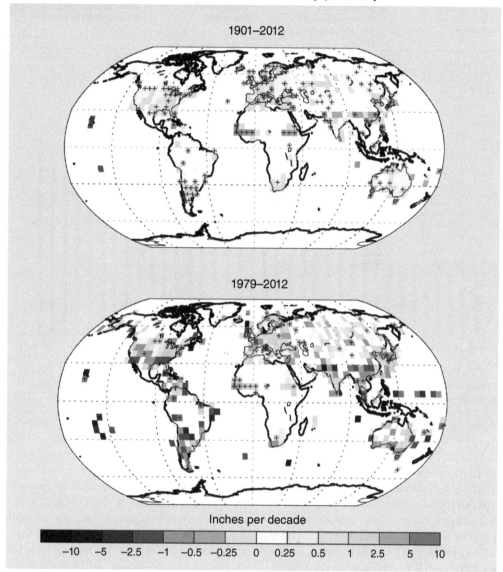

Figure 2.4 Global precipitation trends for the period 1901–2012 (top) and 1979–2012 (bottom). Based on data from NOAA NCDC. From Melillo et al. (2014).

it does rain (Janssen et al., 2014; Melillo et al., 2014; IPCC, 2013).

2.2.3 Climate Change Effects on Severe Weather

Along with the overall changes in climate, there is strong evidence of an increasing trend over recent decades in some types of extreme weather events, including their frequency, intensity, and duration, with resulting impacts on our society. It is becoming clearer that the changing trends in severe weather are already affecting us greatly. The USA has sustained 178 weather/climate disasters since 1980 where damages/costs

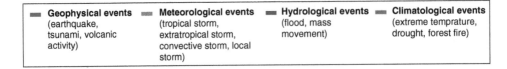

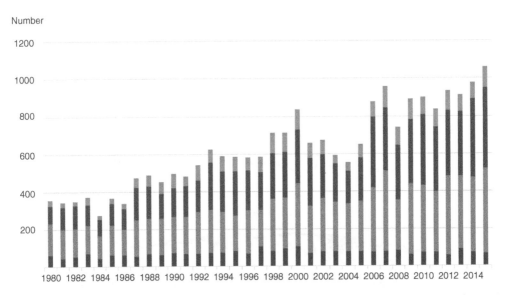

Figure 2.5 The number of severe loss events from natural catastrophes per year since 1980 through 2015 as evaluated by Munich Re. Overall losses totaled $90 billion dollars (2015 was not a high year in terms of total costs; the previous year was $110 billion), of which roughly $27 billion was insured. In 2015, natural catastrophes claimed 23 000 lives (average over the last 30 years was 54 000). *Source:* Munich Re (https://www. munichre.com/us/weather-resilience-and-protection/media-relations/news/160104-natcatstats2015/index. html). Includes copyrighted material of Munich Re and its licensors.

reached or exceeded $1 billion per event (including CPI adjustment to 2013), with an overall increasing trend (see http://www. ncdc.noaa.gov/billions/; also Smith and Katz, 2012). The total cost of these 178 events over the 34 years is well over $1 trillion. In the years 2011 and 2012, there were more such weather events than previously experienced in any given year, with 14 events in 2011 and 11 in 2012, with costs exceeding $60 billion in 2011 and $110 billion during 2012. There were eight billion-dollar-plus events in the USA in 2014. The events in these analyses include major heatwaves, severe storms, tornadoes, droughts, floods, hurricanes, and wildfires. A portion of these increased costs can be attributed to the increase in population and infrastructure near coastal regions. However, even if hurricanes and their large, mostly coastal, impacts were excluded, there still would be an overall increase in the number of billion-dollar events over the last 34 years. Similar analyses by Munich Re and other organizations show that there are growing numbers of severe weather events worldwide causing extensive damage and loss of lives. Figure 2.5 shows the overall increase in the number of severe events since 1980 through 2015. Even though geophysical events like earthquakes are included in Figure 2.5, they are roughly a constant number each year, while the number of severe climate- and weather-related events has increased dramatically. In summary, there is a clear trend in the impacts of severe weather events on human society not only in the USA, but throughout the world.

A series of studies by Kunkel et al. (2013), Peterson et al. (2013), Vose et al. (2014), and Wuebbles et al. (2014a), along with many other journal papers, have led to a collective assessment regarding changes in various weather extremes relative to the changing climate. The adequacy of the existing data to detect trends in severe weather events was examined relative to the current scientific ability to understand what drives those trends, that is, how well the physical processes are understood, and thus how the extremes are expected to change in the future. This assessment shows that there are some events, such as those relating to temperature and precipitation extremes, where there is strong understanding of the trends and the underlying causes of the changes. The adequacy of data for floods, droughts, and extratropical cyclones to detect trends is also high, but there is only medium understanding of the underlying cause of their long-term changes. There is also medium understanding of the observed trends and cause of changes in hurricanes and in snow events. For some events, such as strong winds, hail, ice storms, and tornadoes, there is currently insufficient understanding of the trends or of the causes for the trends to make strong conclusions about these events in a changing climate. These findings also correlate well with global analyses of climate extremes (IPCC, 2012, 2013).

Changing trends in some types of extreme weather events have been observed in recent decades. Modeling studies indicate that these trends are consistent with the changing climate. Much of the world is being affected by changing trends in extreme events, including increases in the number of extremely hot days, less extreme cold days, more precipitation events coming as unusually large precipitation, and more floods in some regions and more drought in others (Min et al., 2011; IPCC, 2012, 2013; Zwiers et al., 2013; Melillo et al., 2014; Wuebbles et al., 2014a, 2014b). High-impact, large-scale extreme events are complex phenomena involving various factors that come together to create a "perfect storm." Such extreme weather obviously does occur naturally. However, the influence of human activities on global climate is altering the frequency and/or severity of many of these events. Observed trends in extreme weather events, such as more hot days, fewer cold days, and more precipitation coming as extreme events, are expected to continue and to intensify over this century.

In most of the USA over the last couple of decades, the heaviest rainfall events have become more frequent (see, e.g., Figure 2.6), and the amount of rain falling in very heavy precipitation events has been significantly above average. This increase has been greatest in the Northeast, Midwest, and upper Great Plains. Similar findings are being found in many other parts of the world. Since basic physics tells us that a warmer atmosphere should generally hold more water vapor, this finding is not so surprising. Analyses indicate that these trends will continue (Janssen et al., 2014; Melillo et al., 2014; Wuebbles et al., 2014a, 2014b).

The meteorological situations that cause heatwaves are a natural part of the climate system. Thus the timing and location of individual events may be largely a natural phenomenon, although even these may be affected by human-induced climate change (Trenberth and Fasullo, 2012). However, there is emerging evidence that most of the increasing heatwave severity over our planet is likely related to the changes in climate, with a detectable human influence for major recent heatwaves in the USA (Meehl et al., 2009; Rupp et al., 2012; Duffy and Tebaldi, 2012), Europe (Stott et al., 2010; Trenberth, 2011), and Russia (Christidis et al., 2011). As an example, the summer 2011 heatwave and drought in Oklahoma and Texas, which cost Texas an estimated $8 billion in agricultural losses, was primarily driven by precipitation deficits, but the human contribution to climate change approximately doubled the probability that the heat was record-breaking (Hoerling et al., 2013). So while an event such as this Texas heatwave and drought could be triggered by a naturally occurring event such

Observed change in very heavy precipitation

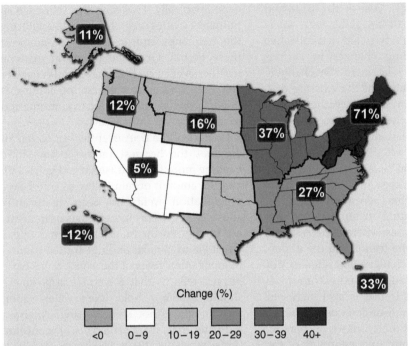

Figure 2.6 Percent increases in the amount of precipitation falling in very heavy events (defined as the heaviest 1% of all daily events) from 1958 to 2012 for each region of the continental USA. These trends are larger than natural variations for the Northeast, Midwest, Puerto Rico, Southeast, Great Plains, and Alaska. The trends are not larger than natural variations for the Southwest, Hawaii, and the Northwest. The changes shown in this figure are calculated from the beginning and end points of the trends for 1958 to 2012. *Source:* Adapted from Karl et al. (2009) in Melillo et al. (2014).

as a deficit in precipitation, the chances for record-breaking temperature extremes have increased and will continue to increase as the global climate warms. Generally, the changes in climate are increasing the likelihood for these types of severe events.

In the tropics, the most important types of storms are tropical cyclones, referred to as hurricanes when they occur in the Atlantic Ocean. Over the 40 years of satellite monitoring, there has been a shift toward stronger hurricanes in the Atlantic, with fewer smaller (category 1 and 2) hurricanes and more intense (category 4 and 5) hurricanes. There has been no significant trend in the global number of tropical cyclones (IPCC, 2012, 2013) nor has any trend been identified in the number of US landfalling hurricanes (Melillo et al., 2014).

Trends remain uncertain in some types of severe weather, including the intensity and frequency of tornadoes, hail, and damaging thunderstorm winds, but such events are under scrutiny to determine if there is a climate change influence. Initial studies do suggest that tornadoes could get more intense in the coming decades (Diffenbaugh et al., 2013).

After at least two thousand years of little change, the world's sea level rose by roughly 0.2 meters (8 inches) over the last century, and satellite data provide evidence that the rate of rise over the past 20 years has roughly doubled. Sea level is rising because ocean water expands as it heats up and because water is added to the oceans from melting glaciers and ice sheets. Also, the observed increase in atmospheric carbon dioxide (CO_2), resulting largely from fossil fuel burning, also results in increasing the amount of CO_2 in the oceans and thus, a larger amount of carbonic acid. The oceans are currently absorbing about a quarter of the carbon dioxide emitted to the atmosphere annually (Le Quéré et al., 2009) and are becoming more acidic as a result, leading to concerns about intensifying impacts on marine ecosystems (Melillo et al., 2014).

2.3 The Basis for a Human Cause for Climate Change

The Earth's climate has long been known to change in response to natural external factors, termed climate forcings. These include variations in the energy received from the Sun, volcanic eruptions, and changes in the Earth's orbit, which affects the distribution of sunlight across the world. The Earth's climate is also affected by factors that are internal to the climate system, which are the result of complex interactions between the atmosphere, ocean, land surface, and living things. These internal factors include natural modes of climate system variability, such as those that form El Niño events in the Pacific Ocean.

Natural changes in external forcings and internal factors have been responsible for past climate changes. At the global scale, over multiple decades, the impact of external forcings on temperature far exceeds that of internal variability, which is less than 0.28 °C (0.5 °F) (Swanson et al., 2009). At the regional scale, and over shorter time periods, internal variability can be responsible for much larger changes in temperature and other aspects of climate. Today, however, the picture is very different. Although natural factors still affect climate, human activities are now the primary cause of the current warming: specifically, human activities that increase atmospheric levels of CO_2 and other heat-trapping gases and various particles that, depending on the type of particle, can have either a heating or cooling influence on climate.

The greenhouse effect is key to understanding how human activities affect the Earth's climate. As the Sun shines on the Earth, the Earth heats up. The Earth then re-radiates this heat back to space. Some gases, including H_2O, CO_2, ozone (O_3), methane (CH_4), and nitrous oxide (N_2O), absorb some of the heat given off by the Earth's surface and lower atmosphere. These heat-trapping gases then radiate energy back toward the surface, effectively trapping some of the heat inside the climate system. This greenhouse effect is a natural process, first recognized in 1824 by the French mathematician and physicist Joseph Fourier and confirmed by British scientist John Tyndall in a series of experiments starting in 1859. Without this natural greenhouse effect (but assuming the same albedo, or reflectivity, as today), the average surface temperature of the Earth would be about 33 °C (60 °F) colder than today.

Over the last five decades, natural drivers of climate such as solar forcing and volcanoes would actually have led to a slight cooling. For example, accurate observations of the Sun from satellites since 1978 show that the solar output has actually decreased slightly from 1978 to now. Natural drivers cannot explain the observed warming over this period. The majority of the warming can only be explained by the effects of human influences (Stott et al., 2010; Gillet et al., 2012; IPCC, 2013; Santer et al., 2013), especially the emissions from burning fossil fuels (i.e., coal, oil, and natural gas), and from changes in land use, such as deforestation. As a result of human activities, atmospheric concentrations of various gases and particles are changing, including those for CO_2, CH_4, and N_2O, and particles such as black carbon (soot), which has a warming influence, and sulfates, which have an overall cooling influence (because they reflect sunlight). The most important changes are occurring in the concentration of CO_2; its atmospheric concentration has now reached 400 ppm (400 molecules per 1 million molecules of air; this small amount is important because of the heat-trapping ability of CO_2). This level of 400 ppm of CO_2 has not been seen on Earth for over one million years, well before the appearance of humans – preindustrial levels of CO_2 were approximately 280 ppm. The increase in CO_2 over the last several hundred years is almost entirely due to burning of fossil fuels and to a lesser extent, from land use change (IPCC, 2013).

The conclusion that human influences are the primary driver of recent climate change is based on multiple lines of independent evidence. The first line of evidence is our fundamental understanding of how certain gases trap heat (these so-called greenhouse gases include H_2O, CO_2, CH_4, N_2O, and some other gases and particles that can all absorb the infrared radiation emitted from the Earth that otherwise would go to space), how the climate system responds to increases in these gases, and how other human and natural factors influence climate.

Another line of evidence is from reconstructions of past climates using evidence such as tree rings, ice cores, and corals. These show that the change in global surface temperatures over the last five decades is clearly unusual, and outside the range of natural variability. These analyses show that the last decade (2000–2009) was warmer than any time in at least the last 1300 years and perhaps much longer (IPCC, 2013; PAGES 2 K Consortium, 2013; Mann et al., 2008). Through 2016, it appears that this decade will be much warmer than the previous decade.

The rate of globally averaged surface air temperature increase was slower in the period from 2000 to 2009 than it was in the prior three decades, but this is not in conflict with our basic understanding of global warming and its primary cause. The decade of 2000 to 2009 was still the warmest decade on record. In addition, global surface air temperature does not always increase steadily and can be influenced by natural variability on the scale of a few decades (for further discussion, see IPCC, 2013; Melillo et al., 2014; Karl et al., 2015). Other climate change indicators, like the decrease in Arctic sea ice and sea level rise, have not seen a slower change in the rate of change during the same period.

Evidence also comes from using climate models to simulate the climate of the past century, separating the human and natural factors that influence climate. As shown in Figure 2.7, when the human factors are removed, these models show that solar and volcanic activity would have tended to slightly cool the earth, and other natural variations are too small to explain the amount of

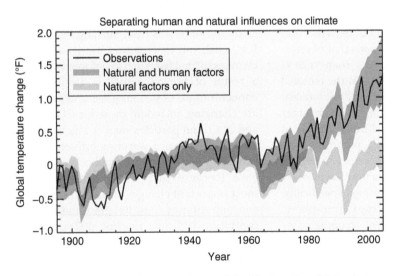

Figure 2.7 Observed global average changes (black line), and model simulations using only changes in natural factors (solar and volcanic) in green, and with the addition of human-induced emissions (blue). Climate changes since 1950 cannot be explained by natural factors or variability, and can only be explained by human factors. *Source:* Adapted from Huber and Knutti (2012) in Melillo et al. (2014).

warming. The range of values accounted for the range of results from the 20+ different models from around the world that were used in these analyses for the international climate assessment (IPCC, 2013). Only when the human influences are included do the models reproduce the warming observed over the past 50 years.

2.4 Twenty-first Century Projections of Climate Change

On the global scale, climate model simulations show consistent projections of future conditions under a range of emissions scenarios (that depend on assumptions of population change, economic development, our continued use of fossil fuels, changes in other human activities, and other factors). For temperature, all models show warming by late this century that is much larger than historical variations nearly everywhere (Figure 2.8). For precipitation, models are in complete agreement in showing decreases in precipitation in the subtropics and increases in precipitation at higher latitudes. As mentioned earlier, extreme weather events associated with extremes in temperature and precipitation are likely to continue and to intensify.

Choices made now and in the next few decades about emissions from fossil fuel use and land use change will determine the amount of additional future warming over this century and beyond. Global emissions of CO_2 and other heat-trapping gases continue to rise. How much climate will change over this century and beyond depends primarily on two factors:

1) Human activities and resulting emissions.
2) How sensitive the climate is to those changes (i.e., the response of global temperature to a change in radiative forcing caused by human emissions).

Uncertainties in how the economy will evolve, what types of energy will be used, or what our cities, buildings, or cars will look like in the future are all important and limit the ability to project future changes in climate. Scientists can, however, develop scenarios – plausible projections of what might happen, under a given set of assumptions. These scenarios describe possible futures in terms of population, energy sources, technology, heat-trapping gas

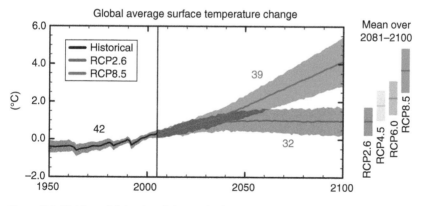

Figure 2.8 Multi-model simulated time series from 1950 to 2100 for the change in global annual mean surface temperature relative to 1986–2005 for a range of future emissions scenarios that account for the uncertainty in future emissions from human activities – as analyzed with the 20+ models from around the world used in the most recent international assessment (IPCC, 2013). The mean and associated uncertainties (1.64 standard deviations (5–95%) across the distribution of individual models (shading)) based on the averaged over 2081–2100 are given for all of the RCP scenarios as colored vertical bars. The numbers of models used to calculate the multi-model mean is indicated. *Source:* IPCC (2013). Reproduced with permission of the IPCC.

emissions, atmospheric levels of carbon dioxide, and/or global temperature change.

A certain amount of climate change is inevitable due to the build-up of CO_2 in the atmosphere from human activities (although there is a rapid exchange of CO_2 with the biosphere, the eventual lifetime for atmospheric CO_2 is dependent on removal to the deep ocean). The Earth's climate system, particularly the oceans, tends to lag behind changes in atmospheric composition by decades, and even centuries due to the large heat capacity of the oceans and other factors. Another 0.2–0.3 °C (about 0.5 °F) increase is expected over the next few decades (Matthews and Zickfeld, 2012) although natural variability could still play an important role over this time period (Hawkins and Sutton, 2011). The higher the human-related emissions of CO_2 and other heat-trapping gases over the coming decades, the higher the resulting changes expected by mid-century and beyond. By the second half of the century, however, scenario uncertainty (i.e., uncertainty about what will be the level of emissions from human activities) becomes increasingly dominant in determining the magnitude and patterns of future change, particularly for temperature-related aspects (Hawkins and Sutton, 2009, 2011).

As seen in Figures 2.8 and 2.9, for a range of scenarios that vary from assuming strong continued dependence on fossil fuels in energy and transportation systems over the twenty-first century (scenario RCP8.5) to assuming major mitigation actions (RCP2.6), global surface temperature change for the end of the twenty-first century is *likely* to exceed an increase of 1.5 °C (2.7 °F) relative to 1850 to 1900 for all projections except for the RCP2.6 scenario (IPCC, 2013). Note that the RCP2.6 scenario is much lower than the other scenarios examined because it not only assumes significant mitigation to reduce emissions, but it also assumes that technologies are developed that can achieve net negative carbon dioxide emissions (removal of CO_2 from the atmosphere) before the end of the century.

A number of research studies have examined the potential criteria for dangerous human interferences in climate where it will be difficult to adapt to the changes in climate without major effects on our society (e.g., Hansen et al., 2007). Most of these studies have concluded that an increase in globally averaged temperature of roughly 1.5 °C (2.7 °F) is an approximate threshold for dangerous human interferences with the climate system (see IPCC, 2013, 2014 for further discussion; earlier studies had proposed 2 °C), but that this threshold is not exact and the changes in climate are geographically diverse and impacts are sector dependent, so there really is no defined threshold by when dangerous interferences are actually reached.

The warming and other changes in the climate system will continue beyond 2100 under all RCP scenarios, except for a leveling of temperature under RCP2.6. In addition, it is fully expected that the warming will continue to exhibit interannual-to-decadal variability and will not be regionally uniform.

Projections of future changes in precipitation show small increases in the global average but substantial shifts in where and how precipitation falls (Figure 2.10). Generally, areas closest to the poles are projected to receive more precipitation, while the dry subtropics (the region just outside the tropics, between 23° and 35° on either side of the Equator) will generally expand toward the poles and receives less rain. Increases in tropical precipitation are projected during rainy seasons (such as monsoons), especially over the tropical Pacific. Certain regions, including the western USA – especially the Southwest (Melillo et al., 2014) and the Mediterranean (IPCC, 2013) – are presently dry and are expected to become drier. The widespread trend of increasing heavy downpours is expected to continue, with precipitation becoming more intense (Gutowski et al., 2007; Boberg et al., 2009; Sillmann et al., 2013). The patterns of the projected changes of precipitation do not contain the spatial details that characterize observed precipitation, especially in mountainous terrain,

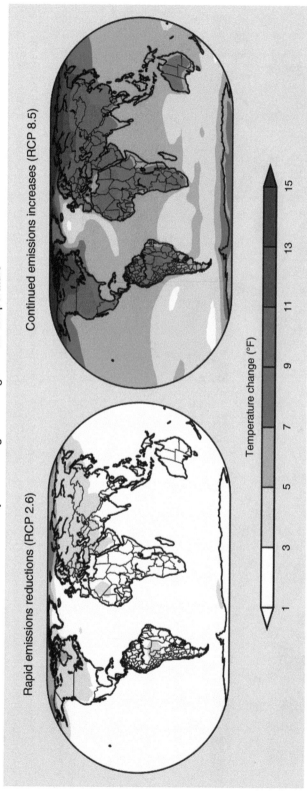

Projected change in average annual temperature

Rapid emissions reductions (RCP 2.6)

Continued emissions increases (RCP 8.5)

Temperature change (°F)

1   3   5   7   9   11   13   15

Figure 2.9 Projected change in average annual temperature over the period 2071–2099 (compared to the period 1971–2000) under a low scenario that assumes rapid reductions in emissions and concentrations of heat-trapping gases (RCP 2.6), and a higher scenario that assumes continued increases in emissions (RCP 8.5). *Source:* Based on data from NOAA NCDC. From Melillo et al. (2014).

Projected change in average annual precipitation

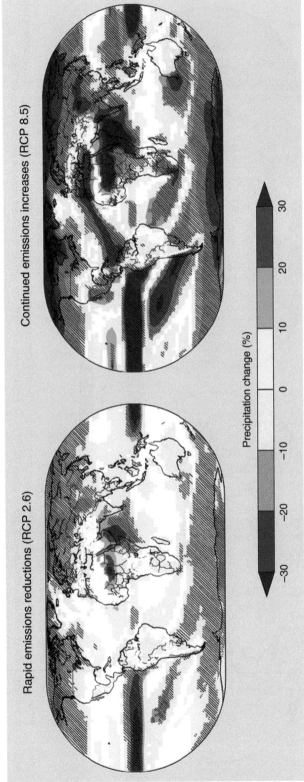

Figure 2.10 Projected change in average annual precipitation over the period 2071–2099 (compared to the period 1971–2000) under a low scenario that assumes rapid reductions in emissions and concentrations of heat-trapping gasses (RCP 2.6), and a higher scenario that assumes continued increases in emissions (RCP 8.5). Hatched areas indicate that the projected changes are significant and consistent among models. White areas indicate that the changes are not projected to be larger than could be expected from natural variability. In general, northern parts of the USA (especially the Northeast and Alaska) are projected to receive more precipitation, while southern parts (especially the Southwest) are projected to receive less. *Source:* Based on data from NOAA NCDC. From Melillo et al. (2014).

because of model uncertainties and their current spatial resolution (IPCC, 2013).

As mentioned earlier, some areas both in the USA and throughout the world are already experiencing climate-related disruptions, particularly due to extreme weather events. These trends are likely to continue throughout this century and perhaps beyond (depending on the actions we take). Existing research indicates the following trends over the coming decades (see Melillo et al., 2014, or IPCC, 2013, for more details):

- It is likely that over the coming decades the frequency of warm days and warm nights will increase in most land regions, while the frequency of cold days and cold nights will decrease. As a result, an increasing tendency for heatwaves is likely in many regions of the world.
- Some regions are likely to see an increasing tendency for droughts while others are likely to see an increasing tendency for floods. This roughly corresponds to the wet getting wetter and the dry getting drier.
- It is likely that the frequency and intensity of heavy precipitation events will increase over land. These changes are primarily driven by increases in atmospheric water vapor content, but also affected by changes in atmospheric circulation.
- Tropical storm (hurricane)-associated storm intensity and rainfall rates are projected to increase as the climate continues to warm.
- Initial studies also suggest that tornadoes are likely to become more intense.
- For some types of extreme events, like wind storms and ice and hail storms, there is too little understanding currently of how they will be affected by the changes in climate.

Around the world, many millions of people and many assets related to energy, transportation, commerce, and ecosystems are located in areas at risk of coastal flooding because of sea level rise and storm surge. Sea level is projected to rise an additional 0.3 to 1.2 meters (1 to 4 feet) in this century (see

Figure 2.11; Melillo et al., 2014; similar findings in IPCC, 2013). The estimates for the range of projected sea level rise over this century remain quite large; this may be due in part to what emissions scenario we follow, but more importantly it depends on just how much melting occurs from the ice on large land masses, especially from Greenland and Antarctica. Recent projections show that for even the lowest emissions scenarios, thermal expansion of ocean waters (Yin, 2012) and the melting of small mountain glaciers (Marzeion et al., 2012) will result in 28 cm (11 inches) of sea level rise by 2100, even without any contribution from the ice sheets in Greenland and Antarctica. This suggests that about 0.3 m (1 foot) of global sea level rise by 2100 is probably a realistic low end. Recent analyses suggest that 1.2 m (4 feet) may be a reasonable upper limit (Rahmstorf et al., 2012; IPCC, 2013; Melillo et al., 2014). Although scientists cannot yet assign likelihood to any particular scenario, in general, higher emissions scenarios would be expected to lead to higher amounts of sea level rise.

Because of the warmer global temperatures, sea level rise will continue beyond this century. Sea levels will likely continue to rise for many centuries at rates equal to or higher than that of the current century. Many millions of people live within areas than can be affected by the effects of storm surge within a rising sea level. The Low Elevation Coastal Zone (less than 10 m elevation) constitutes 2% of the world's land area, yet contains 10% of the world's population (over 600 million people) (McGranahan et al., 2007; Neumann et al., 2015). Most of the world's megacities are within the coastal zone. By 2030, with sea level rise, the area will expand and 800–900 million people will be exposed (Güneralp et al., 2015; Neumann et al., 2015).

As mentioned earlier, CO_2 is dissolving into the oceans where it reacts with seawater to form carbonic acid, lowering ocean pH levels ("acidification") and threatening a number of marine ecosystems (Doney et al., 2009). Over the last 250 years, the oceans have absorbed 560 billion tons of CO_2,

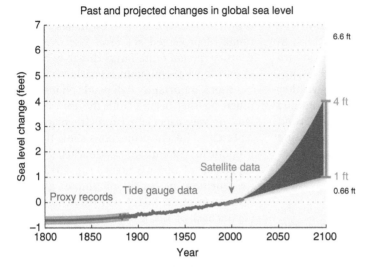

Figure 2.11 Estimated, observed, and projected amounts of global sea level rise from 1800 to 2100, relative to the year 2000. Estimates from proxy data (e.g., based on sediment records) are shown in red (1800–1890, pink band shows uncertainty), tide gauge data in blue for 1880–2009 (Church and White, 2011; Church et al., 2011), and satellite observations are shown in green from 1993 to 2012 (Nerem et al., 2010). The future scenarios range from 0.66 feet (0.20 m) to 6.6 feet (2 m) in 2100 (Parris et al., 2012). These scenarios are not based on climate model simulations, but rather reflect the range of possible scenarios based on scientific studies. The orange line at right shows the currently projected range of sea level rise of 1 to 4 feet (0.3–1.22 m) by 2100, which falls within the larger risk-based scenario range. The large projected range reflects uncertainty about how glaciers and ice sheets will react to the warming ocean, the warming atmosphere, and changing winds and currents. As seen in the observations, there are year-to-year variations in the trend. *Source:* Melillo et al. (2014).

increasing the acidity of surface waters by 30% (Melillo et al., 2014). Although the average oceanic pH can vary on interglacial timescales (Caldeira and Wickett, 2003), the current observed rate of change is roughly 50 times faster than known historical change (Hönisch et al., 2012; Orr, 2011). Regional factors such as coastal upwelling (Feely et al., 2008), changes in discharge rates from rivers and glaciers (Mathis et al., 2011), sea ice loss (Yamamoto-Kawai et al., 2009), and urbanization (Feely et al., 2010) have created "ocean acidification hotspots" where changes are occurring at even faster rates.

The acidification of the oceans has already caused a suppression of carbonate ion concentrations that are critical for marine calcifying animals such as corals, zooplankton, and shellfish. Many of these animals form the foundation of the marine food web. Today, more than a billion people worldwide rely on food from the ocean as their primary source of protein. Ocean acidification puts this important resource at risk.

Projections indicate that in a higher emissions scenario (that assume continuing use of fossil fuels), ocean pH could be reduced from the current level of 8.1 to as low as 7.8 by the end of the century (Orr et al., 2005). Such large rapid changes in ocean pH have probably not been experienced on the planet for the past 100 million years, and it is unclear whether and how quickly ocean life could adapt to such rapid acidification (Hönisch et al., 2012). The potential impact on the human source of food from the oceans is also unclear. Unfortunately, since sustained efforts to monitor ocean acidification worldwide are only beginning, it is currently impossible to quantify this risk or to be able to predict exactly how ocean acidification impacts will cascade throughout the marine food chain and affect the overall structure of marine ecosystems.

2.5 Climate and Health

Climate change threatens human health and well-being in many ways, including impacts from increased extreme weather events, wildfire, decreased air quality, threats to mental health, and diseases transmitted by food, water, and vectors such as mosquitoes, ticks, and fleas (see Figure 2.12 for an overview). Some of these health impacts are already underway in the USA (Melillo et al., 2014). Climate change will, absent other factors, amplify some of the existing health threats we now face. As discussed below, certain people and communities are especially vulnerable, including children, the elderly, the sick, and the poor.

The following eight subsections examine key health concerns of special interest relative to the changing climate.

2.5.1 Temperature-Related Death and Illness

Temperature extremes most directly affect health by compromising the body's ability to regulate its internal temperature. Loss of internal temperature control can result in a cascade of illnesses, including heat cramps, heat exhaustion, heatstroke, and hyperthermia

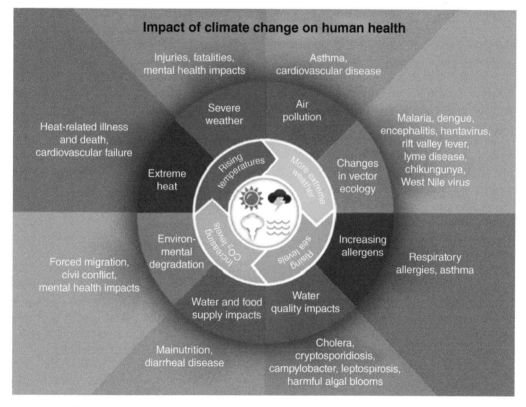

Figure 2.12 The inner circle represents the physical environment. The first ring represents the four primary manifestations of climate change in the physical environment (climate drivers): increasing carbon dioxide concentrations in the atmosphere (yellow), rising temperatures (red), rising sea levels (blue), and more extreme weather (green). The four climate drivers can act through natural and human systems to cause conditions listed in the second ring, such as changes in vector ecology, extreme heat, and changes in water and food supply. Surrounding the second ring are the types of health effects that may result from the conditions listed in the ring. Reproduced courtesy of George Luber, Centers for Disease Control.

in the presence of extreme heat, and hypothermia and frostbite in the presence of extreme cold. Temperature extremes can also worsen chronic conditions such as cardiovascular disease, respiratory disease, cerebrovascular disease, and diabetes-related conditions. The projected changes in climate will likely lead to a decrease in deaths from cold in the winter but could lead to thousands to tens of thousands of additional deaths each year in the USA from heat in the summer, as calculated by extrapolating statistical relationships and without considering potential adaptive changes (USGCRP, 2016). The reduction in deaths is projected to be smaller than the increase in summertime heat-related deaths in most US regions (Luber et al., 2014).

An increase in population tolerance to extreme heat, but not extreme cold, has been observed over time. This could be related to increased use of air conditioning, improved social responses, and/or physiological acclimatization. Including this adaptation trend in human health projections will reduce but not eliminate the increase in future deaths from heat.

Impacts of temperature extremes are geographically varied and disproportionally affect certain populations of concern. Elderly persons and people working outdoors have a higher risk of dying due to increasing frequency, intensity, and duration of future heat and heatwaves. Children and working age adults have increased vulnerability to heat-related illness. The socially isolated, economically disadvantaged, some communities of color (e.g., non-Hispanic black populations), and those with chronic illnesses are also especially vulnerable to death or illness (e.g., Anderson and Bell, 2011).

2.5.2 Air Quality Impacts

The warmer temperatures associated with climate change are likely to increase air quality concerns, especially increasing the production of ozone (by up to 10 ppb in 2050) (Melillo et al., 2014). Slower moving weather systems could also increase the likelihood of higher concentrations of air pollutants and pollens and other allergens. Changes to the climate will tend to make it harder for any given regulatory approach to reduce ground-level ozone pollution in the future as meteorological conditions become increasingly conducive to forming ozone over most of the USA. Unless offset by additional emissions reductions, these climate-driven increases in ozone will cause premature deaths, hospital visits, lost school days, and acute respiratory symptoms. Current estimates suggest that a 1 °C (1.8 °F) rise in global temperature could cause 1000 premature deaths or more each year related to worsened ozone and particle pollution (Melillo et al., 2014). The elderly have been shown to be particularly sensitive to short-term particle exposure, with a higher risk of hospitalization and death (Bell and Dominici, 2008).

Changes in climate, specifically rising temperatures, altered precipitation patterns, and increasing atmospheric carbon dioxide, are expected to contribute to increased production of plant-based allergens (e.g., Ziska et al., 2011), and thus increasing levels of some airborne allergens and associated increases in asthma episodes and other allergic illnesses, compared to a future without climate change. Figure 2.13 shows the lengthening season for ragweed pollens across the central USA since 1995.

2.5.3 Vector-Borne Diseases

Climate is one of the factors that affects the distribution of diseases borne by vectors such as fleas, ticks, and mosquitoes. The geographic and seasonal distribution of vector populations, and the diseases they can carry, depends not only on climate, but also on land use, socioeconomic and cultural factors, pest control, access to healthcare, and human responses to disease risk, among other factors (Melillo et al., 2014). Climate change is expected to alter the geographic and seasonal distributions of existing vectors and vector-borne diseases.

Americans are currently at risk from numerous vector-borne diseases, including

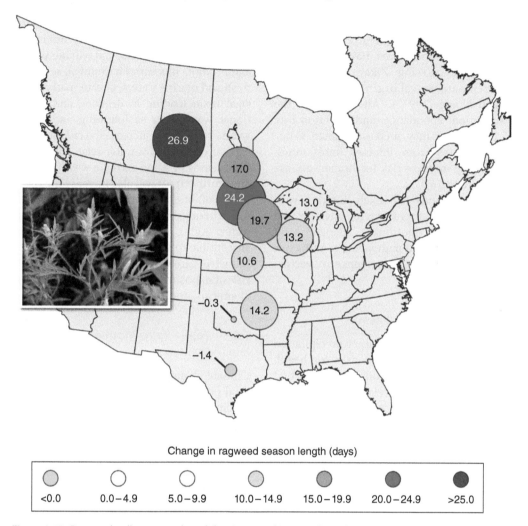

Figure 2.13 Ragweed pollen season length has increased in central North America between 1995 and 2011 by as much as 11 to 27 days in parts of the USA and Canada in response to rising temperatures. Increases in the length of this allergenic pollen season are correlated with increases in the number of days before the first frost. As shown in the figure, the largest increases have been observed in northern cities. *Source:* Data updated from Ziska et al. (2011). Photo credit: Lewis Ziska, U.S. Department of Agriculture. From Melillo et al. (2014).

Lyme disease, dengue fever, West Nile virus, and Rocky Mountain spotted fever. As the climate changes, ticks capable of carrying the bacteria that cause Lyme disease and other pathogens will show earlier seasonal activity and a generally northward expansion in their habitat range in response to increasing temperatures associated with climate change (USGCRP, 2016, and references therein).

Longer seasonal activity and expanding geographic range of these ticks may increase the risk of human exposure to ticks.

Rising temperatures, changing precipitation patterns, and a higher frequency of some extreme weather events associated with climate change will also influence the distribution, abundance, and infection rate of mosquitoes that transmit West Nile virus and other pathogens by altering habitat availability and mosquito and viral reproduction rates. The Zika virus is the latest example of a rapidly spreading epidemic – heavy rain and warm temperatures have helped the mosquitoes carrying Zika thrive (http://www.climatecentral.org/news/zika-virus-climate-change-19970). Alterations in the distribution, abundance, and infection rate of mosquitoes may increase human exposure to bites from infected mosquitoes, which may increase risk for human disease (USGCRP, 2016).

Climate change will likely interact with other driving factors (such as travel-related exposures or evolutionary adaptation of invasive vectors and pathogens) to influence the emergence or re-emergence of vectorborne pathogens.

2.5.4 Water-Related Illnesses

The increasing trend for larger precipitation events can lead to greater risks for health effects (Figure 2.14). Floods are the second deadliest of all weather-related hazards in the USA, accounting for approximately 98 deaths per year (Melillo et al., 2014). Flash floods and flooding associated with tropical storms result in the highest number of deaths. In addition to the immediate health hazards associated with extreme precipitation events when flooding occurs, other hazards can often appear once a storm event has passed. Waterborne disease outbreaks typically result weeks following inundation, and water intrusion into buildings can result in mold contamination that manifests later.

Increases in both coastal and inland water temperatures associated with climate change will expand the seasonal windows of growth and the geographic range of suitable habitat for naturally occurring pathogens and toxin-producing harmful algae. These changes are projected to increase the risk of exposure to waterborne pathogens and algal toxins that can cause a variety of illnesses.

Recreational waters and sources of drinking water will be compromised by increasingly frequent and intense extreme precipitation events. Surface runoff and flooding associated with heavy precipitation and storm surge events increase pathogen loads originating from urban, agricultural, and wildlife sources and promote blooms of harmful algae in both fresh and marine waters. Greater pathogen or algal toxin loading in drinking and recreational water sources following an extreme weather event will increase the risk of human exposure to agents of water-related illness.

Increases in some extreme weather events and storm surges will also increase the risk of failure of, or damage to, water infrastructure for drinking water, wastewater, and stormwater. Aging infrastructure is particularly susceptible to failure. A breakdown in water infrastructure would contribute to increased risk of exposure to water-related pathogens, chemicals, and algal toxins.

2.5.5 Food Safety, Nutrition, and Distribution

Climate change is expected to threaten both food production and certain aspects of food quality. Although there are many practices to safeguard food in the USA, climate change, including rising temperatures and changes in weather extremes, is expected to intensify pathogen and toxin exposure, increasing the risk, if not the actual incidence, of foodborne illnesses. Exposure to a variety of pathogens in water and food causes diarrheal disease. Seasonality, air and water temperature, precipitation patterns, and extreme rainfall events are all known to affect disease transmission. Elderly people are most vulnerable to serious outcomes, and those exposed to inadequately or untreated groundwater will be among those most affected.

Elevated sea surface temperatures and increasing trends in some weather extremes will increase human exposure to water contaminants in food. Climate change will also alter the incidence and distribution of pests, parasites, and microbes, which will lead to increases in the use of pesticides for crop protection, animal agriculture, and aquaculture.

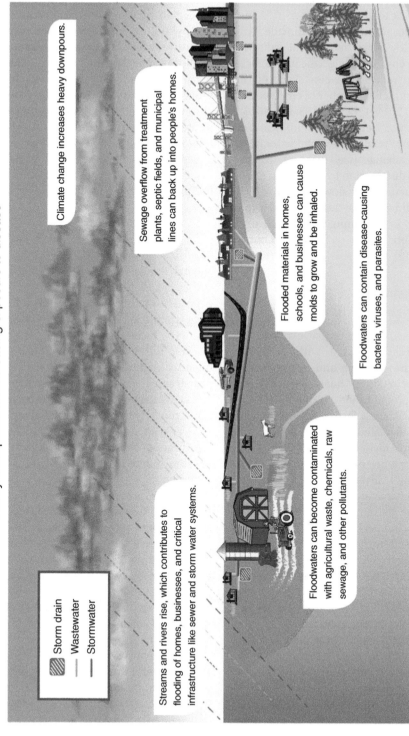

Figure 2.14 Heavy downpours, which are increasing in much of the USA, have contributed to increases in heavy flood events. The figure illustrates how humans can become exposed to waterborne diseases, which typically arise in the weeks following inundation. Human exposures to waterborne diseases can occur via drinking water, as well as recreational waters. *Source:* Based on data from NOAA NCDC. From Melillo et al. (2014).

Increased use of pesticides may result in increased human exposure to chemical contaminants in the food chain.

Rising atmospheric carbon dioxide will continue to lower the nutritional value of most food crops, including wheat and rice, and can also reduce the concentration of essential minerals in a number of crop species (Myers et al., 2014; Erlich and Harte, 2015). Increases in the frequency or intensity of some extreme weather events associated with climate change may increase disruptions of food distribution by damaging existing infrastructure or slowing shipments. These impediments may lead to food damage, spoilage, or contamination, which may limit availability and access to safe and nutritious food.

2.5.6 Extreme Weather-Related Impacts

Climate change may increase exposure to health hazards associated with projected increases in the frequency and/or intensity of extreme precipitation, hurricanes, coastal inundation, drought, and wildfires in some regions of the United States. Adverse health outcomes associated with exposure to extreme events include death, injury, or illness; exacerbation of underlying medical conditions; and adverse effects on mental health. The character and severity of health impacts from extreme events depend not only on the frequency or intensity of the extremes themselves but also on a population's exposure, sensitivity, and adaptive capacity. Many types of extreme events can cause loss of essential infrastructure (such as water, transportation, and power systems) required to safeguard human health.

A key example is wildfires. Climate change has already contributed to increasing concerns about increasing intensity of wildfires. Long periods of record high temperatures associated with droughts can contribute to dry conditions that drive wildfires, especially in the western parts of the USA. Wildfire smoke contains particulate matter, carbon monoxide, nitrogen oxides, and various volatile organic compounds that can significantly reduce air quality, both locally and in areas downwind of wildfires. Resulting smoke exposure can increase respiratory and cardiovascular hospitalizations, emergency department visits and medication dispensations for asthma, bronchitis, chest pain, chronic obstructive pulmonary disease, respiratory infections, and medical visits for lung illnesses. Future climate change is projected to contribute to wildfire risks and associated emissions, with further increasing harmful impacts on health.

2.5.7 Mental Health and Well-being

Mental illness is already one of the major causes of suffering in the USA. Many people exposed to climate-related disasters experience stress and serious mental health consequences. Depending on the type of the disaster, these serious mental health consequences include significant symptoms of post-traumatic stress disorder, depression, and general anxiety, which often occur at the same time. The majority of affected people recover over time on their own, although a significant proportion of exposed individuals develop chronic levels of psychological dysfunction.

Specific groups of people are at higher risk for distress following climate-related events. These groups include children, the elderly, and women (especially pregnant and postpartum women), people with pre-existing mental illness, low-income persons, first-responders, and people who are homeless. Communities that rely on the natural environment for sustenance and livelihood and populations living in areas most susceptible to specific climate change events are at increased risk for adverse mental health outcomes.

Increases in extreme heat will have an impact on the incidence of disease and death of people with mental illness. Significant segments of people with mental illnesses who are most vulnerable to extreme heat, such as the elderly, are also taking medications that impair the body's ability to regulate heat and therefore have increased vulnerability to the effects of heat. The Ohio Department of Mental Health has compiled a list of such commonly used psychotropic medications (http://dbh.dc.gov/sites/default/files/dc/sites/dmh/release_content/attachments/8777/heatadvice.pdf).

2.5.8 Climate–Health Risk Factors and Populations of Concern

People and communities across the USA differ in their exposures, their inherent sensitivity, and their adaptive capacity, affecting their ability to respond to and cope with climate change-related health threats. Vulnerability to climate change varies with time and across geographic areas, across communities, and among individuals within communities. People experience different vulnerabilities at different ages and life stages. The very young and the very old are particularly sensitive to climate-related health impacts.

Climate change-related health risks interact with some of the same non-climate factors that increase the risk of poor health generally. Non-climate factors, such as those related to demographic changes, socioeconomic factors, and pre-existing or chronic illnesses, may amplify, moderate, or otherwise influence climate-related health effects, particularly when they occur simultaneously or close in time or space. Geographic data analyses are increasingly being used to provide more sophisticated mapping of risk factors and social vulnerabilities to identify and protect specific locations and groups of people.

2.6 Summary and a Look Forward

Observations show that climate change is happening, that it is happening rapidly, and that it is primarily due to human activities, especially the emissions occurring from our

dependence on fossil fuels. As a result, there is an increasing level of risks to society from climate change, especially with the associated changing trends in severe weather events and from sea level rise. There is an ever-increasing risk to human health in direct relationship to these changes in climate.

It has become increasingly clear that our future depends on how we act to limit climate change. We must reduce emissions of the heat-trapping gases and particles to avoid unmanageable levels of climate change and the resulting impacts, including those on human health. At the same time we need to adapt to the changes in climate that are unavoidable. Adaptation is not a choice – our choice is whether to adapt proactively or respond to the consequences. Adaptation requires a paradigm shift, focusing on managing risks. Proactively preparing for climate change can reduce impacts while also facilitating a more rapid and efficient response to changes as they happen. Such efforts are beginning in the USA and other parts of the world, to build adaptive capacity and resilience to climate change impacts. Using scientific information to prepare for climate changes in advance can provide economic opportunities, and proactively managing the risks can reduce impacts and costs over time.

Large reductions in global emissions of heat-trapping gases can significantly reduce the risks associated with many of the worst impacts of climate change. The international agreement made in Paris by 195 countries in December 2015 is an important start to achieving this. The 21st annual Conference of Parties (COP21) resulted in a global action plan to reduce emissions of carbon dioxide and other greenhouse gases. The current plan only extends through 2030 but the long-term goal is to keep the increase in global average temperature to well below 2 °C (3.6 °F) above preindustrial levels. This itself will be extremely difficult to do, but the ultimate aim would be to keep the temperature change below 1.5 °C (2.7 °F). This would be roughly equivalent to following the extremely low RCP2.6 scenario discussed earlier (about half of the global climate models used in the 2013 IPCC assessment produced a change of about 1.5 °C).

The current agreement is not sufficient to reach even the 2 °C limit but it is an important step towards getting there and perhaps to 1.5 °C. Its full implementation throughout the world, including the USA, should lead to incentives for the development of new energy and transportation technologies that should further reduce emissions. This is an important step. It is clear that the choices we make to reduce climate change over the next few decades will affect not only us, but also our children, our grandchildren, and future generations.

References

Anderson, G.B. and Bell, M.L. (2011). Heat waves in the United States: Mortality risk during heat waves and effect modification by heat wave characteristics in 43 U.S. communities. *Environmental Health Perspectives* 119, 210–218.

Bell, M.L. and Dominici, F. (2008). Effect modification by community characteristics on the short-term effects of ozone exposure and mortality in 98 US communities. *American Journal of Epidemiology* 167, 986–997.

Boberg, F., Berg, P., Thejll, P., Gutowski, W.J., and Christensen, J.H. (2009). Improved confidence in climate change projections of precipitation evaluating using daily statistics from PRUDENCE ensemble. *Climate Dynamics* 32, 1097–1106.

Caldeira, K. and Wickett, M.E. (2003). Oceanography: anthropogenic carbon and ocean pH. *Nature* 425, 365.

Christidis, N., Stott, P.A., and Brown, S.J. (2011). The role of human activity in the recent warming of extremely warm daytime temperatures. *Journal of Climate* 24, 1922–1930.

Church, J.A. and White, N.J. (2011). Sea-level rise from the late 19th to the early 21st century. *Surveys in Geophysics* 32, 585–602.

Church, J.A., White, N.J., Konikow, L.F., et al. (2011). Revisiting the Earth's sea-level and energy budgets from 1961 to 2008. *Geophysical Research Letters* 38, L18601.

Deser, C., Knutti, R., Solomon, S., and Phillips, A.S. (2012). Communication of the role of natural variability in future North American climate. *Nature Climate Change* 2, 775–779.

Diffenbaugh, N.S, Scherer, M., and Trapp, R.J. (2013). Robust increases in severe thunderstorm environments in response to greenhouse forcing. *Proceedings of the National Academy of Sciences of the USA* 110, 16361–16366.

Doney, S.C., Fabry, V.J., Feely, R.A., and Kleypas, J.A. (2009). Ocean acidification: the other CO2 problem. *Annual Review of Marine Science* 1, 169–192.

Duffy, P.B. and Tebaldi, C. (2012). Increasing prevalence of extreme summer temperatures in the U.S. *Climatic Change* 111, 487–495.

Erlich, P.R. and Harte, J. (2015). Opinion: To feed the world in 2050 will require a global revolution. *Proceedings of the National Academy of Sciences of the USA* 112(48), 14743–14744.

Feely, R.A., Sabine, C.L., Hernandez-Ayon, J.M., Ianson, D., and Hales, B. (2008). Evidence for upwelling of corrosive "acidified" water onto the continental shelf. *Science* 320, 1490–1492.

Feely, R.A., Alin, S.R., Newton, J., et al. (2010). The combined effects of ocean acidification, mixing, and respiration on pH and carbonate saturation in an urbanized estuary. *Estuarine, Coastal and Shelf Science* 88, 442–449.

Gillett, N.P., Arora, V.K., Flato, G.M., Scinocca, J.F., and Salzen, K.V. (2012). Improved constraints on 21st-century warming derived using 160 years of temperature observations. *Geophysical Research Letters* 39, L01704.

Güneralp, B., Güneralp, İ., and Liu, Y. (2015). Changing global patterns of urban exposure to flood and drought hazards. *Global Environmental Change*, 31, 217–225.

Gutowski, W.J., Takle, E.S., Kozak, K.A., Patton, J.C., Arritt, R.W., and Christensen, J.H. (2007). A possible constraint on regional precipitation intensity changes under global warming. *Journal of Hydrometeorology* 8, 1382–1396.

Hansen, J., Sato, M., Ruedy, R., et al. (2007). Dangerous human-made interference with climate: A GISS modelE study. *Atmospheric Chemistry and Physics* 7, 2287–2312.

Hawkins, E. and Sutton, R. (2009). The potential to narrow uncertainty in regional climate predictions. *Bulletin of the American Meteorological Society* 90, 1095–1107.

Hawkins, E. and Sutton, R. (2011). The potential to narrow uncertainty in projections of regional precipitation change. *Climate Dynamics* 37, 407–418.

Hoerling, M., Chen, M., Dole, R., et al. (2013). Anatomy of an extreme event. *Journal of Climate* 26, 2811–2832.

Hönisch, B., Ridgwell, A., Schmidt, D.M., et al. (2012). The geological record of ocean acidification. *Science* 335, 1058–1063.

Huber, M. and Knutti, R. (2011). Anthropogenic and natural warming inferred from changes in Earth's energy balance. *Nature Geoscience* 5, 31–36.

IPCC (Intergovernmental Panel on Climate Change) (2012). *Managing the Risks of Extreme Events and Disasters to Advance Climate Change Adaptation*. A Special Report of the Intergovernmental Panel on Climate Change (eds Field, C.B.,, Barros, V., Stocker, T.F., et al.). Cambridge, UK: Cambridge University Press.

IPCC (Intergovernmental Panel on Climate Change) (2013). *Climate Change 2013: The Physical Science Basis. Contribution of Working Group I to the Fifth Assessment Report of the Intergovernmental Panel on Climate Change* (eds Stocker, T.F., Qin, D., Plattner, G-K., et al.). Cambridge/New York: Cambridge University Press.

IPCC (Intergovernmental Panel on Climate Change) (2014). *Climate Change 2014: Synthesis Report. Contribution of Working Groups I, II and III to the Fifth Assessment Report of the Intergovernmental Panel on Climate Change* (eds Core Writing Team, Pachauri, R.K., and Meyer, L.A.). Geneva, Switzerland: IPCC.

Janssen, E., Wuebbles, D.J., Kunkel, K.E., Olsen, S.C., and Goodman, A. (2014). Trends and projections of extreme precipitation over the contiguous United States. *Earth's Future* 2, 99–113.

Karl, T.R., Melillo, J.T., and Peterson, T.C. (eds) (2009). *Global Climate Change Impacts in the United States*. New York: Cambridge University Press. Available online at: http://downloads.globalchange.gov/usimpacts/pdfs/climate-impacts-report.pdf (accessed November 15, 2017).

Karl, T.R., Arguez, A., Huang, B., et al. (2015). Possible artifacts of data biases in the recent global surface warming hiatus. *Science*, 348, 1469–1472.

Kunkel, K.E., Karl, T.R., Brooks, H., et al. (2013). Monitoring and understanding changes in extreme storm statistics: State of knowledge. *Bulletin of the American Meteorological Society* 94, 499–514.

Le Quéré, C., Raupach, M.R., Canadell, J.G., and Marland, G. (2009). Trends in the sources and sinks of carbon dioxide. *Nature Geoscience* 2, 831–836.

Luber, G., Knowlton, K., Balbus, J., et al. (2014). Human health. In: Melillo, J.M., Richmond, T.C., and Yohe, G.W. (eds), *Climate Change Impacts in the United States: The Third National Climate Assessment*. U.S. Global Change Research Program, pp. 220–256. Available online at: http://nca2014.globalchange.gov/report/sectors/human-health (accessed November 15, 2017).

Mann, M.E., Zhang, Z., Hughes, M.K., et al. (2008) Proxy-based reconstructions of hemispheric and global surface temperature variations over the past two millennia. *Proceedings of the National Academy of Sciences of the USA* 105, 13252–13257.

Marzeion, B., Jarosch, A.H., and Hofer, M. (2012) Past and future sea level change from the surface mass balance of glaciers. *The Cryosphere Discussions* 6, 3177–3241.

Matthews, H.D. and Zickfeld, K. (2012) Climate response to zeroed emissions of greenhouse gases and aerosols. *Nature Climate Change* 2, 338–341.

Mathis, J.T., Cross, J.N., and Bates, N.R. (2011) Coupling primary production and terrestrial runoff to ocean acidification and carbonate mineral suppression in the eastern Bering Sea. *Journal of Geophysical Research* 116, C02030.

McGranahan, G., Balk, D., and Anderson, B. (2007) The rising tide: assessing the risks of climate change and human settlements in low elevation coastal zones. *Environment and Urbanization* 19, 17–37.

Meehl, G.A., Tebaldi, C., Walton, G., Easterling, D., and McDaniel, L. (2009) Relative increase of record high maximum temperatures compared to record low minimum temperatures in the U.S. *Geophysical Research Letters* 36, L23701.

Melillo, J.M., Richmond, T.C., and Yohe, G.W. (eds) (2014). *Climate Change Impacts in the United States: The Third National Climate Assessment*. U.S. Global Change Research Program. Available at: http://nca2014.globalchange.gov. (accessed November 15, 2017).

Min, S., Zhang, X., Zwiers, F., and Hegerl, G. (2011). Human contribution to more-intense precipitation extremes. *Nature* 470, 378–381.

Myers, S.S., Zanobetti, A., Kloog, I., et al. (2014). Increasing CO2 threatens human nutrition. *Nature* 510, 139–142.

Nerem, R.S., Chambers, D.P., Choe, C., and Mitchum, G.T. (2010). Estimating mean sea level change from the TOPEX and Jason altimeter missions. *Marine Geodesy* 33, 435–446.

Neumann, B., Vafeidis, A.T., Zimmermann, J., and Nicholls, R.J. (2015). Future coastal population growth and exposure to sea-level rise and coastal flooding—A global assessment. *PLoS ONE*, 10(3): e0118571.

Orr, J.C. (2011). Recent and future changes in ocean carbonate chemistry. In: Gattuso, J-P.

and Hansson, L. (eds), *Ocean Acidification*. Oxford University Press, pp. 41–66.

Orr, J.C., Fabry, V.J., Aumont, O., et al. (2005). Anthropogenic ocean acidification over the twenty-first century and its impact on calcifying organisms. *Nature* 437, 681–686.

PAGES 2K Consortium (2013). Continental-scale temperature variability during the past two millennia. *Nature Geoscience* 6, 339–346.

Parris, A., Bromirski, P., Burkett, V., et al. (2012). *Global Sea Level Rise Scenarios for the United States National Climate Assessment*. NOAA Tech Memo OAR CPO-1, National Oceanic and Atmospheric Administration. Available at: http://scenarios.globalchange.gov/sites/default/files/NOAA_SLR_r3_0.pdf (accessed November 15, 2017).

Peterson, T.C., Heim, R.R. Jr, Hirsch, R., et al. (2013). Monitoring and understanding changes in heat waves, cold waves, floods and droughts in the United States: State of knowledge. *Bulletin of the American Meteorology Society* 94, 821–834.

Rahmstorf, S., Perrette, M., and Vermeer, M. (2012). Testing the robustness of semi-empirical sea level projections. *Climate Dynamics* 39, 861–875.

Rupp, D.E., Mote, P.W., Massey, N., Rye, C.J., Jones, R., and Allen, M.R. (2012). Did human influence on climate make the 2011 Texas drought more probable? Explaining extreme events of 2011 from a climate perspective. *Bulletin of the American Meteorological Society* 93, 1052–1054.

Santer, B.D., Painter, J.F., Mears, C.A., et al. (2013). Identifying human influences on atmospheric temperature. *Proceedings of the National Academy of Sciences of the USA* 110, 26–33.

Sillmann, J., Kharin, V.V., Zwiers, F.W., Zhang, X., and Bronaugh, D. (2013). Climate extremes indices in the CMIP5 multimodel ensemble: Part 2. Future climate projections. *Journal of Geophysical Research: Atmospheres* 118, 2473–2493.

Smith, A.B. and Katz, R.W. (2013). U.S. Billion-dollar weather and climate disasters:

data sources, trends, accuracy and biases. *Natural Hazard* 67, 387–410.

Stott, P.A., Gillett, N.P., Hegerl, G.C., et al. (2010). Detection and attribution of climate change: a regional perspective. *Wiley Interdisciplinary Reviews: Climate Change* 1, 192–211.

Swanson, K.L., Sugihara, G., and Tsonis, A.A. (2009). Long-term natural variability and 20th century climate change. *Proceedings of the National Academy of Sciences of the USA* 106, 16120–16123.

Trenberth, K.E. (2011). Changes in precipitation with climate change. *Climate Research*, 47, 123.

Trenberth, K.E. and Fasullo, J.T. (2012). Climate extremes and climate change: The Russian heat wave and other climate extremes of 2010. *Journal of Geophysical Research: Atmospheres* 117, D17103.

UKRS (UK Royal Society) and NAS (National Academy of Sciences) (2014). *Climate Change: Evidence and Causes*. Washington, DC: National Academy Press.

USGCRP (2016). *The Impacts of Climate Change on Human Health in the United States: A Scientific Assessment* (eds Crimmins, A., Balbus, J., Gamble, J.L., et al.). Washington, DC: U.S. Global Change Research Program.

Vose, R.S., Applequist, S., Menne, M.J., Williams, C.N. Jr, and Thorne, P. (2012). An intercomparison of temperature trends in the US Historical Climatology Network and recent atmospheric reanalyses. *Geophysical Research Letters* 39, L10703.

Vose, R.S., Applequist, S., Bourassa, M.A., et al. (2014). Monitoring and understanding changes in extremes: Extratropical storms, winds, and waves. *Bulletin of the American Meteorological Society* doi:10.1175/BAMS-D-12-00162.1.

Wuebbles, D.J., Meehl, G., Hayhoe, K., et al. (2014a). CMIP5 climate model analyses: Climate extremes in the United States. *Bulletin of the American Meteorological Society* doi: http://dx.doi.org/10.1175/BAMS-D-12-00172.1.

Wuebbles, D.J., Kunkel, K., Wehner, M., & Zobel, Z. (2014b). Severe weather in the United States under a changing climate. *EOS* 95, 149–150.

Yamamoto-Kawai, M., McLaughlin, F.A., Carmack, E.C., Nishino, S., and Shimada, K. (2009). Aragonite undersaturation in the Arctic Ocean: Effects of ocean acidification and sea ice melt. *Science* 326, 1098–1100.

Yin, J. (2012). Century to multi-century sea level rise projections from CMIP5 models. *Geophysical Research Letters* 39, L17709.

Ziska, L.H. (2011). Climate change, carbon dioxide and global crop production: food security and uncertainty. In: Dinar, A. and Mendelsohn, R. (eds), *Handbook on Climate Change and Agriculture*. Edward Elgar Publishing, pp. 9–31.

Ziska, L., Knowlton, K. Rogers, C., *et al.* (2011). Recent warming by latitude associated with increased length of ragweed pollen season in central North America. *Proceedings of the National Academy of Sciences of the USA* 108, 4248–425.

Zwiers, F., Alexander, L., Hegerl, G., et al. (2013). Climate extremes: challenges in estimating and understanding recent changes in the frequency and intensity of extreme climate and weather events. In: Asrar, G. and Hurrell, J. (eds), *Climate Science for Serving Society*. Springer, pp. 339–389.

3

Food Safety and Security

Megin Nichols, Lauren Stevenson, Casey Barton Behravesh, and Robert V. Tauxe

Centers for Disease Control and Prevention, Atlanta, GA, USA

3.1 Evolution of Food Production

Over time, agricultural practices have evolved and changed in response to influences from the environment and climate, advancing technologies, and dietary demands of the population (Gurven and Kaplan, 2007). Reliable food sources produced through advancing agricultural practices have supported the increasing global human population. However, inequity in food safety and security have continued through to modern times. The Food and Agriculture Organization of the United Nations (FAO) estimates that about 795 million people around the globe were chronically undernourished during 2012–2014 (FAO et al., 2014). A One Health approach is needed to protect and promote food safety and food security, address the rapid growth and transformation of the livestock sector, and ensure sustainability of the environment and the natural resources used to produce a global food supply (Figure 3.1).

Food system industrialization through the last century, especially in the USA and Europe, involved specialization, simplification, routinization, mechanization, standardization, and consolidation of many agriculture systems (Ikerd, 1996; Lang, 2003). As agriculture became more specialized, producers focused on farming one crop or raising one animal species, rather than growing multiple crops and raising different types of livestock on a farm. This focus changed food production processes as producers accumulated the equipment and resources required to produce larger quantities of one crop or animal product. With specialized machinery and more intensive production systems, agriculture moved toward production of more uniform types of crops and standardization of breeds and animal body conformation to allow for more efficient processing. However, the industrialization of food systems has had unintended consequences on human, animal, and environmental health; for example, plants and animals have become more susceptible to certain diseases resulting from a lack of diversity (Keesing et al., 2010). Concentration of animals into often smaller areas such as confined animal feeding operations for swine and poultry, can allow for increased spread of pathogens, and virulence and resistance genes among them, which can contribute to new One Health challenges.

More efficient production increased food surpluses, which spurred trade and shipment of food and fiber overseas. The globalization of the food trade has led to increased availability and diversification of food throughout the

Beyond One Health: From Recognition to Results, First Edition.
Edited by John A. Herrmann and Yvette J. Johnson-Walker.

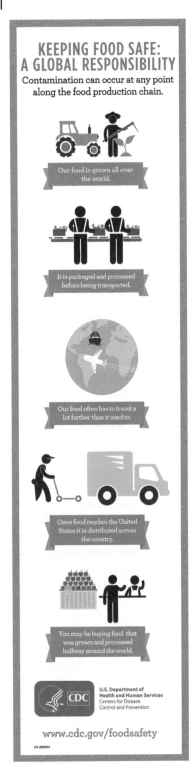

**KEEPING FOOD SAFE:
A GLOBAL RESPONSIBILITY**
Contamination can occur at any point
along the food production chain.

Our food is grown all over
the world.

It is packaged and processed
before being transported.

Our food often has to travel a
lot farther than it used to.

Once food reaches the United
States it is distributed across
the country.

You may be buying food that
was grown and processed
halfway around the world.

CDC
U.S. Department of
Health and Human Services
Centers for Disease
Control and Prevention

www.cdc.gov/foodsafety

CS 255504

Figure 3.1 A brief depiction of the global food
production chain.

world (Tritscher et al., 2013). As a result, food products served in a given country are often produced or sourced from other countries. This also means that it is possible for contaminated food items to lead to illness among consumers in multiple countries (Tauxe et al., 2010). Therefore, it is important to develop and promote uniform standards and requirements that ensure a safe supply of food. The unequal distribution of food globally can be a barrier to food security for countries that do not have full access to advances in food production, processing, and preparation. Global food safety and food security initiatives based on scientific evidence are needed across borders and industries to address the impact that a globalized food system has on human, animal, and environmental health.

Foodborne disease occurs when a food is contaminated with a pathogen or toxin that harms the individual consuming it. Contamination can occur during production as the animal or plant is being raised, during or after harvest as it is being processed into food, and during preparation before it is eaten. More than 250 different pathogens or toxins can contaminate food, some with human reservoirs, and some with animal reservoirs (Bryan, 1982). The spectrum of implicated foods is complex and ever changing, reflecting changes in consumer tastes and preparation techniques, changes in food industry technologies and sources, and the varied food trade and production chains, which might range from a few meters to thousands of kilometers in length. Many advances in food production and processing technology have greatly improved food safety and minimized the contamination of food by harmful biological and chemical agents (Sanders, 1999). An understanding of how transmission of pathogens occurs through our food supply that is sufficient to interrupt contamination requires a One Health approach that considers the behavior of the microbes, plants, animals, and people in the production environment.

Policy measures designed to minimize food safety hazards and thereby help enhance food security have evolved over time (Tauxe and Esteban, 2006). Over 50 years ago, in 1963, the Codex Alimentarius Commission was established as the principal body for the FAO and the World Health Organization (WHO) Food Standards Programme, with the intent of developing international food safety and nutrition standards and guidance to protect consumer health and trade (FAO, 2001). Independent initiatives have also arisen to assist with food safety. One example, is the Global Food Safety Initiative (GFSI), which is a collaboration among food safety experts throughout the food industry including retail, manufacturing, and foodservice companies. The GFSI sets requirements for food safety schemes through a benchmarking process to improve cost efficiency in the food supply chain, develop mechanisms to exchange information, increase consumer awareness, and review good food safety practices (Consumer Goods Forum, 2015).

Consumers are demanding safe and affordable food, indicating to government and agricultural industries the need to implement policies and programs that promote best practices in food safety (Tauxe et al., 2010). Countries that export food should implement a variety of processes to ensure food safety, to reduce pesticide residues, and to ensure wholesome products free from pests and other contaminants, to meet requirements of importing countries. In the USA, the Food and Drug Administration (FDA) oversees importation of produce and seafoods while the US Department of Agriculture (USDA) ensures that foreign animal diseases and pests are not imported on meat and other food items. Both agencies apply the *equivalency principle*, namely that imported foods must meet safety standards that are equivalent to those required of products from the USA. Ensuring the safety of a food product from point of origin to point of sale can be very challenging given the complex path food travels from farm to fork (Figure 3.2). Occasionally, a process put in place to mitigate one hazard can result in unintended consequences. The case study in Box 3.1 demonstrates the need to minimize food safety risks through environmental control measures while recognizing the unintended consequences of processing designed to mitigate and control pests.

3.2 Foodborne Illness

Worldwide, approximately 2.2 million deaths annually result from foodborne and waterborne illnesses (Havelaar et al., 2015). More than 60% of newly emerging and re-emerging pathogens of humans, including those that are transmitted by food and water, are zoonotic (Jones et al., 2008). A 2010 evaluation of 31 foodborne hazards found that the global burden of foodborne disease resulted in 33 million Disability Adjusted Life Years (DALYs), with children aged up to 5 years accounting for 40% of this burden (Havelaar et al., 2015). The burden was not equally distributed worldwide. The greatest burden of foodborne disease occurred in regions in Africa, Southeast Asia, and a region of the Eastern Mediterranean (Havelaar et al., 2015). Some infections were similar among regions; for example, non-typhoidal *Salmonella enterica* resulted in foodborne illness worldwide.

Among people who are exposed to foodborne pathogens such as *Salmonella* in the USA, only a proportion of these exposed people become ill. Of these, only some ill people seek medical care and have a specimen obtained and submitted to a clinical laboratory. Laboratories test some of these specimens for a given pathogen and identify the causative organism in some of these tested specimens and thereby confirm the case. The laboratory-confirmed case is subsequently reported to a local or state health department (Figure 3.3). Most people who develop illness from *Salmonella* and other foodborne pathogens recover with mild signs of illness; however, in some people who are very young (<5 years), older (>65 years), or who have a weakened immune system, illness can be severe

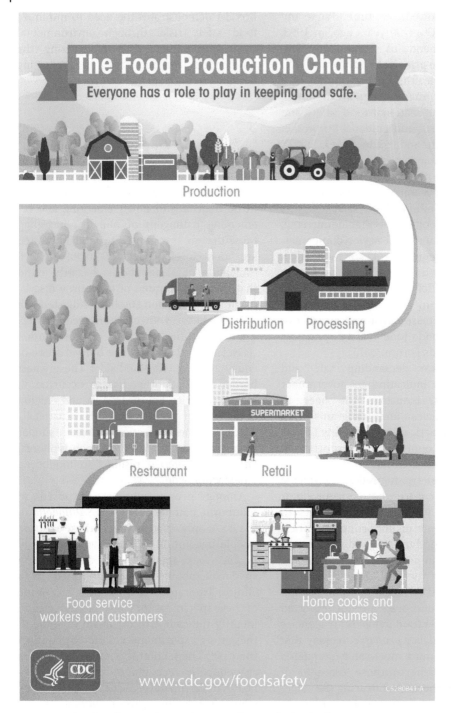

Figure 3.2 Food production chain with potential points for food safety interventions.

Box 3.1 Case study of an outbreak linked to food sourced globally
(Sivapalasingam et al., 2003)

In January 2000, public health officials in Virginia identified an outbreak of *Salmonella* Newport after noting an increase in a specific pulsed field gel electrophoresis (PFGE) pattern among five ill patients during November and December of 1999. The geographic and temporal clustering of this PFGE pattern was highly suggestive of an outbreak. Other health departments and Centers for Disease Control and Prevention (CDC) were queried regarding any change in the prevalence of this pattern of *Salmonella* Newport. An increase was detected nationally by CDC using the *Salmonella* Outbreak Detection Algorithm (SODA), a computer algorithm that can flag significant increases in the frequency of specific *Salmonella* serotypes. This suggested a nationwide outbreak was occurring. On January 11, 2000, CDC requested that additional testing be performed for all *Salmonella* Newport isolates received at state laboratories that were received since November 1, 1999. Information regarding this increase in a particular strain of *Salmonella* Newport was shared with 15 European Union members who participated in an international system for laboratory-based *Salmonella* surveillance. The laboratory investigation was accompanied by an epidemiologic investigation. Investigators defined a case as diarrhea in a person with onset occurring during November 1 through 31 December 1999, with a *Salmonella* Newport isolate with the outbreak PFGE pattern. Seventy-eight patients from 13 states were infected with the outbreak strain. Fifteen patients were hospitalized; two died. Interviews were conducted with case patients to investigate potential common food items or other means of exposures. Initial interviews revealed that many case patients were Asian or Latino.

A case-control study was then initiated by selecting two non-ill "controls" for every one case-patient; cases and controls were matched by race/ethnicity. Among 28 patients enrolled in the matched case-control study, 14 (50%) reported that they ate mangoes in the five days before illness onset, compared with four (10%) of the control subjects during the same period. This exposure was statistically significant, and the traceback investigation to determine the origin of the mangoes consumed by ill people was initiated.

Traceback was conducted by the FDA, which regulates produce, by using information on venue locations where case patients reported purchasing or eating mangoes during the five days before illness onset. A regulatory traceback ensued, which consisted of traceback data from patients who remembered purchasing mangoes from a single location on a single day; of these, only those who remembered the name and address of the purchase location, date of purchase or who had a receipt of purchase for mangoes eaten during the five days before illness onset were included in the traceback investigation. Four of the ill people remembered the purchase location and date or had a receipt for mangoes consumed in the five days prior to illness onset. Initial traceback failed to yield a common store of purchase, common distributor, or a common importer or shipment of mangoes. However, the traceback investigation converged when a single common farm in Brazil was shown to have supplied mangoes to all four purchase locations. Once this farm was identified, FDA, the US Department of Agriculture (USDA) Animal Plant Health Inspection Service (APHIS), and CDC investigated at the farm. Mango farms that export to the USA have oversight by USDA APHIS, which is responsible for preventing importation of plant pests, such as the Mediterranean fruit fly. Farm workers were interviewed regarding farming practices, mango processing, and transport. Water samples were collected and tested, and remaining true to One Health investigation principles, cloacal samples were obtained from a toad found near mango processing tanks.

(Continued)

Box 3.1 (Continued)

The farm processed approximately 11 tons of mangoes during the last quarter of 1999; 60% of these mangoes were exported to the USA; 30% were exported to Europe; 5% were exported to Argentina; and 5% were consumed in Brazil. Investigators determined that the mangoes were harvested by hand and processed onsite. To kill Mediterranean fruit flies, mangoes imported into the USA from Brazil were dipped in hot water, and then chilled in a cold-water bath. The cold water was not treated and was contaminated with *Salmonella* Newport, which infected people in the USA. When hot fruit is placed in a cold water bath, the internal spaces of the fruit contract and the fruit takes up fluid through the stem scar, the calyx, or other pores, and any bacteria in the water can be drawn in (Institute of Medicine (US) Food Forum, 2009, Sivapalasingam et al.,

2003). All dip tanks were unenclosed, and toads, birds, and bird feces were noted in or near the tanks.

The water for processing mangoes came from a nearby river. Testing of the water and the toad did not yield the outbreak strain of *Salmonella* Newport. However, *Escherichia coli* and other strains of *Salmonella* were detected. This investigation altered the way mango producers processed water for use in washing fruit. After this investigation, USDA APHIS recommended that mango producers who export to the USA ensure that processing water is filtered and adequately chlorinated, that chlorine levels are measured, and, if hot and cold water dips are used, that they should be at least 30 minutes apart. In addition, irradiation was approved as an alternative treatment for Mediterranean fruit fly control.

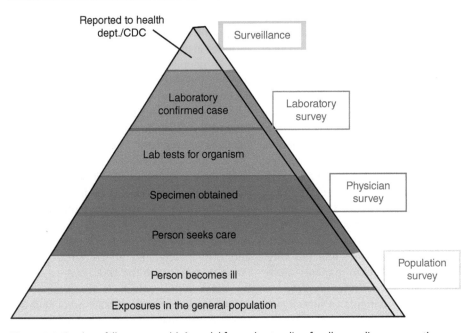

Figure 3.3 Burden of illness pyramid: A model for understanding foodborne disease reporting.

resulting in hospitalization or death. To prevent foodborne illness, it is important to prepare, store, and handle food in a safe manner. This process might vary according to location and food items. However, some of the basic principles of safe food handling,

when applied, can greatly reduce risk of foodborne illness (Figure 3.4). The ability to detect specific foodborne pathogens has benefited greatly from cross-disciplinary learning. For example, two Department of Agriculture researchers, Smith and Salmon,

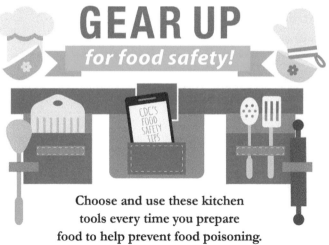

GEAR UP
for food safety!

Choose and use these kitchen
tools every time you prepare
food to help prevent food poisoning.

Kitchen Sink

- Wash your hands for **20 seconds** with soap and running water.
- Wash fruits and vegetables before peeling.
- Do not wash meat, poultry, or eggs.

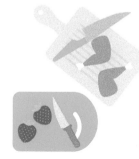

Cutting Board and Utensils

- Use separate cutting boards, plates, and knives for produce and for raw meat, poultry, seafood, and eggs.
- Clean with hot, soapy water or in dishwasher (if dishwasher-safe) after each use.

Thermometer

- Use a food thermometer to make sure food cooked in the oven, stove or on the grill reaches a temperature hot enough to kill germs.
  - All poultry, including ground: **165°F**
  - Ground beef, pork, lamb, and veal: **160°F**
  - Beef, pork, lamb, and veal chops, roasts and steaks: **145°F**
  - Fish: **145°F**

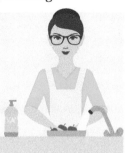

Figure 3.4 Examples of how consumers can practice good food safety techniques.

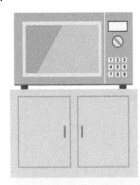

Microwave

- Know your microwave's wattage.
  - Check inside the door, owner's manual, or manufacturer's website. Lower wattage means longer cooking time.
- Follow recommended cooking and standing times, to allow for additional cooking after microwaving stops.
- When reheating, use a food thermometer to make sure food reaches 165°F.

Refrigerator

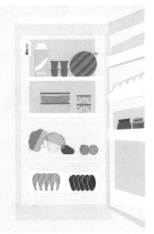

- Keep your refrigerator between 40°F and 32°F, and your freezer at 0°F or below.
- Refrigerate fruits, vegetables, milk, eggs, and meats within 2 hours; (1 hour if the temperature is 90°F or higher).
- Store raw meat on the bottom shelf away from fresh produce and ready-to-eat food.
- Throw out foods left unrefrigerated for over 2 hours.
- Thaw or marinate foods in the refrigerator.

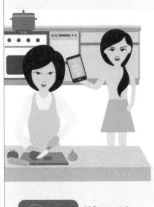

Computer or mobile devices

- Look for more tips to keep food safe at www.cdc.gov/foodsafety
- Stay up to date on food recalls at www.foodsafety.gov/recalls

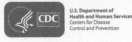

U.S. Department of Health and Human Services
Centers for Disease Control and Prevention

www.cdc.gov/foodsafety

Figure 3.4 (*Continued*)

were investigating a fatal diarrheal disease of swine, when they discovered a bacterial pathogen. Though this was not the cause of that fatal diarrhea, it was a serious pathogen of swine and many other species, that was subsequently named *Salmonella* (Salmon, 1885). The microbiologist van Ermengen, investigating an outbreak of fatal paralytic botulism that affected a village in Belgium, reproduced the symptoms by feeding the suspected food and an organism isolated from it to guineas pigs, identifying both *Clostridium botulinum* and its toxin (van Ermengem, 1897). To this day, the mouse assay remains a standard diagnostic technique for detecting botulism toxin. More recently, a veterinary pathologist taught a pediatric infectious disease specialist how to isolate *Campylobacter* easily from diarrheic stools, leading to the discovery that these bacteria were a common cause of diarrhea in children in Brussels, and elsewhere (Dekeyser et al., 1972).

Identifying sources and developing control measures that target specific pathogen food combinations has also been informed by multidisciplinary perspectives. Pasteurization of milk was initially driven both by concern about animals infected with bovine tuberculosis (caused by *Mycobacterium bovis*) and the organism that causes "septic sore throat" (a bovine streptococcus), as well as by fear of typhoid fever and other diseases of human origin that might be introduced by contaminated water or workers (Rosenau, 1926). The US meat inspection system has its roots in the hazards posed by ill animals entering the meat and poultry supply, and since 1906, has been based on peri-mortem inspection of the animals. More recently, meat inspection has been updated to focus on processes that reduce the unseen contamination of meat and poultry with microbes (Tauxe and Esteban, 2006). The great strides made in controlling or eliminating anthrax, brucellosis, trichinosis, and other zoonoses that caused severe illness in food animal populations have now brought the developed world to a new stage. Now our food animals often silently carry human pathogens that cause few or no symptoms in the animals themselves. *Salmonella* sv. Enteritidis silently colonizes the ovaries of many laying and broiler chickens; *Campylobacter jejuni* is present in the intestines and feces of many healthy chickens; Shiga toxin-producing *E. coli* can be found in the rectums of many ruminants; and *Yersinia enterocolitica* colonizes the throats and tonsils of many pigs (Zdolec et al., 2015; Wesley et al., 2008; O'Sullivan et al., 2011; Low et al., 2005).

A One Health perspective can help unite the concern for human health with finding specific measures to reduce the frequency of foodborne pathogens in animals. A decades-long collaboration among public health, several agencies in the USDA, and the egg industry found that *Salmonella* sp. infection was often transmitted vertically from the infected hen through internal contamination of the egg to the next generation of birds, or to unwitting consumers of the eggs (Angulo and Swerdlow, 1999). Innovative field investigations led to several control measures from the flock to the table, and ultimately largely controlled the epidemic (Wright et al., 2016). They included eliminating the infection from the source flocks using methods first developed to control *Salmonella* Pullorum and *Salmonella* Gallinarum, serious pathogens of poultry (Gast, 1999). They also included regulating refrigeration during transport and storage, changing practices in restaurants and institutions to eliminate egg pooling, and developing new commercial technologies to pasteurize eggs in the shell.

Recent investigations into the relationships among human pathogens and fruits and vegetables suggest that an even broader perspective is appropriate. Although it is believed that enteric bacteria are particularly adapted to the animal gut, some of them also have specific properties, likely acquired over millions of years, that adapt them to life in plants (Meric et al., 2013). Plant pathologists observe that plants close the respiratory pores on their leaves (stomata) on exposure to *Salmonella* flagella (Melotto et al., 2006). Yet some salmonellae can force the pores back open again, using specific molecular "crowbars," then enter the pores, where they suppress the plant's own innate immune response, and persist inside the leaf indefinitely (Melotto et al., 2014). Some salmonellae can easily enter tomato or melon plants through the root hairs, and make their way to the growing fruits (Gu et al., 2013; Gautam et al., 2014). Some strains of *E. coli* O157 are also able to manipulate the stomatal openings and gain entry to the interior of leaves (Saldana et al., 2011). These intriguing properties would mean the pathogen excreted by an animal could then colonize a protected site inside the plant and persist until it is eaten by a roaming herbivore (Fletcher, 2013). A two-host cycle like this between herbivores and the plants they eat may pre-date humanity by many millions of years. Humans then may be the accidental host who is infected sometimes after eating the animal and sometimes after eating the plant (Fletcher et al., 2013). Produce contaminated by animals near or in growing fields has resulted in outbreaks of human illness (Jay et al., 2007; Gardner et al., 2011). Understanding and intervening in these complex cycles is a multidisciplinary challenge.

3.3 A One Health Approach to Foodborne Illness Detection and Response

How are foodborne illnesses detected and investigated using a One Health approach? A One Health approach to food safety involves a science-based strategy to conducting interdisciplinary surveillance for foodborne illness. Foodborne disease detection is performed by epidemiologists, laboratorians, environmental health specialists, veterinarians, physicians, and many other One Health professionals. To ensure food safety through detection of contaminated food products leading to illness, professionals in all disciplines must routinely share information through coordinated, cross-sector surveillance and communication. For example, many health surveillance systems rely on laboratory information. Astute medical professionals recognize human illness and perform appropriate testing, such as stool culture, to detect pathogens. Once a laboratory detects an enteric pathogen such as *Salmonella* or *E. coli*, the illness is reported to a local public health authority. Information reported often includes patient demographics and contact information. Ill persons are then interviewed regarding potential risk factors for foodborne illness using a hypothesis-generating questionnaire including questions on foods eaten, grocery stores or restaurants where food was purchased, animal exposures in the home and away from home, drinking water sources, recreational water exposures, and travel history (Figure 3.5).

In addition to collection of epidemiologic information from ill people, the microbial isolates obtained through culture of stool, blood, or other body tissues/fluids are sent to reference laboratories, which perform additional testing and characterization. PulseNet, a partnership between the CDC, the Association of Public Health Laboratories (APHL), federal regulatory agency partners (e.g., FDA, USDA), and public health laboratories in all 50 US states, was created to maintain a central repository for DNA fingerprints extracted from bacteria of patients with foodborne disease (Swaminathan et al., 2001; Scharff et al., 2016; Centers for Disease Control and Prevention, 2016a) (Figure 3.6). Since 1996, these DNA fingerprints are obtained through PFGE and increasingly through whole genome sequencing (WGS) (Figure 3.7). Public health laboratories around the USA submit these DNA fingerprints to PulseNet, which is routinely searched by participants for clusters of ill people whose pathogens share the same genetic pattern. The underlying assumption of the analysis is that bacterial isolates with indistinguishable PFGE patterns or isolates that are closely genetically related by WGS likely had a common source. Food, animal, and environmental isolates are also included in PulseNet, and genetic relatedness to isolates from any source can suggest potential linkages to ill patients. The PulseNet network has been replicated in Canada, Europe, the Asia Pacific region, and Latin America. These independent networks work together through PulseNet International and allow public health officials and laboratorians to share molecular epidemiologic information enabling rapid recognition and investigation of international foodborne disease outbreaks. Communication between the various international PulseNet networks provides the opportunity to exchange information and detect foodborne disease outbreaks across country borders (Swaminathan et al., 2006). Surveillance conducted across borders is a critical part of monitoring and evaluating the impact a globalized food system has on human, animal, and environmental health.

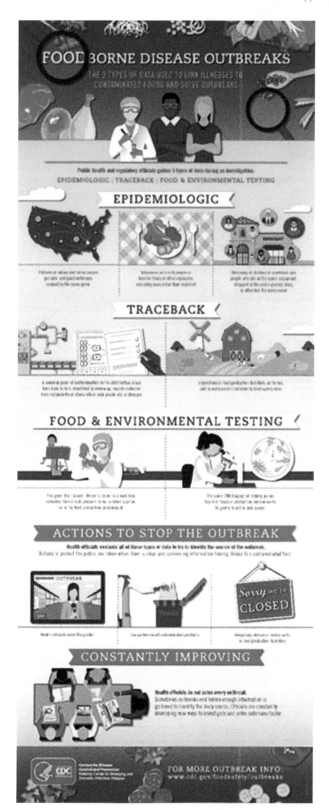

Figure 3.5 Three legs of evidence used in outbreak investigations to determine food vehicles.

PulseNet is a national laboratory network that connects foodborne illness cases to detect outbreaks. PulseNet uses DNA fingerprinting, or patterns of bacteria making people sick, to detect thousands of local and multistate outbreaks. Since the network began in 1996, PulseNet has improved our food safety systems through identifying outbreaks early. This allows investigators to find the source, alert the public sooner, and identify gaps in our food safety systems that would not otherwise be recognized.

1982
E. coli O157:H7 is first recognized as a significant human pathogen.

1984
Pulsed-field gel electrophoresis (PFGE), the current gold standard for DNA fingerprinting, is developed by Schwartz and Cantor.

1993
E. coli O157:H7 causes a major outbreak in the Western US states.

1994
CDC and several state health laboratories demonstrate the utility of PFGE for detecting and investigating outbreaks of foodborne disease.

1995
» The concept of PulseNet takes shape in discussions between CDC, the Association of Public Health Laboratories (APHL), state public health laboratories and federal partners.

» CDC provides $150,000 to PulseNet to conduct an initial project demonstrating its effectiveness.

1996
» CDC launches PulseNet with the APHL, federal partners, and the original area public health laboratories in Massachusetts, Minnesota, Texas, and Washington.

» The first PulseNet training for standardized PFGE and analysis of patterns is organized at CDC. The area laboratories and the U.S. Department of Agriculture Food Safety and Inspection Service (USDA) laboratories attend.

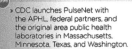

1997
» PulseNet detects an outbreak of *E. coli* O157:H7 in Colorado linked to frozen ground beef from a Nebraska processing plant. Twenty-five million pounds of potentially contaminated ground beef are recalled.

» CDC establishes the Epidemiology Laboratory Capacity (ELC) building program. This program funds public health laboratories to join PulseNet.

1998
PulseNet is honored by the Vice President of the United States at a White House ceremony.

» The U.S. Food and Drug Administration's (FDA) Center for Food Safety and Applied Nutrition (CFSAN) laboratory joins PulseNet.

1999
PulseNet wins the Innovations in American Government Award, recognizing excellence and creativity in the public sector.

» The National Food Safety Initiative is established, detailing how $43.2 million is to be used to strengthen food safety in the US. PulseNet becomes one of the first CDC-established networks that this initiative supports.

2000
PFGE analysis software is provided by APHL to all existing PulseNet laboratories allowing the creation of organized databases.

2001
PulseNet becomes a nationwide system: all 50 state public health laboratories are trained and certified in PFGE.

2002
PulseNet wins the prestigious Innovations in American Government Award for the second time.

2004
CDC pilots the *Listeria* Initiative in 10 states to aid in the investigation of listeriosis clusters detected by PulseNet, decreasing the time from detection to stopping the outbreak.

2005
» Manufacturers introduce the first commercially available next-generation DNA sequencing system. Next-generation sequencing technologies will shape the future of PulseNet and accelerate outbreak detection.

» PulseNet integrates multiple locus variable number tandem repeat analysis (MLVA) as a genotyping tool for *E. coli* O157:H7 and *Salmonella enterica* serotype Typhimurium.

2006
PulseNet links contaminated bagged spinach to a large multistate outbreak of *E. coli* O157:H7, prompting a nationwide recall. The outbreak sickens 225 people in 27 states and causes 39 cases of kidney failure and 5 deaths.

Figure 3.6 PulseNet timeline.

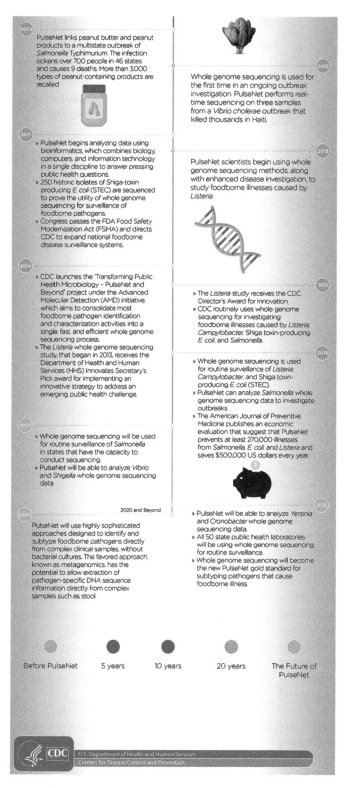

2009
PulseNet links peanut butter and peanut products to a multistate outbreak of *Salmonella* Typhimurium. The infection sickens over 700 people in 46 states and causes 9 deaths. More than 3,000 types of peanut-containing products are recalled.

2010
Whole genome sequencing is used for the first time in an ongoing outbreak investigation. PulseNet performs real-time sequencing on three samples from a *Vibrio cholerae* outbreak that killed thousands in Haiti.

2011
» PulseNet begins analyzing data using bioinformatics, which combines biology, computers, and information technology in a single discipline to answer pressing public health questions.
» 250 historic isolates of Shiga-toxin producing *E. coli* (STEC) are sequenced to prove the utility of whole genome sequencing for surveillance of foodborne pathogens.
» Congress passes the FDA Food Safety Modernization Act (FSMA) and directs CDC to expand national foodborne disease surveillance systems.

2013
PulseNet scientists begin using whole genome sequencing methods, along with enhanced disease investigation, to study foodborne illnesses caused by *Listeria*.

2014
» CDC launches the "Transforming Public Health Microbiology – PulseNet and Beyond" project under the Advanced Molecular Detection (AMD) initiative, which aims to consolidate most foodborne pathogen identification and characterization activities into a single, fast, and efficient whole genome sequencing process.
» The *Listeria* whole genome sequencing study, that began in 2013, receives the Department of Health and Human Services (HHS) Innovates Secretary's Pick award for implementing an innovative strategy to address an emerging public health challenge.

2015
» The *Listeria* study receives the CDC Director's Award for Innovation
» CDC routinely uses whole genome sequencing for investigating foodborne illnesses caused by *Listeria*, *Campylobacter*, Shiga toxin-producing *E. coli*, and *Salmonella*.

2016
» Whole genome sequencing is used for routine surveillance of *Listeria*, *Campylobacter*, and Shiga toxin-producing *E. coli* (STEC).
» PulseNet can analyze *Salmonella* whole genome sequencing data to investigate outbreaks.
» The American Journal of Preventive Medicine publishes an economic evaluation that suggest that PulseNet prevents at least 270,000 illnesses from *Salmonella*, *E. coli*, and *Listeria* and saves $500,000 US dollars every year.

2017
» Whole genome sequencing will be used for routine surveillance of *Salmonella* in states that have the capacity to conduct sequencing.
» PulseNet will be able to analyze *Vibrio* and *Shigella* whole genome sequencing data.

2018
» PulseNet will be able to analyze *Yersinia* and *Cronobacter* whole genome sequencing data.
» All 50 state public health laboratories will be using whole genome sequencing for routine surveillance.
» Whole genome sequencing will become the new PulseNet gold standard for subtyping pathogens that cause foodborne illness.

2020
2020 and Beyond
PulseNet will use highly sophisticated approaches designed to identify and subtype foodborne pathogens directly from complex clinical samples, without bacterial cultures. The favored approach, known as metagenomics, has the potential to allow extraction of pathogen-specific DNA sequence information directly from complex samples such as stool.

Before PulseNet   5 years   10 years   20 years   The Future of PulseNet

CDC
U.S. Department of Health and Human Services
Centers for Disease Control and Prevention

Figure 3.6 (*Continued*)

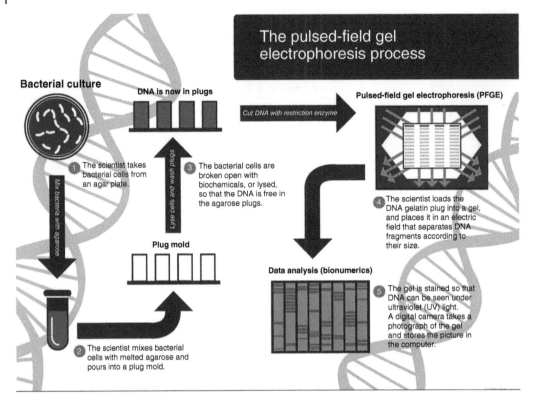

The pulsed-field gel electrophoresis process

Bacterial culture

DNA is now in plugs

Cut DNA with restriction enzyme

Pulsed-field gel electrophoresis (PFGE)

Mix bacteria with agarose

Lyse cells and wash plugs

1. The scientist takes bacterial cells from an agar plate.

3. The bacterial cells are broken open with biochemicals, or lysed, so that the DNA is free in the agarose plugs.

4. The scientist loads the DNA gelatin plug into a gel, and places it in an electric field that separates DNA fragments according to their size.

Plug mold

Data analysis (bionumerics)

5. The gel is stained so that DNA can be seen under ultraviolet (UV) light. A digital camera takes a photograph of the gel and stores the picture in the computer.

2. The scientist mixes bacterial cells with melted agarose and pours into a plug mold.

Figure 3.7 Pulsed-field gel electrophoresis (PFGE) workflow.

During outbreak investigations, epidemiologic data are compared for people with matching isolates to look for common food items, restaurants, animal contact, or other potential sources of illness. Foods that appear to be associated with illnesses can be traced back to their sources, looking for points of shared origin. Once a suspected source is identified, a One Health investigative approach can be taken and environmental testing can be performed to look for contamination with the outbreak strain that might have been introduced during production, processing, or preparation. Sharing of this information across multiple sectors involved in One Health helps to identify gaps in production processes and lessons learned for prevention of future outbreaks and illnesses. Genetic analysis of bacterial isolates from food processing, animals, the environment, and human illnesses can provide additional information about environmental bacterial reservoirs and can be used for surveillance purposes. Environmental testing can also be used to improve agricultural practices, food inspection, and regulatory activities.

In 2013, CDC began using WGS to detect outbreaks caused by *Listeria*. WGS reveals all the genetic material, or the genome, of an organism (like bacteria and viruses) in one efficient process. CDC is partnering with other federal agencies and state and local health departments to analyze *Listeria* from human cases, and possible food sources, to detect outbreaks earlier to prevent illnesses, and to link illnesses to food sources. By sequencing all *Listeria* isolates and interviewing all listeriosis patients in detail, the number of solved outbreaks per year increased from two to nine (Jackson et al., 2016). WGS is expanding and is being used to investigate illnesses caused by other foodborne pathogens such as *Campylobacter, E. coli,* and *Salmonella* (Figure 3.8).

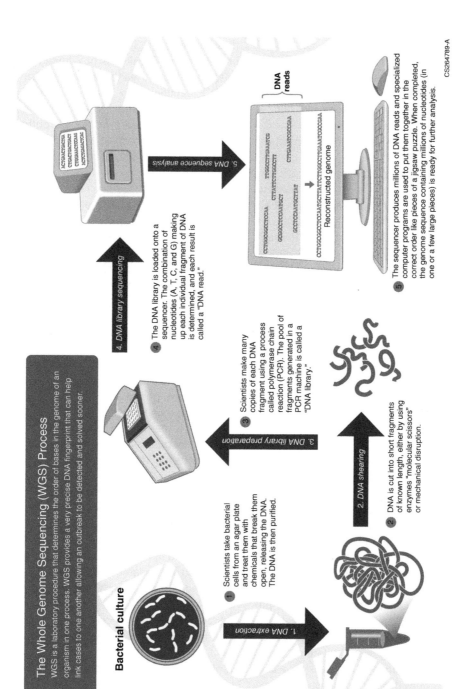

The Whole Genome Sequencing (WGS) Process

WGS is a laboratory procedure that determines the order of bases in the genome of an organism in one process. WGS provides a very precise DNA fingerprint that can help link cases to one another allowing an outbreak to be detected and solved sooner.

Bacterial culture

1. DNA extraction

① Scientists take bacterial cells from an agar plate and treat them with chemicals that break them open, releasing the DNA. The DNA is then purified.

2. DNA shearing

② DNA is cut into short fragments of known length, either by using enzymes "molecular scissors" or mechanical disruption.

3. DNA library preparation

③ Scientists make many copies of each DNA fragment using a process called polymerase chain reaction (PCR). The pool of fragments generated in a PCR machine is called a "DNA library."

4. DNA library sequencing

④ The DNA library is loaded onto a sequencer. The combination of nucleotides (A, T, C, and G) making up each individual fragment of DNA is determined, and each result is called a "DNA read."

5. DNA sequence analysis

DNA reads

CCTGCGGCCTCCGA
TTGGCCTTGAAATCG
CTTATTCTTGGCCTT
GGGGCCTCCAATGCT
GCCTCCAAATGCTAT
CCTGGAAATCGCCGA

Reconstructed genome

CCTTGGCGGGCCTCCGATTATTCTTGGCCTTGAAATCGCCGGA

⑤ The sequencer produces millions of DNA reads and specialized computer programs are used to put them together in the correct order like pieces of a jigsaw puzzle. When completed, the genome sequence containing millions of nucleotides (in one or a few large pieces) is ready for further analysis.

CS264789-A

Figure 3.8 Whole genome sequencing (WGS) workflow.

Box 3.2 Caramel apple case study

Listeriosis is a rare but serious illness caused by eating food contaminated with the bacterium *Listeria monocytogenes*. Listeriosis can be fatal, especially in certain high-risk groups, including the elderly, and people with weakened immune systems and certain chronic medical conditions (such as cancer). In pregnant women, listeriosis can cause miscarriage, stillbirth, premature labor, and serious illness or death in newborn babies.

In October 2014, people in multiple states began developing illness with *Listeria monocytogenes*. The PulseNet surveillance system identified illnesses that were part of this outbreak. Both PFGE and WGS were used to examine *Listeria* bacteria isolated from ill people; WGS was used because it provides a more detailed DNA fingerprint than PFGE. Two outbreak clusters were identified by PFGE; when WGS was used, the two *Listeria* illness clusters were distinct and isolates within each cluster were found to be highly related. CDC investigated the two clusters together because one person was infected with both *Listeria* strains simultaneously and because illnesses in the two clusters occurred during a similar time period and in similar regions of the country.

By January 2015, public health investigators identified 35 people from 12 states infected with the outbreak strains. Thirty-four (97%) of the ill people were hospitalized; listeriosis contributed to at least three of seven reported deaths. Eleven (31%) illnesses were pregnancy-associated, with one illness resulting in a fetal loss.

During interviews of ill people, 28 (90%) of the 31 people with available information reported eating commercially produced, prepackaged caramel apples in the 28 days before illness onset. The caramel apples people reported consuming were different brands. Only 1 (3%) of 36 non-outbreak-associated cases interviewed reported consuming caramel apples during the same time period. The three ill people who did not report eating caramel apples did report eating whole or sliced apples. The source of the whole or sliced apples was unknown, and it is unknown whether these apples were linked to the patients' illnesses. This outbreak was not limited to the USA; the Public Health Agency of Canada (PHAC) identified two cases of listeriosis in Canada with the same DNA fingerprints, or PFGE patterns, as seen in the US outbreak; additional testing via WGS showed that only one case was genetically related to the US outbreak.

CDC and FDA issued a recommendation that consumers should not eat *any* commercially produced, prepackaged caramel apples until more detailed information was available. A traceback investigation was conducted using caramel apple purchase locations for 11 outbreak cases. Subsequently, three caramel apple manufacturers received notice from an apple supplier headquartered in California, that there may be a connection between the listeriosis outbreak and the apples supplied to them (Supplier X). The three companies issued voluntary recalls of caramel apples because they had the potential to be contaminated with *Listeria monocytogenes*.

Although the manufacturers of the brands reported by these cases received apples from other growers, the traceback investigation confirmed that Supplier X was the only apple grower that supplied apples to each company. A call was held with Supplier X to inform them of the findings of the investigation and Supplier X issued a voluntary recall of whole apples it sold in 2014 used for caramel apples; about two weeks later, Supplier X recalled all Gala and Granny Smith apples produced in 2014.

State and FDA specialists conducted a joint investigation at the apple packing facility. Environmental samples were taken by swabbing surfaces likely to come into contact with apples; several of these samples resulted in growth of *Listeria monocytogenes*. Twenty days after the investigation at the packing facility, PFGE analysis of the *Listeria*

Box 3.2 (Continued)

monocytogenes isolated from environmental samples collected at Supplier X confirmed that the DNA fingerprints of the pathogen matched the outbreak strains of *Listeria monocytogenes* isolated from people affected by the outbreak. WGS analysis of the *Listeria monocytogenes* isolated from environmental samples and whole apples collected at Supplier X also confirmed that the genomes of the pathogens were highly related to the outbreak strains. After an FDA review, the recall of Gala and Granny Smith apples from Supplier X was complete.

Source: Angelo et al., 2017.

The case study in Box 3.2 demonstrates how advanced molecular detection (AMD) methods, such as whole genome sequencing (WGS), can be applied during outbreak investigations to examine relatedness of bacterial isolates. In this investigation, what initially appeared to be two distinct outbreaks by PFGE analysis turned out to be a single outbreak.

Laboratory-based surveillance can track changes in testing practices over time, supply information about populations impacted by foodborne illness, and provide incentives for improvement of food safety and policy development. This includes tracking the increased use of culture-independent diagnostic tests (CIDTs) to detect enteric pathogens such as *Salmonella*, *E. coli*, and *Campylobacter*. CIDTs are tests that can detect the DNA of bacteria directly from patient samples like stool. As their name implies, CIDTs do not need a culture (e.g., growing bacterial cells on agar in a lab) to identify the species that caused a patient's illness. Clinical laboratories are increasing their use of CIDTs because they save costs and diagnose illnesses faster; however, they do not provide a bacterial isolate. This alters the way public health surveillance is conducted and the type of information that can be obtained. Without a bacterial isolate, it is not possible to subtype by serotyping or PFGE, nor to sequence bacterial DNA, so the outbreak detection capacity of PulseNet may be lost. Bacterial isolates are needed to test for antimicrobial resistance to guide treatment and to track the reservoirs of resistance. Without bacterial isolates, other methods of antimicro-

bial susceptibility testing will have to be developed. Serotyping and subtyping can help target interventions such as serotype-specific vaccines to administer to animals, which can assist with prevention of illness in humans. In the short term, the solution is to encourage the culture by traditional methods of the specimen that tests positive for a key pathogen by CIDT, so-called "reflex culture." In the longer term, a new generation of culture-independent tests is needed that provide the information required by public and animal health agencies.

Some human pathogens with reservoirs in food animals have spread around the globe in silent pandemics. Early in the 1970s, a particular rare type of *Salmonella*, serotype Agona, appeared suddenly in outbreaks of human illness on several continents (Clark et al., 1973). Investigation of one such outbreak in Arkansas traced it from a restaurant back to a chicken farm, and to the feed the chickens had been eating, and ultimately to one ingredient of the chicken feed, a fishmeal made from Peruvian anchovies. This feed ingredient had been used globally, and reminds us of how the feed supply can be a route of rapid dissemination (Crump et al., 2002). In the 1970s, the incidence of recognized *Yersinia enterocolitica* infections in some parts of Europe increased rapidly and illness was traced to eating or handling undercooked pork (Mollaret et al., 1979; Tauxe et al., 1987). Later, those same serogroups of *Yersinia enterocolitica* became frequent in US swine, and caused illness in the USA (Lee et al., 1990; Jones, 2003). It seems likely, though not well documented, that it spread across the Atlantic through trade in live animals. In the 1990s one serotype of *Vibrio parahaemolyticus* O3:K6, a pathogen associated with eating raw shellfish, emerged in Southeast Asia and ultimately arrived in North America. It most likely was transferred from one harbor to another in the ballast water of commercial shipping vessels (Daniels et al., 2000). The appearance and spread of poultry-associated *Salmonella* Enteritidis was particularly well studied around the world in the 1980s and 1990s. It appears that a global pandemic occurred with a small number of strains that can transmit vertically from progenitor flocks (Rodrigue et al., 1990). This pandemic may have been mediated by the global trade in chicks or fertile eggs, rather than by human travelers, migrating birds, or other routes, as Australia remains free of egg-associated *Salmonella* Enteritidis (Moffatt et al., 2016). Strict animal quarantine laws restrict importation of chicks or eggs into that country (Tanner, 1997).

3.4 Antibiotic Resistance and Food Safety

The One Health nature of managing the safety of our food supply is well illustrated by the challenge posed by antibiotic resistance in enteric pathogens like *Salmonella* and *Campylobacter*. In the USA it has been estimated that 400 000 antibiotic-resistant infections occur each year, representing about 20% of the 2.3 million resistant infections that occur annually (Centers for Disease Control and Prevention, 2013b). Antibiotics are important in the treatment and management of infections in humans and animals, and wherever they are used, they may select for bacteria that are resistant to them. The selection can involve pathogens and non-pathogens alike; when the resistance genes appear on mobile genetic elements, such as plasmids, then bacteria can rapidly acquire a suite of resistance genes from other bacteria. Such transferable multidrug resistance was first

documented in *Shigella* in Japan in the 1950s, soon after antibiotics were introduced to treat widespread dysentery in the human population (Watanabe, 1963). Since then, defining the principles of judicious antibiotic use and stewardship has been a growing challenge in both human and animal medicine, and even in plant pathology, where antibiotics are used to treat or prevent bacterial infections of fruit trees.

Multidrug resistant bacteria have been detected in food products, including meat and fresh produce. In numerous foodborne outbreaks, *Salmonella* bacteria carrying resistance-coding genes for multiple antibiotics have been detected (Doyle, 2015). Resistance to antimicrobials has also been detected in environmental bacteria (Finley et al., 2013). Fresh produce may be contaminated by irrigation or wash water containing bacteria (Steele and Odumeru, 2004; Allende and Monaghan, 2015). Antibiotics are widely used in food-producing animals, and according to data published by FDA, there are more kilograms of antibiotics sold in the USA for food-producing animals than for people (Food and Drug Administration, 2014). Use of antibiotics can contribute to the emergence of antibiotic-resistant bacteria in food-producing animals. Resistant bacteria in food-producing animals are of concern because these animals can serve as carriers. Antibiotic use in food-producing animals can harm public health through the following sequence of events: use of antibiotics in food-producing animals allows antibiotic-resistant bacteria to thrive while susceptible bacteria are suppressed or die (Figure 3.9). Resistant bacteria can be transmitted from food-producing animals to humans through the food supply or through direct contact and handling of infected animals. Resistant bacteria can contaminate the foods that come from those animals, and people who consume these foods can potentially develop antibiotic-resistant infections (Centers for Disease Control and Prevention, 2013b). Resistant bacteria can cause infections in humans and these infections might result in adverse health consequences (Centers for Disease Control and Prevention, 2013b).

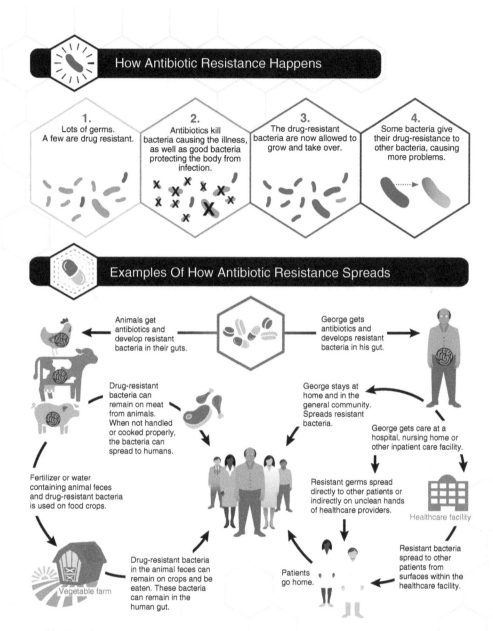

Figure 3.9 Some examples of how antibiotic resistance can spread.

Well-documented investigations have linked specific uses of antibiotics in animals with increases in resistant organisms, the contamination of food with those organisms, and resulting human illnesses. For example, in 1985, chloramphenicol-resistant *Salmonella* Newport caused hundreds of cases of illness in California, and was linked to eating ground beef (Spika et al., 1987). The ground beef was traced back to dairy cattle from two counties in California, and a survey of dairy farms showed a strong relationship between the presence of chloramphenicol-resistant *Salmonella* on those farms and the use of that drug in those dairy cattle (Pacer et al., 1989). This drug was not approved for use in cattle. Following the approval of fluoroquinolones (FQ) for use in poultry, the frequency of FQ-resistant *Campylobacter* infections increased rapidly in the 1990s (Smith et al., 1999). An epidemiologic investigation showed that the resistant infections were associated with eating poultry, and with international travel, and that *Campylobacter* illnesses tended to last longer if the infecting organism was resistant, than if it was susceptible (Kassenborg et al., 2004; Nelson et al., 2004). As a result, FDA withdrew approval for the use of this class of drugs in poultry (Nelson et al., 2007). In Canada, resistance monitoring captured a sharp decline in ceftriaxone resistance in human infections with *Salmonella* Heidelberg (a poultry-associated serotype) after the broiler industry stopped using that agent to treat eggs prophylactically, and documented a rebound when the practice was reintroduced (Dutil et al., 2010). In Taiwan, severe infections with multidrug-resistant *Salmonella* Choleraesuis occurred in humans simultaneously with an outbreak of the same infections in swine that were being treated with a variety of antibiotics. In humans, these infections often affected the aortic cardiac valve, causing catastrophic and often fatal shock, and could also be fatal in the swine (Yan et al., 2003; Hsueh et al., 2004). The epidemic continued for years, the progressive increase in resistance made infections more difficult to treat, and the same resistance gene cassette has appeared in other *Salmonella* serotypes (Su et al., 2011). The epidemic appears finally to be decreasing with better animal disease control measures, including remuneration to farmers for sending ill pigs for disposal, rather than rushing them to market (Su et al., 2014).

Antibiotics must be used judiciously in humans and animals because both uses contribute to the emergence and the persistence and spread of antibiotic-resistant bacteria. Preserving the effectiveness of antibiotics is vital to protecting human and animal health. To aid in this effort, FDA has limited the use of "Medically Important" antimicrobials in food animals, including antimicrobial drugs that are considered important for therapeutic use in humans (Food and Drug Administration, 2015). Measures that can also aid in illness prevention include cooking foods to adequate temperatures to kill bacteria, and washing hands with soap and water after handling pets and livestock.

Much of the antimicrobial resistance encountered in human medicine is related to the use of antibiotics to treat humans, both in the developed and the developing world. In many places, the number of agents that remain effective to treat severe infections has decreased. This means it is important to consider the broader impacts of selective pressure inherent wherever antibiotics are used. Some resistant infections cause severe illness. People with infections that are resistant to antibiotics might require increased recovery time, incur increased medical expenses, and can die if the infection cannot be treated. Additionally, physicians might have to recommend second- or third-choice drugs for treatment when the bacteria that cause infections are resistant to the drug of choice and this drug doesn't work. But the alternative drugs might be less effective, more toxic, and more expensive. To conduct surveillance for antimicrobial resistance, a One Health approach is needed. One such surveillance system for antimicrobial resistance is the National Antimicrobial Resistance Monitoring

System for Enteric Bacteria (NARMS). NARMS is a collaboration among state and local public health departments, CDC, FDA, and the USDA (Figure 3.10). Since 1996, this surveillance system has tracked changes in the antimicrobial susceptibility of certain enteric bacteria found in ill people (CDC), retail meats (FDA), and food

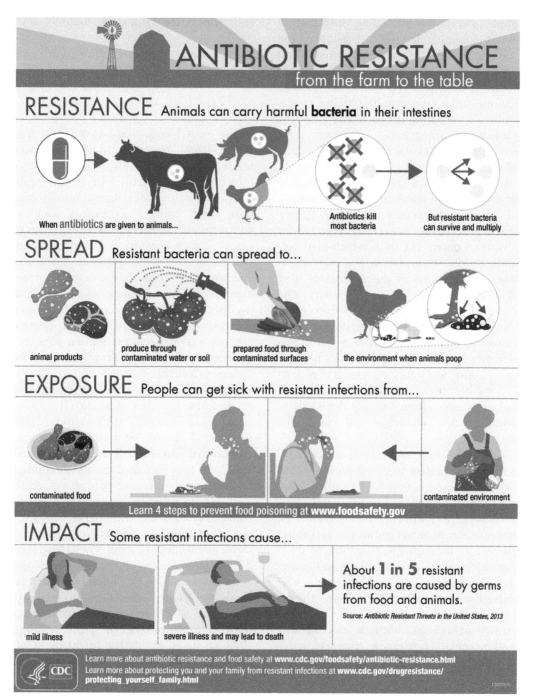

Figure 3.10 Antibiotic resistance from farm to fork.

animals at slaughter (USDA Food Safety Inspection Service) in the USA (Centers for Disease Control and Prevention, 2016b). The information collected through this One Health program helps protect public health by providing information about emerging bacterial resistance, the ways in which resistance is spread, and how resistant infections differ from susceptible infections (Centers for Disease Control and Prevention, 2016b). In Canada, similar monitoring is conducted by the Canadian Integrated Program for Antimicrobial Resistance (CIPARS) (Public Health Agency of Canada, 2007). In Europe, integrated resistance information is assembled by each country and assembled by the European Food Safety Agency (EFSA) and the European Centre for Disease Control (ECDC), which also collects routine information on the indications and volumes of the antibiotics used (European Food Safety Authority and European Centre for Disease Prevention and Control, 2016). However, data on antimicrobial use in agriculture are not systematically collected in the USA or in many other countries. Routine systems of reporting and benchmarking antibiotic use could help to inform future policy decisions to address the challenge of antibiotic resistance.

Currently, there is no systematic global surveillance system to detect antimicrobial resistance threats in the food supply. Today, the international identification of antibiotic resistance threats occurs through domestic importation of novel antibiotic resistance threats or through identification of overseas outbreaks (Centers for Disease Control and Prevention, 2013b). A comprehensive surveillance system for these threats is needed and should include the use of AMD technologies, which can identify antimicrobial resistance threats much faster than current practice. However, these technologies are not being used widely in the USA or in other countries. Integrated One Health surveillance systems can facilitate sharing of information on emerging disease threats, including antimicrobial resistance (Uchtmann et al., 2015).

3.5 Zoonotic Disease and Foodborne Pathogens

While most human *Salmonella* infections result from exposure to contaminated foods, an estimated 11% of all *Salmonella* infections are attributed to animal exposures, including both direct animal handling and indirect exposures such as contact with areas where an animal lives or roams (i.e., a habitat) and handling contaminated pet food (Hale et al., 2012). Human infections have resulted from exposure to a wide range of animals including pet reptiles such as small turtles, bearded dragons, and crested geckos; amphibians; hedgehogs; guinea pigs; pet rodents; and live poultry (Centers for Disease Control and Prevention, 2013a; Mettee Zarecki et al., 2013; Bartholomew et al., 2014; Lowther et al., 2011; Centers for Disease Control and Prevention, 2005; Bosch et al., 2016). Salmonellae are part of the normal intestinal flora for these animals, and they can shed the bacteria intermittently in their feces or droppings. Areas where these animals live and roam can be contaminated with salmonellae and be a source of infection to people exposed to those environments, even when there is no direct contact between animals and people (Lowther et al., 2011). Contact with dry pet foods and feeder rodents used to feed reptiles have also been implicated in large multistate outbreaks of human illness (Behravesh et al., 2010; Imanishi et al., 2014; Cartwright et al., 2016).

Certain animal foods, such as commercially prepared pet food, can cause human illness when contaminated with *Salmonella*, because humans handle these foods. The association between human outbreaks of salmonellosis and *Salmonella*-contaminated pet foods is well established. Children may put pet food contaminated with *Salmonella* into their mouths (Behravesh et al., 2010; Imanishi et al., 2014). Animals can be asymptomatically or clinically infected with *Salmonella* from contaminated pet food, thus increasing the risk of human exposure. CDC reported that from January 1, 2006 to October 31, 2008, 79 human cases of salmonellosis were linked to *Salmonella* Schwarzengrund in dry dog food manufactured by a company in the USA (Behravesh et al., 2010). In 2005, Canadian public health officials reported that cases of salmonellosis in Canada and the USA were linked to pet treats contaminated with *Salmonella* Thompson (Centers for Disease Control and Prevention, 2006; Behravesh et al., 2010). In addition, Canadian outbreaks of human salmonellosis linked to pet treats have been documented, including *Salmonella* Newport in beefsteak-patty dog treats manufactured in Texas in 2002, and *Salmonella* Infantis in pig-ear dog treats manufactured in Canada in 1999 (Food and Drug Administration, 2013; Centers for Disease Control and Prevention, 2006). Live and frozen mice or rats may be fed to carnivorous reptiles and amphibians; some companies raise and sell these "feeder rodents" for use as food for reptiles or amphibians. If the feeder rodents are colonized with *Salmonella*, the bacteria can be transmitted to reptiles as well as to the humans handling the rodents and reptiles and to the environment where the feeder rodents are stored or handled (Goupil et al., 2012; Cartwright et al., 2016) (Box 3.3).

3.6 Outbreak Response Communication

Communicating the lessons learned through outbreak investigation and surveillance for foodborne illness will lead to further understanding of food safety and may be done through a coordinated One Health approach. The news media can be valuable partners in communicating improvements in food production, processing, and preparation. Communication regarding unsafe food can prevent illnesses and motivate changes in behaviors such as cooking food to temperatures that result in sufficient reduction of bacteria to prevent illness. A One Health approach to communication is often needed, as communication about foodborne illness can also impact the agricultural industry and public action might not be commensurate with public health risk. The need to communicate with the public is based on the need to convey public health action that can be taken to prevent illness, and must be timely to be effective. This type of communication can be found during outbreak investigations and communications regarding recalls of food products. When a product cannot be easily recalled, as is the case with pets, public health messaging can focus on prevention measures that can be taken to reduce the risk of illness through improving animal husbandry, biosecurity, reducing environmental contamination and cross-contamination, and handwashing. Overall, food safety is improved when consumers know what they can do to prevent foodborne illness. Sharing lessons learned across multiple sectors, including human and animal health, industry, and agriculture, is essential to ensuring that healthful food is available. In the future, a platform for global communication of food safety and security issues could be very useful, particularly if it considers a collaborative One Health approach to reach the relevant stakeholders (Uchtmann et al., 2015).

Box 3.3 **Investigation of antibiotic-resistant** *Salmonella enterica* **serotype I 4,[5],12:i:–** (Cartwright et al., 2016)

In December 2008, the UK's Health Protection Agency (HPA) detected 3 *Salmonella enterica* I 4,[5],12:i:–, which had not previously been reported in England or Wales (Harker et al., 2011; Hopkins et al., 2012). The HPA investigated and found that a high percentage of people infected with this *Salmonella* serotype kept a reptile at home. In addition, most of the ill people who owned reptiles fed those reptiles imported frozen feeder mice. Rodents can carry *Salmonella* and appear healthy and clean while shedding the organism, which can contaminate cages and bedding, leading to indirect human exposure; direct exposure via handling of the animal can also occur. The process of producing frozen feeder rodents may contribute to external contamination of the rodent with *Salmonella*. During CO_2 chamber euthanasia, the bowels and bladders of the rodents are evacuated. Exposure to the evacuated feces and urine may further contribute to external contamination of the animals, which could increase the risk of human *Salmonella* exposure, especially if safe handling practices are not followed. Samples of frozen feeder mice from several major suppliers were tested; the outbreak strain was identified in samples from a single supplier (Company A), which was located in the USA (Harker et al., 2011). HPA notified CDC of their investigation in March 2009.

Upon notification, the PulseNet database was searched for isolates with PFGE patterns that were indistinguishable from the HPA isolates. CDC identified 35 *Salmonella* I 4,[5],12:i:– isolates with PFGE patterns that were indistinguishable; however, reptile and rodent exposures were only reported by 4 (14%) of the 29 persons interviewed. The pattern was monitored by CDC epidemiologists and by June 2010, PulseNet USA identified an additional 29 isolates matching the outbreak

strains, this time, a review of case patient interviews noted 12 (80%) of the 15 interviewed cases reported reptile exposure. A One Health outbreak investigation was initiated.

A case-control study was conducted to examine reptile ownership among ill persons and practices involved with handling of frozen feeder rodents. The case-control study found that case patients were more likely than controls to have reptile exposure. Reptiles were commonly fed rodents, and case patients reported storing frozen rodents in the same freezer with human food and thawing frozen rodents in their kitchen. About half of the case patients interviewed were aware of the association between *Salmonella* and reptiles or amphibians; however, very few were aware of the association between *Salmonella* and rodents (Cartwright et al., 2016).

State partners collected samples of droppings from bearded dragons in the home of a case-patient; *Salmonella* I 4,[5],12:i:– was isolated from the droppings of one reptile with a PFGE pattern indistinguishable from the outbreak strain. The bearded dragons were fed mice sourced from three stores; one store procured mice from a distributor who purchased frozen mice in bulk from Company A. The distributor repackaged the mice into smaller quantities for resale by the pet store.

Environmental investigations were conducted at Company A by FDA, which regulates animal food that enters state commerce. Company A raises and produces frozen feeder mice and rats onsite. FDA inspected Company A in early July 2010 and collected samples from their facility, including rodent feed, frozen feeder mice, and swabs of the environment. During a second inspection in late July 2010, samples of frozen rats, environmental samples, and samples of irradiated frozen mice were collected. During a third inspection in March 2011, samples collected included irradiated

Box 3.3 (Continued)

frozen feeder mice, nonirradiated frozen rats, and swabs of the room where irradiated product is stored prior to shipment. *Salmonella* I 4,[5],12:i:– isolates with a PFGE pattern indistinguishable from the outbreak strain were obtained from all the frozen feeder mice (*n* = 13) and environmental samples (*n* = 19) collected during FDA's initial inspection in early July 2010. These findings prompted an international voluntary recall of all frozen feeder animals produced by Company A between May 2009 and July 2010; an estimated 6 million frozen feeder rodents were subject to the recall. In late July 2010, Company A began irradiating all frozen feeder mice at a certified food irradiation facility. Samples of irradiated mice collected during the late July–August inspection did not yield *Salmonella*; however, swabs taken in the room where irradiated product was stored prior to distribution, including the table used for packing irradiated product for shipment, yielded the outbreak strain of *Salmonella*. The irradiated frozen feeder mice samples collected during the March 2011 follow-up inspection by FDA again did not yield *Salmonella*. However, environmental samples obtained from the irradiated finished product storage area yielded the outbreak strain of *Salmonella*.

NARMS routinely tests at least three isolates from multistate outbreaks for antibiotic susceptibility. In this outbreak three human isolates from the outbreak demonstrated resistance to tetracycline (3/3 isolates), ceftriaxone (1 of 3 isolates), and ampicillin (1 of 3 isolates). Among the samples collected during the July 2010 inspection, tetracycline resistance was demonstrated in 12 of the 13 *Salmonella* isolates obtained from frozen mice, and in all 19 isolates obtained from environmental sampling. An additional environmental isolate collected during the March 2011 follow-up inspection also demonstrated resistance to tetracycline. None of the environmental samples demonstrated resistance to ceftriaxone or ampicillin. Company A used feed containing chlortetracycline and a sulfonamide antibiotic for nontherapeutic purposes. Use of antibiotics can contribute to

resistance; therefore, it is possible the prior use of antibiotics in the feed by Company A helped select for, or maintain, the tetracycline-resistant strain of *Salmonella* in this outbreak. Because antimicrobial drug use in both humans and animals can contribute to the development of antimicrobial resistance, it is important to use antimicrobials judiciously.

This international outbreak of tetracycline-resistant *Salmonella* I 4,[5],12:i:– infections had over 500 cases occurring from 2008 to 2010 throughout the USA, the UK, and Canada. A case-control study conducted in the USA found that cases were significantly associated with exposure to reptiles and feeder rodents. Although Company A recalled all frozen feeder animals produced during the time period and initiated irradiation of frozen feeder mice prior to sale, cases with this PFGE pattern continued to be reported in all three affected countries throughout 2012. In the USA, a decrease in cases was not reported in the 6 months immediately following the recall. The protracted nature of this outbreak might have resulted from a variety of factors, including that distributors typically purchase frozen rodents in bulk and repackage them in smaller quantities prior to selling them to local stores. Both the initial shipments and the repackaged rodents have minimal package labeling, making traceback of purchases to the distributor or producer challenging. Frozen feeder rodent producers, suppliers, and distributors should follow the animal food labeling requirements as described in 21 CFR §501.5, and all packages of frozen feeder rodents should include safe handling instructions. Persons should wash their hands thoroughly with soap and water after handling live or frozen feeder rodents, as well as reptiles or anything in the area where the animals live (Cartwright et al., 2016). Continued One Health opportunities exist for public health officials, the pet industry, veterinarians, and consumers to work together to prevent salmonellosis associated with pet food, pets, and other animals.

References

Allende, A. and Monaghan, J. (2015). Irrigation water quality for leafy crops: A perspective of risks and potential solutions. *Int J Environ Res Public Health* 12, 7457–7477.

Angelo, K., Conrad, A., Saupe, A., et al. (2017). Multistate outbreak of Listeria monocytogenes infections linked to whole apples used in commercially produced, prepackaged caramel apples: United States, 2014–2015. *Epidemiol Infect* 145(5), 848–856.

Angelos, J., Arens, A., Johnson, H., Cadriel, J., and Osburn, B. (2016). One Health in food safety and security education: A curricular framework. *Comp Immunol Microbiol Infect Dis* 44, 29–33.

Angulo, F. and Swerdlow, D. (1999). Epidemiology of human *Salmonella enterica* Serovar Enteritidis infections in the United States. In: Gast, R., Potter, M., Wall, P., and Saeed, A. (eds), *Salmonella enterica serovar Enteritidis in Humans and Animals: Epidemiology, Pathogenesis, and Control*, 1st edn. Ames, IA: Iowa State University Press.

Bartholomew, M.L., Heffernan, R.T., Wright, J.G., et al. (2014). Multistate outbreak of Salmonella enterica serotype enteritidis infection associated with pet guinea pigs. *Vector Borne Zoonotic Dis* 14, 414–421.

Behravesh, C.B., Ferraro, A., Deasy, M. 3rd, et al. (2010). Human Salmonella infections linked to contaminated dry dog and cat food, 2006–2008. *Pediatrics* 126, 477–483.

Bosch, S., Tauxe, R.V., and Behravesh, C.B. (2016). Turtle-associated salmonellosis, United States, 2006–2014. *Emerg Infect Dis* 22, 1149–1155.

Boyce, B. (2013). Trends in farm-to-table from a sociological perspective. *J Acad Nutr Diet* 113, 892–8.

Bryan, F. (1982). *Disease transmitted by foods (A classification and summary)*, 2nd edn. Atlanta, GA: Centers for Disease Control, HHS Publication No. (CDC) 83–8237.

Cartwright, E.J., Nguyen, T., Melluso, C., et al. (2016). A multistate investigation of antibiotic-resistant Salmonella enterica serotype I 4,[5],12:i:– infections as part of an international outbreak associated with frozen feeder rodents. *Zoonoses Public Hlth* 63, 62–71.

Centers for Disease Control and Prevention (2005). Outbreak of multidrug-resistant Salmonella typhimurium associated with rodents purchased at retail pet stores–– United States, December 2003–October 2004. *MMWR Morb Mortal Wkly Rep* 54, 429–433.

Centers for Disease Control and Prevention (2006). Human salmonellosis associated with animal-derived pet treats––United States and Canada, 2005. *MMWR Morb Mortal Wkly Rep* 55, 702–705.

Centers for Disease Control and Prevention (2013a). Notes from the field: Multistate outbreak of human Salmonella typhimurium infections linked to contact with pet hedgehogs – United States, 2011–2013. *MMWR Morb Mortal Wkly Rep* 62, 73.

Centers for Disease Control and Prevention (2013b). Antibiotic Resistance Threats in the United States, 2013. Atlanta, GA: CDC.

Centers for Disease Control and Prevention (2016a). Announcement: 20th Anniversary of PulseNet: the National Molecular Subtyping Network for Foodborne Disease Surveillance – United States, 2016. *MMWR Morb Mortal Wkly Rep* 65, 636.

Centers for Disease Control and Prevention (2016b). National Antimicrobial Resistance Monitoring System for Enteric Bacteria (NARMS) [Online]. Available at: https://www.cdc.gov/narms/index.html (accessed July 24, 2016).

Clark, G., Kauffman, A., Gangarosa, E., and Thompson, M. (1973). Epidemiology of an international outbreak of *Salmonella agona*. *Lancet* ii, 490–493.

Consumer Goods Forum (2015). The Global Food Safety Initiative. Available at: http://www.mygfsi.com/files/Information_Kit/Fact_Sheets/1_GFSI_Overview_NAmerica.pdf (accessed December 14, 2016).

Crump, J., Griffin, P., and Angulo, F. (2002). Bacterial contamination of animal feed and its relationship to human foodborne illness. *Clin Infect Dis* 35, 859–865.

Daniels, N., Ray, B., Easton, A., Marano, N., et al. (2000). Emergence of new *Vibrio parahaemolyticus* serotype in raw oysters: A prevention quandary. *JAMA* 284, 1541–1545.

Dekeyser, P., Gossuin-Detrain, M., Butzler, J.P., and Sternon, J. (1972). Acute enteritis due to related vibrio: first positive stool cultures. *J Infect Dis* 125, 390–392.

Doyle, M.E. (2015). Multidrug-resistant pathogens in the food supply. *Foodborne Pathog Dis*, 12, 261–279.

Dutil, L., Irwin, R., Finley, R., et al. (2010). Ceftiofur resistance in Salmonella enterica serovar Heidelberg from chicken meat and humans, Canada. *Emerg Infect Dis* 16, 48–54.

European Food Safety Authority and European Centre For Disease Prevention And Control (2016). The European Union Summary report on antimicrobial resistance in zoonotic and indicator bacteria from humans, animals and food in 2014. *EFSA J* 14.

FAO (Food and Agriculture Organization of the United Nations) (2001). *Codex Alimentarius Commission – Procedural Manual – Twelfth Edition*. Rome: Secretariat of the Joint FAO/WHO Food Standards Programme.

FAO (Food and Agriculture Organization of the United Nations), International Fund for Agricultural Development, and World Food Programme (2014). Strengthening the enabling environment for food security and nutrition. In: *The State of Food Insecurity in the World 2014*. Rome: FAO.

Finley, R.L., Collignon, P., Larsson, D.G., et al. (2013). The scourge of antibiotic resistance: the important role of the environment. *Clin Infect Dis* 57, 704–710.

Fletcher, J., Leach, J., Eversole, K., and Tauxe, R. (2013). Human pathogens on plants: Designing a multidisciplinary strategy for research. *Phytopathology* 103, 306–315.

Food and Drug Administration (2013). Compliance Policy Guide Sec. 690.800 Salmonella in Food for Animals. Federal Register.

Food and Drug Administration (2014). Antimicrobials sold or distributed for use in food-producing animals.

Food and Drug Administration (2015). Veterinary Feed Directive. Department of Health and Human Services. Available at: https://www.gpo.gov/fdsys/pkg/FR-2015-06-03/pdf/2015-13393.pdf (accessed December 18, 2017).

Gardner, T.J., Fitzgerald, C., Xavier, C., et al. (2011). Outbreak of campylobacteriosis associated with consumption of raw peas. *Clin Infect Di*, 53, 26–32.

Gast, R. (1999). Applying experimental infection models to understand the pathogenesis, detection and control of Salmonella enterica serovar Enteritidis in poultry. In: Saeed, A., Gast, R., Potter, M., and Wall, P. (eds), *Salmonella enterica Serovar Enteritidis in Humans and Animals: Epidemiology, Pathogenesis, and Control*. Ames, IA: Iowa State University Press, chapter 22.

Gautam, D., Dobhal, S., Payton, M.E., Fletcher, J., and Ma, L.M. (2014). Surface survival and internalization of salmonella through natural cracks on developing cantaloupe fruits, alone or in the presence of the melon wilt pathogen Erwinia tracheiphila. *PLoS One* 9, e105248.

Goupil, B.A., Trent, A.M., Bender, J., Olsen, K.E., Morningstar, B.R., and Wunschmann, A. (2012). A longitudinal study of Salmonella from snakes used in a public outreach program. *J Zoo Wildl Med* 43, 836–841.

Gu, G., Cevallos-Cevallos, J.M., and Van Bruggen, A.H. (2013). Ingress of Salmonella enterica Typhimurium into tomato leaves through hydathodes. *PLoS One* 8, e53470.

Gurven, M. and Kaplan, H. (2007). Longevity among hunter-gatherers: a cross-cultural examination. *Popul Dev Rev* 33, 321–365.

Hale, C.R., Scallan, E., Cronquist, A.B., et al. (2012). Estimates of enteric illness attributable to contact with animals and their environments in the United States. *Clin Infect Dis* 54(Suppl. 5), S472–479.

Harker, K.S., Lane, C., De Pinna, E., and Adak, G.K. (2011). An outbreak of Salmonella Typhimurium DT191a associated with reptile feeder mice. *Epidemiol Infect* 139, 1254–1261.

Havelaar, A.H., Kirk, M.D., Torgerson, P.R., et al. (2015). World Health Organization global estimates and regional comparisons of the burden of foodborne disease in 2010. *PLoS Med* 12, e1001923.

Hopkins, K.L., de Pinna, E., and Wain, J. (2012). Prevalence of Salmonella enterica serovar 4,[5],12:i:– in England and Wales, 2010. *Euro Surveill*, 17.

Hsueh, P., Teng, L., Tseng, S., et al. (2004). Ciprofloxacin-resistant *Salmonella enterica* Typhimurium and Choleraesuis from pigs to humans, Taiwan. *Emerg Infect Dis* 10, 60–68.

Ikerd, J. (1996). Maintaining the profitability of agriculture. American Agricultural Economics Association Pre-Conference, July 27, 1996, San Antonio, TX. University of Missouri, pp. 27–38.

Imanishi, M., Rotstein, D.S., Reimschuessel, R., et al. (2014). Outbreak of Salmonella enterica serotype Infantis infection in humans linked to dry dog food in the United States and Canada, 2012. *J Am Vet Med Assoc* 244, 545–553.

Institute of Medicine (US) Food Forum (2009). *Managing Food Safety Practices from Farm to Table: Workshop Summary*. Washington (DC): The National Academies Collection: Reports funded by National Institutes of Health.

Jackson, B.R., Tarr, C., Strain, E. et al. (2016). Implementation of nationwide real-time whole-genome sequencing to enhance listeriosis outbreak detection and investigation. *Clin Infect Dis* 63(3), 380–386.

Jay, M.T., Cooley, M., Carychao, D., et al. (2007). Escherichia coli O157:H7 in feral swine near spinach fields and cattle, central California coast. *Emerg Infect Dis* 13, 1908–1911.

Jones, K.E., Patel, N.G., Levy, M.A., et al. (2008). Global trends in emerging infectious diseases. *Nature* 451, 990–993.

Jones, T.F. (2003). From pig to pacifier: chitterling-associated yersiniosis outbreak among black infants. *Emerg Infect Dis* 9, 1007–1009.

Kassenborg, H., Smith, K., Vugia, D., et al. (2004). Fluoroquinolone-resistant Campylobacter infections: Eating poultry outside of the home and foreign travel are risk factors. *Clin Infect Dis* 38, S279–S284.

Keesing, F., Belden, L.K., Daszak, P., et al. (2010). Impacts of biodiversity on the emergence and transmission of infectious diseases. *Nature* 468, 647–652.

Lang, T. (2003). Food industrialisation and food power: implications for food governance. *Dev Policy Rev* 21, 555–568.

Lee, L.A., Gerber, A.R., Longsway, D.R., et al. (1990). *Yersinia enterocolitica* O:3 infections in infants and children, associated with the household preparation of chitterlings. *N Engl J Med* 322, 984–987.

Low, J.C., McKendrick, I.J., McKechnie, C., et al. (2005). Rectal carriage of enterohemorrhagic Escherichia coli O157 in slaughtered cattle. *Appl Environ Microbiol* 71, 93–97.

Lowther, S.A., Medus, C., Scheftel, J., Leano, F., Jawahir, S., and Smith, K. (2011). Foodborne outbreak of Salmonella subspecies IV infections associated with contamination from bearded dragons. *Zoonoses Public Hlth* 58, 560–566.

Melotto, M., Underwood, W., Koczan, J., Nomura, K., and He, S.Y. (2006). Plant stomata function in innate immunity against bacterial invasion. *Cell* 126, 969–980.

Melotto, M., Panchal, S., and Roy, D. (2014). Plant innate immunity against human bacterial pathogens. *Front Microbiol* 5, 411.

Meric, G., Kemsley, E.K., Falush, D., Saggers, E.J, and Lucchini, S. (2013). Phylogenetic distribution of traits associated with plant colonization in Escherichia coli. *Environ Microbiol* 15, 487–501.

Mettee Zarecki, S.L., Bennett, S.D., Hall, J., et al. (2013). US outbreak of human Salmonella infections associated with aquatic frogs, 2008–2011. *Pediatrics* 131, 724–731.

Moffatt, C.R., Musto, J., Pingault, N., et al. (2016). Salmonella typhimurium and outbreaks of egg-associated disease in Australia, 2001 to 2011. *Foodborne Pathog Dis* 13, 379–385.

Mollaret, H.H., Bercovier, H., and Alonso, J.M. (1979). Summary of the data received at the WHO Reference Center for Yersinia enterocolitica. *Contrib Microbiol Immunol* 5, 174–184.

Nelson, J., Smith, K., Vugia, D., et al. (2004). Prolonged diarrhea due to ciprofloxacin-resistant *Campylobacter* infection. *J Infect Dis* 190, 1150–1157.

Nelson, J., Chiller, T., Powers, J., and Angulo, F. (2007). Fluoroquinolone-resistant *Campylobacter* species and the withdrawal of fluoroquinolones from use in poultry; A public health success story. *Clin Infect Dis* 44, 977–980.

O'Sullivan, T., Friendship, R., Blackwell, T., et al. (2011). Microbiological identification and analysis of swine tonsils collected from carcasses at slaughter. *Can J Vet Res* 75, 106–111.

Pacer, R.E., Spika, J.S., Thurmong, M.C., Hargrett-Bean, N., and Potter, M.E. (1989). Prevalence of *Salmonella* and multiple-resistant *Salmonella* in California dairies. *J Am Vet Med Assn* 195, 59–63.

Poppy, G.M., Chiotha, S., Eigenbrod, F., et al. (2014). Food security in a perfect storm: using the ecosystem services framework to increase understanding. *Phil Trans R Soc Lond B Biol Sci* 369, 20120288.

Public Health Agency of Canada (2007). Canadian Integrated Program for Antimicrobial Resistance Surveillance (CIPARS). Available at: http://www.phac-aspc.gc.ca/cipars-picra/index-eng.php (accessed August 10, 2016).

Rodrigue, D.C., Tauxe, R.V., and Rowe, B. (1990). International increase in *Salmonella enteritidis*: A new pandemic? *Epidemiol Infect* 105, 21–27.

Rosenau, M.J. (1926). *Preventative Medicine and Hygiene*, New York: D. Appleton and Co.

Saldana, Z., Sanchez, E., Xicohtencatl-Cortes, J., Puente, J.L., and Giron, J.A. (2011). Surface structures involved in plant stomata and leaf colonization by shiga-toxigenic *Escherichia coli* O157:H7. *Front Microbiol* 2, 119.

Salmon de, S.T. (1885). Report on swine plague. U.S. Bureau of Animal Industry.

Sanders, T.A. (1999). Food production and food safety. *BMJ* 318, 1689–1693.

Scharff, R.L., Besser, J., Sharp, D.J., Jones, T.F., Peter, G.S., and Hedberg, C.W. (2016). An economic evaluation of PulseNet: A network for foodborne disease surveillance. *Am J Prev Med* 50, S66–73.

Sivapalasingam, S., Barrett, E., Kimura, A., et al. (2003). A multistate outbreak of Salmonella enterica Serotype Newport infection linked to mango consumption: impact of water-dip disinfestation technology. *Clin Infect Dis* 37, 1585–1590.

Smith, K., Besser, J., Hedberg, C., et al. (1999). Quinolone-resistant infections of Campylobacter jejuni in Minnesota, 1992–1998. *N Engl J Med* 340, 1525–1532.

Spika, J.S., Waterman, S.H., Hoo, G.W., et al. (1987). Chloramphenicol-resistant Salmonella newport traced through hamburger to dairy farms. A major persisting source of human salmonellosis in California. *N Engl J Med* 316, 565–570.

Steele, M. and Odumeru, J. (2004). Irrigation water as source of foodborne pathogens on fruit and vegetables. *J Food Prot* 67, 2839–2849.

Su, L., Teng, W., Chen, C., et al. (2011). Increasing ceftriaxone resistance in *Salmonella*, Taiwan. *Emerg Infect Dis* 17, 1086–1090.

Su, L.H., Wu, T.L. and Chiu, C.H. (2014). Decline of Salmonella enterica serotype Choleraesuis infections, Taiwan. *Emerg Infect Dis* 20, 715–716.

Swaminathan, B., Barrett, T.J., Hunter, S.B., Tauxe, R.V. and CDC PulseNet TAsk Force (2001). PulseNet: the molecular subtyping network for foodborne bacterial disease surveillance, United States. *Emerg Infect Dis* 7, 382–389.

Swaminathan, B., Gerner-Smidt, P., Ng, L.K., et al. (2006). Building PulseNet International: an interconnected system of laboratory networks to facilitate timely public health recognition and response to foodborne disease outbreaks and emerging foodborne diseases. *Foodborne Pathog Dis* 3, 36–50.

Tanner, C. (1997). Principles of Australian quarantine. *Aust J Agr Resour Econ* 41, 541–558.

Tauxe, R. and Esteban, E. (2006). Advances in food safety to prevent foodborne diseases in the United States. In: Ward, J. and Warren, C. (eds), *Silent Victories: The History and Practice of Public health in Twentieth-Century America*. Oxford: Oxford University Press, chapter 2.

Tauxe, R. V., Vandepitte, J., Wauters, G., et al. (1987). Yersinia enterocolitica infections and pork: the missing link. *Lancet* i, 1129–1132.

Tauxe, R.V., Doyle, M.P., Kuchenmuller, T., Schlundt, J., and Stein, C.E. (2010). Evolving public health approaches to the global challenge of foodborne infections. *Int J Food Microbiol* 139(Suppl. 1), S16–28.

Tritscher, A., Miyagishima, K., Nishida, C., and Branca, F. (2013). Ensuring food safety and nutrition security to protect consumer health: 50 years of the Codex Alimentarius Commission. *Bull World Health Org* 91, 468–8A.

Uchtmann, N., Herrmann, J.A., Hahn, E.C., and Beasley, V.R. (2015). Barriers to, efforts in, and optimization of integrated One Health surveillance: A review and synthesis. *Ecohealth* 12, 368–384.

van Ermengem, E. (1897). Ueber einen neuen anaeroben Bacillus und seine Beziehungen zum Botulismus. *Zeitschrift fur den Hygiene und Infektionskrankheiten* 26, 1–56.

Watanabe, T. (1963). Infective heredity of multiple drug resistance in bacteria. *Bacteriol Rev* 27, 87–115.

Wesley, I.V., Bhaduri, S., and Bush, E. (2008). Prevalence of Yersinia enterocolitica in market weight hogs in the United States. *J Food Prot* 71, 1162–1168.

Wright, A.P., Richardson, L., Mahon, B.E., Rothenberg, R., and Cole, D.J. (2016). The rise and decline in Salmonella enterica serovar Enteritidis outbreaks attributed to egg-containing foods in the United States, 1973-2009. *Epidemiol Infect* 144(4), 810–819.

Yan, J., Ko, W., Chiu, C., Tsai, S., Wu, H., and Wu, J. (2003). Emergence of ceftriaxone-resistant Salmonella isolates and rapid spread of plasmid-encoded CMY-2-like cephalosporinase, Taiwan. *Emerg Infect Dis* 9, 323–328.

Zdolec, N., Dobranic, V.., and Filipovic, I. (2015). Prevalence of Salmonella spp. and Yersinia enterocolitica in/on tonsils and mandibular lymph nodes of slaughtered pigs. *Folia Microbiol (Praha)* 60, 131–135.

4

Water Security in a Changing World

Jeffrey M. Levengood[1], Ari Hörman[2], Marja-Liisa Hänninen[2], and Kevin O'Brien[1]

[1] University of Illinois at Urbana-Champaign, Urbana, IL, USA
[2] University of Helsinki, Helsinki, Finland

4.1 Introduction

Water is at the core of sustainable development
The Future We Want, Rio + 20
United Nations Conference on
Sustainable Development

The global human population, currently estimated at 7.3 billion, is expected to increase by 33% to 9.7 billion by 2050. Under present conditions and policies, this is projected to require a 60% concomitant increase in agricultural production and 15% increased demand for water to meet the food needs of a projected world population of 9 billion people (World Bank, 2017). And the United Nations (UN) has estimated that, under current practices, the global water demand in developing nations alone will have increased by 400% by 2050 (United Nations World Water Assessment Programme, 2015). Combined with rising gross domestic product (GDP) in virtually all nations, which leads to increased demand for electricity, these increasing needs for water come at a time when long-term droughts are having impacts in highly (e.g., southwestern USA, western Canada), moderately (e.g., Brazil, Columbia), and less-developed (e.g., Malawi) nations alike. Global climate change adds additional uncertainly to the future regional availability of water. Often, poor policies and lack of regulations promoting water conservation lead to wasteful use, exacerbating droughts caused by natural phenomena and disproportionately affecting the poor and disenfranchised.

Herein we address two aspects of water security: water quality and water quantity. Recent decades have seen increased access to safe drinking water. By 2010, 89% of the global population were using potable water, which was an increase in over two billion people in the previous 20 years. Still, nearly one billion people lack access to sufficient quantities of safe water for drinking, food preparation, and hygiene. The UN Committee on Economic, Social and Cultural Rights, through the adoption of General Comment No. 15 (United Nations, 2002), recognized the human right to water, further defined as "the right to sufficient, safe, acceptable and physically accessible and affordable water for personal and domestic uses." More recently, the UN General Assembly, through adoption of Resolution 64/292, recognized the human right to clean drinking water and sanitation (United Nations, 2010). Access to safe water goes hand in hand with proper sanitation and treatment, which is lacking in some regions.

Beyond One Health: From Recognition to Results, First Edition.
Edited by John A. Herrmann and Yvette J. Johnson-Walker.

As we will show, exposure to water contaminated with pathogens and toxicants is not limited to underdeveloped nations.

Sustainable population and economic growth into the future will require that industry, energy, and agriculture make smarter use of a smaller share of finite water resources. We examine the water/energy/food nexus and discuss how improvements in efficiency and waste reduction are needed on both ends of the supply chain. Ensuring the sustainability of global water resources will require multidisciplinary consideration of region-specific needs, resources, and limitations in the production of energy and food.

4.2 Waterborne Pathogens and Contaminants: Technologies for Drinking Water Treatment and Management of Water Safety

Safe drinking water, which is free from harmful microorganisms and substances, is essential for public health and linked with adequate sanitation. At the global level, the access to safe drinking water has improved remarkably during the last 25 years and now more than 91% of the world's population has access to safe drinking water (http://www.who.int/wsportal/casestudies/en/). This improvement has also contributed to the 50% decrease in deaths due to communicable diseases of children younger than 5 years of age during the 15 last years. However, at the same time the target level set for sanitation improvement by the UN's Millennium Development Goals (MDGs) has not been met (United Nations, 2015). One-third (2.4 billion) of the world's population is still without proper sanitation, and more than 900 million do not have access to designated toilets or latrines (http://www.who.int/wsportal/casestudies/en/).

Despite many positive achievements, people still get ill and die because of unsafe drinking water, primarily in developing countries, but also in countries having organized and controlled drinking water supplies and sanitation systems. Unsafe drinking water is still an important single source of gastroenteric diseases, mainly due to fecally contaminated raw water, failures in water treatment processes, or recontamination of treated drinking water (Medema et al., 2003; WHO, 2011). It has been estimated that, across the globe, 842 000 deaths every year are attributable to unsafe water supply and poor sanitation and hygiene. The World Health Organization (WHO) has estimated that a total of 3.5% of all disability-adjusted life years (DALYs) are caused by unsafe drinking water and water-related diarrheal diseases.

A significant portion of the water-related disease burden, primarily vector-borne diseases, is attributable to the problems in management and use of water resources. Additionally, many water sources are also used for leisure and recreational activities, agriculture, and food production, which can be microbiologically or chemically contaminated and pose health risks through those endeavours (Cabelli et al., 1982; van Asperen et al., 1998; Schönberg-Norio et al., 2004). Access to safe water, sanitation, and hygiene is also critical in the prevention and management of 16 out of the 17 neglected tropical diseases, including trachoma, soil-transmitted helminths, and schistosomiasis. These diseases affect more than 1.5 billion people in 149 countries, causing blindness, disfigurement, permanent disability, and death. The One Health approach – the recognition that human, animal, and ecosystem health are inextricably linked – combines expertise in public health, human and veterinary medicine, and drinking water management and provides a strong network for reaching the goal of safe drinking water (Courtenay et al., 2015).

4.2.1 Waterborne Pathogens

Surface water sources (e.g., lakes and rivers) are often contaminated microbiologically by treated or untreated sewage water or fecal discharges of domestic or wild animals, often exacerbated by extreme weather conditions, like heavy rains or floods. *Ground water* sources (e.g., wells, borehole wells) are usually of good microbiological quality. However, ground water can also become contaminated, either by surface water containing animal or human fecal material after heavy rain or snow melt, or by sewage leakages, and become the source of community-based outbreaks, especially if improper or no disinfection treatment has been applied (WHO, 2011).

The most important waterborne microbial pathogens include:

- bacteria (e.g., *Campylobacter* spp., *Escherichia coli*, *Salmonella* spp., *Shigella* spp., *Vibrio cholerae*, and *Yersinia enterocolitica*);
- viruses (adenoviruses, enteroviruses, hepatitis A, hepatitis E, noroviruses, sapoviruses, and rotaviruses); and
- protozoa (*Cryptosporidium parvum*, *Dracunculus medinensis*, *Cyclospora cayetanensis*, *Entamoeba histolytica*, *Giardia duodenalis*, and *Toxoplasma gondii*) (WHO, 2011).
- nematodes (*Dracunculus medinensis*).

Selected microbial pathogens and their characteristics are presented in Table 4.1.

In the mid-1800s, large waterborne disease outbreaks in Europe were caused by *V. cholerae*. The famous outbreak investigations done in London in 1854 by John Snow greatly expanded understanding of the epidemiology and prevention of waterborne diseases (Vinten-Johansen et al., 2003). *V. cholerae* is still a significant cause of waterborne infections, especially in developing countries, where most of the victims are often children under 5 years of age (WHO, 2002, 2003; Ashbolt, 2004). In developed regions, such as the northern European countries, the most important waterborne pathogens are noroviruses and *Campylobacter jejuni* (Guzman-Herrador et al., 2015). Noroviruses and several other waterborne viruses have low or extremely low infectious doses to cause gastroenteritis and they are shed in feces in very high numbers even if the infected person remains or becomes asymptomatic.

Viruses do not multiply in the environment but they can persist in water for long periods. Therefore, inadequate disinfection of fecally contaminated drinking water could easily lead to large outbreaks (Gall et al., 2015).

Enteric parasites, such as *Giardia* spp. and *Cryptosporidium* spp., are well recognized as emerging pathogens transmitted through drinking water and being able to cause severe waterborne gastroenteritis, especially in immunocompromised persons (Franzen and Muller, 1999; Szewzyk et al., 2000; Stuart et al., 2003). One of the largest waterborne outbreaks ever seen was caused by *Cryptosporidium parvum* in Milwaukee, USA, in 1993, where 403 000 persons were infected. Also countries such as the UK and Sweden have experienced large *Cryptosporidium*-associated waterborne outbreaks (Chalmers, 2012).

4.2.2 Antibiotic-Resistant Bacteria in Source and Drinking Water

As a result of decades of usage of antibiotics and other antimicrobial agents in human and veterinary medicine, antimicrobial-resistant bacteria and their resistance genes are common and widespread contaminants of raw water. Many enteric bacterial pathogens and fecal bacteria, such as *E. coli.*, *Klebsiella*, and fecal enterococci, carry genes associated with multiple resistances. Currently, special interest is directed to extended-spectrum beta-lactamase producing *Enterobacteriaceae* (ESBL) or carbamase-producing Gram-negative bacteria, which are especially common in countries where antibiotic usage is uncontrolled (Zurfluh et al., 2013; WHO, 2014). In these countries, resistant bacteria are common in sewage water and surface water causing the risk of further spread. However, these bacteria are also detected in surface waters in highly developed countries (Zurfluh et al., 2013) and they are spreading globally by travel, thus posing an increased human health risk worldwide (WHO, 2014). Antibiotic-resistant bacteria, among other bacteria, are destroyed by adequate drinking water treatment (see Table 4.1).

Table 4.1 Selected waterborne pathogens and their characteristics.

Pathogen	Health significance				Examples of reduction by various water treatment technologies	
	Relative infectivity	Persistence in water supply[a]	Important animal source	Resistance to chlorine	Chlorine (time for 2-log/99% reduction using 1 mg/L at pH 7.5, $T=20°C$)	UV (dose for 4-log/99.99% reduction)
Viruses						
Hepatitis A	High	Long	No	Moderate	~16 min	7–186 mJ/cm^2 for all viruses
Hepatitis E	High	Long	Potentially/yes	Moderate		
Polioviruses	High	Long	No	Moderate		
Adenoviruses	High	Long	No	Moderate		
Noroviruses	High	Long	No/potentially	Moderate		
Rotaviruses	High	Long	No	Moderate		
Bacteria						
Campylobacter jejuni	Moderate	Moderate	Yes	Low		0.65–230 mJ/cm^2 for all bacteria
Escherichia coli	Low	Moderate	Yes	Low	<1 min	
E. coli, EHEC	High	Moderate	Yes	Low		
Shigella spp.	High	Short	No	Low		
Vibrio cholerae	Low	Short/Long	No	Low		
Yersinia enterocolitica	Low	Long	Yes	Low		
Protozoa						
Cryptosporidium parvum	High	Long	Yes	High	~9600 min	<1–60 mJ/cm^2 for all protozoa
Entamoeba histolytica	High	Moderate	No	High		
Giardia intestinalis	High	Moderate	Yes	High	~45 min	
Toxoplasma gondii	High	Moderate	Yes	High		
Helminths						
Dracunculus medinensis	High	Moderate	No	Moderate		
Schistosoma spp.	High	Short	Yes	Moderate		

Data based on WHO, 2011.

a) Short means that infective stages have been detected in water at 20 °C for up to a 1-week period, moderate is 1 week to 1 month; and long is over 1 month.

4.2.3 Chemical Hazards in the Drinking Water

A wide array of hazardous toxic compounds can be present in raw source water as well as in drinking water. According to their suspected toxicity, permitted concentrations of chemicals are regulated in national drinking water regulations, which are commonly based on the guideline values evaluated and published by WHO (2011). The toxicants and other chemicals affecting water utility originate from various sources. To develop control measures to decrease their concentrations to acceptable levels, it is necessary to recognize the major sources of contaminants. Chemical contaminants are often grouped according to their origins:

- Naturally occurring in rock or soils characterized by geology (e.g., arsenic, aluminum, uranium, fluorine, iron, and manganese).
- Industrial activities (e.g., organic solvents, benzene, a large group of organic chlorinated compounds, and cadmium).
- Agricultural activities (e.g., nitrates, pesticides, antibiotics and other pharmaceuticals).
- Human activities, such as pharmaceuticals and cosmetics.
- Formation during water treatment, such as disinfection by-products (DBPs) – often organic halogen-containing compounds and residues of coagulation chemicals (aluminum).
- Leakage or dissolution from water storage or distribution materials (e.g., acrylamide, lead).

Some toxins are also produced by microbes, such as microcystins produced by cyanobacterial growth in surface waters.

4.2.4 Pharmaceuticals in Wastewater and Raw Water Sources

Residues of pharmaceuticals and their metabolites have been present in waters for decades but the monitoring for their levels in wastewater, wastewater effluents, and water-bodies has only recently started. These compounds are acknowledged as emerging hazards to ecosystems and human health since they may enter into drinking water from contaminated raw water source (WHO, 2012; Rivera-Utrilla et al., 2013). Pharmaceutical compounds originate from both human usage and agriculture. In addition, through their manufacturing processes pharmaceutical industries release these compounds into wastewaters and the environment. Pharmaceuticals and personal care products, and their metabolites, are also excreted by people or by domesticated animals through feces and urine into wastewater or directly into the environment. Recent advances in sensitive analytical techniques have ensured detection of trace concentrations (usually present in nanograms per liter) of these chemicals and their transformation products (Riviera-Utrilla et al., 2013). However, there are limited data available on the occurrence and concentrations of these compounds in drinking water (WHO, 2012) and even full-scale wastewater treatment systems do not have the capacity to remove these residues. Their significance for ecosystem and human health is largely unknown and more research is warranted. Discussion for the need and feasibility for regulation of pharmaceutical compound has started in international organizations and in national authorities (WHO, 2012).

4.2.5 Water Treatment Methods

The general purpose of drinking water treatment is to make it safe (potable) by removing or inactivating the pathogenic organisms, their toxins and other hazardous chemicals entirely or to a level that causes no harmful effects (Backer, 2002). *Disinfection* is a process in which harmful microbes are inactivated, chemically or physically, while *purification* refers to removal of harmful substances from drinking water. The aim of water treatment is also to remove unwanted odor, taste, and color and to make water physically and chemically fit for distribution and use (e.g., hardness and pH).

The multiple barrier approach is essential in water treatment, since only in exceptional cases is a single treatment step capable of removing or inactivating all different types of pathogenic microbes or toxins (Stanfield et al., 2003; LeChevallier and Au, 2004). In practice, the multiple barrier concept means a combination of two or more different treatment methods to minimize the possibility that harmful microbes or toxins will enter the drinking water through ineffectiveness or failure in some treatment stages (WHO, 2011). Traditionally, a large-scale water treatment process includes pre-treatment steps using various filter methods and storage, followed by coagulation, flocculation, and sedimentation of impurities, continued by final filtration, and ending with chemical or UV disinfection. Some of the treatment techniques are described below in more detail. The choice of methods will depend on the source water quality, the cost of the treatment process, and the quality and safety standards for the processed water.

4.2.5.1 Thermal Treatment

Thermal treatment, that is, letting the water (rolling) boil at 100 °C for some minutes, is the oldest means of killing microbes and is a simple way to treat smaller amounts of water under field and emergency conditions (Backer, 2002). The "boil water" advice is also a common practice when contaminated drinking water is suspected to cause an acute waterborne outbreak in a community. At 100 °C, all pathogenic vegetative bacteria, protozoa, and viruses are destroyed; only microbial spores, for example, spores of *Clostridium* and *Bacillus*, and heat-resistant toxins, such as some cyanobacterial toxins, survive or maintain their toxicity (Backer, 2002). *Distillation* is a method for producing pure (deionized) water through boiling and then condensing the steam in a clean container; the temperature of boiling water is also effective against microbes and heat-sensitive toxins. *Vacuum distillation* is a method

for distilling the water under negative pressure (and therefore a temperature lower than 100 °C is needed). This method is used to produce drinking water from seawater but due to the low temperature it may not be effective against pathogenic microbes (Al-Kharabshed and YogiGoswami, 2003).

4.2.5.2 Chemical Disinfection

Chemical disinfection of drinking water includes the use of chlorine, iodine, silver, or ozone. The efficiency of chemical treatment is a function of dose, contact time, temperature, and pH (Stanfield *et al.* 2003). The efficiency is described usually by the concentration time (CT) concept, which is a product of the residual chemical concentration and the contact time (Stanfield et al., 2003). The efficiency of all chemicals is reduced by organic material such as humic substances in water. A proportion of the added chemical is bound to the organic material (so-called chemical demand) and cannot act against microbes; only the free residual chemical is effective in microbial inactivation. All chemicals are most effective at moderate temperature (15–20 °C) and at a pH of 6–9 (Backer, 2002). In addition to their antimicrobial effect, certain chemicals, especially ozone, can act as strong oxidants and also oxidize and remove harmful chemicals from drinking water.

Chlorination is the oldest and most commonly used disinfection method in both the developed and developing world (Stanfield et al., 2003; WHO, 2011). It is used as compressed elemental gas, sodium hypochlorite solution (NaOCl), or solid calcium hypochlorite ($Ca(OCl)_2$. It is relatively simple to use as hypochlorite solution also in emergence situations. However, chlorines are also highly toxic and their use requires that personnel should know and follow the handling and safety instructions.

In general, chlorination is effective against bacteria and viruses but less effective or even ineffective against protozoa and algae at the concentrations normally used in drinking water, typically 0.5–1 mg/L (parts per million, ppm) of free residual chlorine (Table 4.1). So-called *shock chlorination* can be done using high doses of chlorine (e.g., 10–50 mg/L) for disinfecting drinking water pipelines or storage tanks. Chlorine combined with amine (chloramine) ensures protection against recontamination of treated drinking water under storage and distribution. Chlorine can react with organic material, especially with humus in the water, and mutagenic (carcinogenic) by-products can be formed. However, the antimicrobial benefits of the chlorination have been estimated to exceed the negative health effects, namely, production of DBPs (Ashbolt, 2004). The formation of by-products can be minimized by removing organic material (humus) before chlorination and controlling the chlorine concentrations used (WHO, 2011).

Iodine can also be used as a water disinfection chemical and its performance is mainly similar to chlorine (Backer and Hollowell, 2000; Goodyer and Behrens, 2000). The *silver* ion has some bactericidal effects, but the use of silver ion products is better suited for preserving previously treated water (Backer, 2002). The silver ion is also used in many filtering devices as an antimicrobial coating (Backer, 1995).

Ozone is a powerful oxidant and effective against bacteria, viruses, and even protozoa. In addition to microbes, ozonation is also effective against cyanobacterial toxins, such as microcystins (Hoeger et al., 2002; LeChevallier and Au, 2004). Ozonation may produce bromate as a harmful by-product (WHO, 2011).

4.2.5.3 Filtration

Filtration is a physical method to remove organisms and other particulate matter from drinking water based on particle and sieve size (Figure 4.1). Particle (also referred to as granular or sand media) filtration is a widely used drinking water treatment, usually combined with coagulation, using organic (e.g., polyamine) or inorganic (e.g., alum) compounds, flocculation using anionic or cationic compounds, and sedimentation. For primitive conditions, a simple sand filter can be easily constructed, for example, from a bucket and fine-grained,

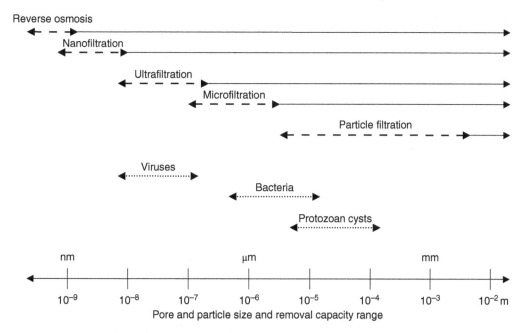

Figure 4.1 Pore size (dashed lines) and range of removal capacity (solid lines) of various filtration methods and general size range of microbial particles (dotted lines).

heated and washed sand. Primitive filters can also be constructed, for example, from used woven and multilayered fabrics.

In addition to particle granular media, filtration media can be made of ceramics or special membranes. A smaller pore size and thus removal of smaller particles can be achieved by ultra- or nanofiltration and reverse osmosis (RO) technology. The RO technique is also effective for removal of monovalent ions and organic compounds of molecular weight greater than 50 (WHO, 2011). RO is the most commonly used technique for desalination of seawater.

4.2.5.4 Other Treatment Methods

Ultraviolet (UV) radiation, especially in the UV-A and UV-B bands, is effective against microorganisms; the optimal wavelength is approximately 265 nm (LeChevallier and Au, 2004). The permeability of UV radiation is reduced by, for example, organic and cloudy material and humus in water (LeChevallier and Au, 2004). Under primitive conditions solar UV radiation can be utilized for drinking water treatment, for example, by exposing the water bottles to direct sunlight for some hours (McGuigan et al., 1998).

Activated carbon is used, for example, in water filters, usually in either powdered or granular form (WHO, 2011). Activated carbon absorbs taste and odor compounds, cyanobacterial toxins, and other organic chemicals (WHO 2011). Removal of microbes is only minimal and occurs through adhesion of the microbes on the surface of activated carbon particles (Backer, 1995).

Electrochemical technologies have been investigated for the removal of organic and inorganic contaminants. Key challenges facing these technologies are related to formation of toxic by-products (e.g., perchlorate and halogenated organic compounds). Technologies may be promising but the mechanisms involved in the oxidation of organic compounds and the corresponding environmental impacts have not been fully addressed (Chaplin, 2014).

Ion-exchange techniques are based on the charge exchange between the water phase and the solid resin phase. These techniques can be used to reduce the hardness and remove contaminants such as nitrate, fluoride, arsenic, selenium, and uranium (WHO, 2011).

4.2.6 Surveillance for Waterborne Diseases

Surveillance of waterborne diseases and outbreak investigation is usually the responsibility of the local, state, regional, or national public health authorities. A successful investigation requires close collaboration between public health, medical, and environmental authorities together with laboratory, veterinary medical, and water treatment plant management expertise applying the One Health concept.

The WHO defines a waterborne outbreak as an episode in which two or more persons experience a similar illness after ingestion of the water from the same source and when the epidemiologic and laboratory evidence implicates the water as the source of the illness (WHO, 2011). The main concern of water safety is focused on the acute illnesses that are typically caused by pathogenic microbes. However, chemical toxicants may also cause acute illnesses (intoxications), for example, after chemical accidents or industrial releases. But, more typically, they cause chronic diseases like cancers after prolonged exposure to elevated concentrations. Based on the strength of the epidemiologic and laboratory findings, the source of the outbreak can be classified as suspected or confirmed. A sufficient number and volume of samples collected from the suspected drinking water at *the early stages of investigation* are essential to catch the possible cause and prove the connection between the exposure and the outbreak (Hunter et al., 2003).

4.2.7 Requirements for Drinking Water Quality

The WHO has established revised guidelines for drinking water quality that can be applied to national standards and legislation, taking into account the national climatic, geographic, socioeconomic, and infrastructural characteristics, as well as national health-based targets (WHO, 2011). In general, water intended for human consumption "must be free from any micro-organisms and parasites and from any substances which, in numbers or concentrations, constitute a potential danger to human health" at the point of compliance (Council of the European Union, 1998).

Since the analysis of all possible enteropathogens can be laborious and require special analytical techniques, several indicator organisms have been proposed, among the earliest being *E. coli* (Ashbolt et al., 2001), which is abundant in human and animal feces. Total coliform and *E. coli* counts are used worldwide as indicators for fecal contamination of drinking and recreational bathing water (Edberg et al., 2000; Havelaar et al., 2001; Rompre et al., 2002; Scott et al., 2002). A microbiological criterion for drinking water hygiene used commonly worldwide requires that *E. coli* or fecal enterococci should not be detected in a 100-mL water sample. Requirements for sampling and limits for tolerated concentrations of various chemical toxicants are given in international or national regulations and are based on the national risk assessment and WHO guidelines (WHO, 2011).

4.2.8 Water Safety Plans (WSPs)

The purpose of drinking water treatment and drinking water hygiene is to minimize the adverse health effects for the consumer, although in practice it is impossible to reduce the risks to zero under all circumstances (Hunter and Fewtrell, 2001). The acceptability of risk is dependent on the given population, circumstances, and time; a risk accepted in a community is not necessarily accepted in another community.

In 2004 the WHO introduced the Water Safety Plans (WSP) approach for ensuring safe drinking water supply. The WSPs draw on many of the principles and concepts from other risk management approaches, in particular from the multi-barrier concept and from the Hazard Analysis of Critical Control Points (HACCP) approach. The WSP should

be developed and implemented for individual drinking water supply systems by using a comprehensive risk assessment and risk management approach that includes all steps in the water supply from catchment to consumer (Figure 4.2) (WHO, 2011). The WSP strategy has recently been adopted as a regulatory requirement in many countries.

Water Safety Plans combined with Quantitative Microbiological Risk Analysis (QMRA) will help drinking water producers and public health authorities set and manage health-based targets for drinking water. Only a few countries, among them The Netherlands and the USA, have set quantitative guideline values for the acceptable annual risk. In The Netherlands, health regulators have set requirements for drinking water companies such that the annual risk for water-associated gastrointestinal illness is less than one person affected per 10 000, 95% of the time (Smeets et al., 2009, 2010; Schijven et al., 2011). The US Environmental Protection Agency (USEPA) has introduced a health-based target in which less than one new infection per 10 000 persons should occur annually, using *Giardia* as a reference organism (Macler and Regli, 1993). The logic behind this requirement is that *Giardia* is more resistant to drinking water disinfection than other microbial pathogens. The requirement is based on the numbers of annually reported cases of giardiasis in the USA at present.

Even though the WSP concept was implemented more than 10 years ago, only limited scientific evidence is available on its impact in improving water safety and health (Dyck et al., 2007; Mudaliar, 2012). In Iceland, a WSP was adopted into legislation in 1995. Recent Icelandic surveillance data showed that both the microbiological quality of tap water was improved (heterotrophic counts < 10 CFU/mL) and the incidence of diarrhea in the population was decreased significantly (Gunnarsdottir, 2012), thus demonstrating the positive impact of an implemented WSP.

The WSP concept can be implemented in all water treatment systems, both large and

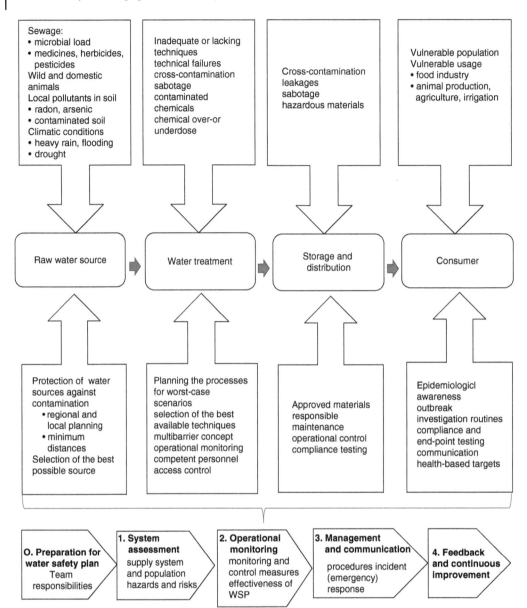

Figure 4.2 Schematic illustration of the water supply system from raw water source to water consumer (in the middle) combined with the hazards and risk factors (arrow boxes downwards) and risk management options (arrow boxes upwards). Hazards and risk factors may have direct or indirect impacts on drinking water safety and increase the risk consequences and severity. Risk management includes actions that intend to reduce and manage the hazards and risk factors. Steps 0–4 of the Water Safety Plan (WSP) represent fundamental parts of the WSP taking into account the whole water supply system from the raw water to the water consumer.

small, and in developed and developing regions, since it is based on the local infrastructure, socioeconomic and environmental conditions, and on nationally decided health-based targets (WHO, 2011). However,

the development and adoption of the WSP system may require education, improved knowledge of the water supply system, and improved cooperation between different stakeholders and experts. Furthermore, technical and financial resources are required to improve the treatment and distribution infrastructure, even in developed regions. Designing and ensuring a safe drinking water supply system is a multi- and interdisciplinary challenge, where close collaboration and cooperation between veterinary, public health, and medical professionals, together with experts on security and quality, water engineering and communication, is essential (Rose, 2002; IWA, 2004; Meinhardt, 2005; Courtenay et al., 2015).

4.3 The Water/Energy/ Food Nexus: Mitigating Global Risks

Water is vital not only for human consumption, but also for agricultural production, electricity generation, and manufacturing. The accelerated global population increase in the past century combined with the acceleration of gross domestic product (GDP) growth (especially in developing nations) has placed significant stress on global water supplies. This discussion surrounding the water/energy/food nexus attempts to highlight these stresses in an effort to mitigate the risks associated with stressed global water supplies. Ignoring these risks can have catastrophic consequences from both social and economic perspectives.

There are a number of challenges that hamper the ability to mitigate threats to this nexus on a global scale. These challenges are due to myriad factors, including the characteristics of the global economy combined with the need for different solutions for different regions, depending on the nature of the challenges specific to those regions. For example, many manufacturing processes are being shifted to developing nations due to their lower labor costs. These processes can stress existing water supplies, thus diverting water from agricultural uses. Agriculture in many regions utilizes large quantities of water: as much as 90% of the water usage in

some Gulf Cooperation Council (GCC) countries is for agriculture (Dziuban, 2011). Water is also vital in most areas of the world for the production of electricity.

Water issues can cross boundaries and regions across the globe. For example, the Middle East has 5% of the world's population, but only 1% of the world's renewable water resources. Per capita availability of water is the lowest, rates of withdrawal already the highest, and more water storage has been installed than in any other region of the world (Granit, 2010). On the other hand, the state of Illinois would seem to have abundant water sources (e.g., it is bordered by one of the Great Lakes and the Mississippi River). However, despite its location and typical climate, Illinois has been susceptible to drought (Figure 4.3; Illinois State Water Survey, 2015). In some other areas, especially the western states of the USA, the issue is related to groundwater recharge rates for aquifers (Meixner et al., 2016). Average declines of 10–20% are expected across the southern High Plains aquifers (Figure 4.4; Meixner et al., 2016).

4.3.1 Water/Energy Nexus

Before we examine the water/energy nexus, it is important to recognize that there is a direct relationship between electrical energy consumption and GDP. This energy-GDP nexus has been recognized by a number of authors for a variety of countries. Mohanty and Chaturvedi (2015) provided clear evidence of this nexus in the growth of the Indian economy (Figure 4.5). The results from this study clearly demonstrated that electrical energy leads economic growth, that is, increase in GDP, and that growth in economies leads to increased electricity consumption (Figure 4.6). However, this relationship is changing over time for more developed nations such as the USA (USEIA, 2013). It is projected that by 2040 growth in electricity consumption (0.9%) will be less than half the growth in GDP (2.4%). This projection reflects a change as compared to

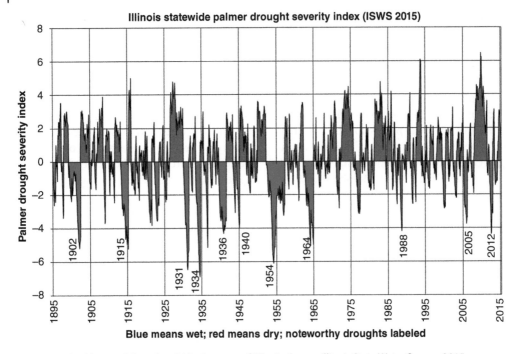

Figure 4.3 Incidence of drought within the state of Illinois. *Source:* Illinois State Water Survey, 2015. Reproduced with permission of Dr Jim Angel.

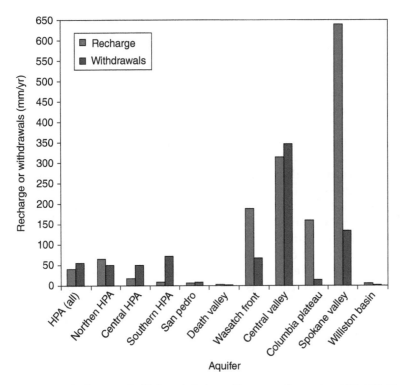

Figure 4.4 Recharge and withdrawals from aquifers across the western USA. HPA, High Plains aquifers. *Source:* Meixner et al., 2016. Reproduced with permission of Elsevier.

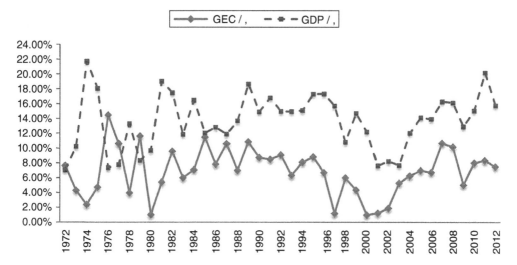

Figure 4.5 Annual growth in electricity consumption (GEC) and nominal gross domestic product (GDP) for India. *Source:* Mohanty and Chaturvedi, 2015. Reproduced with permission of Dr Asit Mohanty.

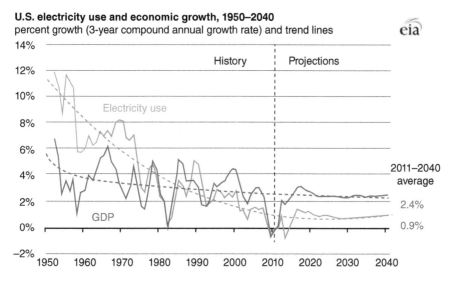

Figure 4.6 Relationship between energy consumption and gross domestic product (GDP) for the USA. *Source:* USEIA, 2013.

the time frame prior to 1975 when growth in electricity consumption outpaced GDP, and between 1975 and 1995 when the growth rate for these factors were nearly identical. This change for the USA is attributed to a number of factors including aggressive energy efficiency policy and investments along with shifts toward less energy-intensive industries.

Now let us bring water into the energy equation. A prominent component of this nexus is the amount of water required for electricity generation. Large quantities of water are typically withdrawn from the environment in traditional methods to generate electricity. *Withdrawal* is defined as water removed from the ground or diverted from a surface-water source for use (Kenny et al., 2009). This water is typically used as a heat-exchanging medium. In other words, it is used to absorb waste heat and is then discharged back into the environment. *Consumption* of water for these applications is defined as water that has been withdrawn and is not returned to the environment after use. This consumption could be due to evaporation, process loss, and so forth (Faeth and Sovacool, 2014).

Faeth and Sovacool (2014) compared water consumption (m^3) per megawatt hour (MWh) of electricity produced from a variety of sources (Table 4.2). Using renewable energy sources in place of nuclear, coal, and natural gas to generate electricity significantly reduces the amount of water required for electricity generation. Nuclear generation of electricity both withdraws and consumes the greatest amount of water. Coal and natural gas generation of electricity both withdraw orders of magnitude more water than solar photovoltaic (PV) and wind. Water consumption for coal and natural gas is approximately the same and is four times greater than solar PV, while wind is exponentially less as water consumption is negligible (Faeth and Sovacool, 2014; Li et al., 2012). This is a major advantage for renewables and provides a means to reduce the amount of water used in the generation of electricity, thereby reducing risks to food and water security.

The implication of the water/energy nexus can be illustrated by examining trends in the Gulf Cooperation Council (GCC). Electricity needs in the GCC have been growing at a rate of 5–8% per year. Electricity consumption per capita (10 000 kWh/capita) and water consumption per capita ($850\,m^3$/year/capita) within the GCC are exceptionally high (Economist Intelligence Unit, 2010). Based on these facts, it is critical to reduce the amount of water used in the generation of electricity. For example, if approximately 1000 MWh of electricity was produced using renewable energy, the amount of water saved would be equivalent to the amount of water produced by two to three desalination plants! There are a number of projections, based on revising the global portfolio for energy generation, that would significantly impact global risks surrounding the water/energy nexus. It is important to note that water consumption as well as carbon emission reductions should be considered when altering existing electricity generation portfolios. Many of the positive scenarios listed below will require a combination of technological advancements along with policy initiatives.

4.3.1.1 Nuclear

Nuclear power is the largest source of low-carbon electricity generation, yet it suffers from the stigma of such disasters as Chernobyl (1986, Ukraine), Three Mile Island (1979, Pennsylvania, USA), Stationary Low-Power Reactor Number One (1961, Idaho, USA), and more recently the Fukushima Daiichi nuclear power plant accident in 2011 (International Energy Agency and Nuclear Energy Agency, 2015). In addition, the management of the nuclear waste generated from plant operation creates the issue of where, how, and for how long to dispose of the spent fuel rods that are still highly radioactive. Even with its torrid history, nuclear power is expected to account for 17% of global electricity production by 2050 (World Nuclear Association, 2016). Major growth of the nuclear generation market is expected to occur in China, India, the Middle East, and the Russian Federation. Increased research and development (R&D) in nuclear safety, advanced fuel cycles, waste management, and innovative designs are necessary to achieve the projected growth.

As pointed out earlier, another significant issue with nuclear generation of electricity is that, whereas the carbon emissions are low, it is one of the worst in terms of water withdrawal and consumption (Table 4.2). The majority of water used by a nuclear power plant is withdrawn for cooling and about 98% is returned but, due to the large volumes withdrawn, there is still a substantial amount of water consumed. It will be critical to implement technologies that reduce these water consumption and withdrawal requirements. A few examples of water reducing

Table 4.2 Water usage per electricity generation method.

	Withdrawal (m^3/MWh)	Consumption (m^3/MWh)
Nuclear	168	1
Natural gas	43	0.4
Coal	86	0.4
Solar PV	0.1	0.1
Wind	0	0

Source: Faeth and Sovacool, 2014. Reproduced with permission of Paul Faeth.

methods include using reclaimed wastewater for cooling such as the Palo Verde nuclear power station near Phoenix, AR, USA, and dry cooling such as the Bilibino power plant which is above the arctic circle in Russia (International Atomic Energy Agency, 2012).

4.3.1.2 Coal

Currently, coal-based electricity generation is the predominant method globally, and often the cheapest form of energy generation in many regions, because the coal is easy and cheap to mine and burn to create electricity (*The Economist*, 2014). But a global slowdown in coal demand has been observed and is projected to continue due to stringent environmental policies designed to reduce CO_2 emissions (International Energy Agency, 2017). Because electricity generation from coal requires large quantities of water, this trend would decrease global water demand for electricity generation.

There are a number of R&D initiatives underway to deploy High-Efficiency Low-Emission (HELE) technologies to improve the efficiencies of coal plants along with decreasing primary pollutants (e.g., SOx, NOx, etc.) (International Energy Agency, 2012). It will also be necessary to deploy carbon capture and sequestration systems to reduce CO_2 emissions to meet future required levels (International Energy Agency, 2013a). However, another challenge is that many coal-fired plants are old,

inefficient, and beyond their designed lifetimes, in addition to using especially high volumes of water.

4.3.1.3 Natural Gas

Electricity generation through the use of natural gas is displacing coal-based electricity production in certain regions of the globe. Relatively low costs for natural gas have also aided this trend. This trend looks promising from the standpoint of reduced CO_2 emissions from electricity generation, yet it will have a relatively small impact on water usage because both coal and natural gas have similar water consumption. And consideration needs to be given to the broader environmental footprint of natural gas production through hydraulic fracturing or hydrofracking, which can cause problems with water contamination and disposal (Vaidyanathan, 2016; Llewellyn et al., 2015).

4.3.1.4 Renewables

At the same time, due to technological advances, electricity generation from renewables is predicted to rise substantially. Some report that photovoltaic (PV)-based electricity generation could achieve a global share of electricity generation of 16% by 2050 (International Energy Agency, 2014). In fact, combining PV (panels directly convert solar energy to electricity) and solar thermal (solar energy used to create heat to run heat engines to create electricity), solar technologies could become the leading source for electricity even earlier, by 2040 (International Energy Agency, 2014). These scenarios would significantly reduce the stress of electricity generation on water sources, but there are a number of caveats for these scenarios. It is assumed that transitional policy support mechanisms are put in place in some markets to enable PV electricity costs to reach competitive levels with existing technologies. In addition, the variability of solar generation needs to be addressed through a number of means. This requires advances in interconnection to the grid, demand-side response, flexible generation, and energy storage

(Kenny et al., 2009). The proportion of electricity generated from renewable sources has varied widely across European countries, though on the whole it has steadily increased from 2004 through 2014 (Figure 4.7).

Electricity generation by wind is predicted to reach 15–18% by 2050 (International Energy Agency, 2013b). This scenario again would reduce stress on global water sources. The caveats surrounding this scenario are that a significant amount of R&D must be funded to improve design, materials, manufacturing technology, and reliability to optimize performance and reduce uncertainties for plant output (International Energy Agency and Nuclear Energy Agency, 2015). Just as with solar, transitional policy support mechanisms will need to be put in place. The issue of intermittence and changes to grid infrastructure will also need to be addressed in order for wind to reach the levels predicted. It will also be important to adapt wind plant design to cold climates and low-wind velocity sites.

4.3.1.5 Water/Energy Nexus Summary

The challenge of the water/energy nexus becomes apparent when the results from the studies above are compared:

- Electricity consumption drives economic growth. And although for developed nations growth rates of energy consumption might be less than GDP growth, the relationship still exists.
- It is important to have reliable and low-cost electricity in order to drive economic growth. This requirement has hampered the penetration of renewables in certain regions of the globe.
- Water consumption in electricity generation is highly reliant on the means of generation.
- Non-renewable sources for electricity generation tend to consume higher quantities of water than renewable resources.
- Renewable resources have the greatest potential to reduce water usage during electricity generation.

- While the amount of renewable generation capacity has increased worldwide, the majority of generation is still accomplished through use of resources (e.g., coal and nuclear) that require large quantities of water.
- Solutions to the water/energy nexus must include a combination of demand-side reductions, as well as further efforts to drive down the costs for renewable energy sources.

4.3.2 Water/Food Nexus

An example of the water/food nexus and its relationship to regional water supply and demand can be illustrated by again examining trends in the Gulf Corporation Council (GCC). The combination of a growing population and increased food production has resulted in great demands on water supplies in the GCC. For example, Saudi Arabia (KSA) quadrupled its domestic food production during the 1980s and early 1990s with a major focus on wheat production, a grain that relies on heavy use of water resources (World Bank, 2016a; Elhadj, 2014). Much of this production has now been moved outside KSA because of the severe depletion of the ground-water supply (Sfakianakis et al., 2010). The impact of agriculture on water is especially evident by the fact that, within KSA, dairy farms require on average 2300 gallons ($8.7\,m^3$) of water to produce one gallon of milk (Dziuban, 2011).

This example illustrates how water supply and demand can directly impact food production and supply chains. This direct supply-demand relationship is analogous to the one observed for water/energy. Just as regions with low water supplies should consider electricity generation methods that require low water demands (i.e., solar PV and wind), regions with low water supplies should focus on regional food supplies that have low water demands.

Despite these similarities, there are some differences between the water/energy and water/food nexus. Energy efficiency methods

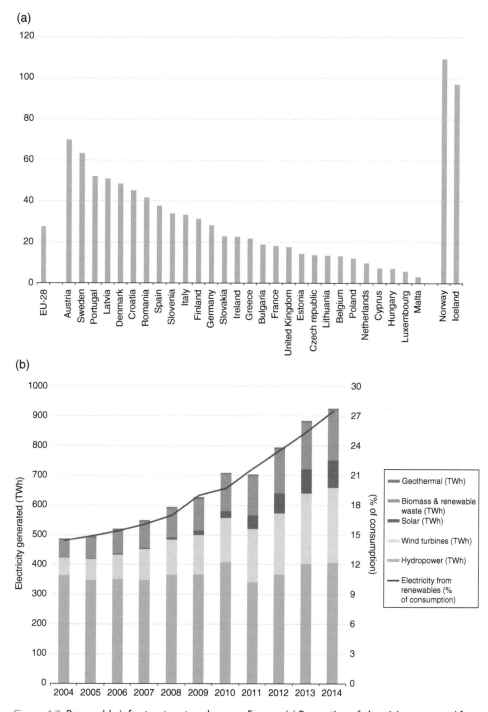

Figure 4.7 Renewable infrastructure trends across Europe. (a) Proportion of electricity generated from renewable sources, 2014 (% of gross electricity consumption). (b) Electricity generated from renewable energy sources, EU-28, 2004–14 YB16. *Source:* Eurostat, 2016.

can reduce water consumption for electricity production, thereby directly reducing water demand. However, the introductions of efficiencies within the food supply chain impacts water in a more indirect fashion. The magnitude of current inefficiencies (or losses) in the food chain can best be understood by considering that "one-third of all food produced for human consumption in the world is lost or wasted" (FAO, 2013a).

The Food and Agriculture Organization (FAO) of the United Nations goes on to say:

The global volume of food wastage is estimated to be 1.6 gigatonnes of "primary product equivalents", while the total wastage for the edible part of food is 1.3 gigatonnes. This amount can be weighed against total agricultural production (for food and non-food uses), which is about 6 gigatonnes. ... The blue water footprint (i.e., the consumption of surface and groundwater resources) of food wastage is about $250\,km^3$, which is equivalent to the annual water discharge of the Volga River, or three times the volume of Lake Geneva.

FAO, 2013a

The FAO defines food wastage as "any food loss due to deterioration or waste" (FAO, 2013a). They explain:

Food loss refers to a decrease in mass (dry matter) or nutritional value (quality) of food that was originally intended for human consumption. These losses are mainly caused by inefficiencies in the food supply chains, such as poor infrastructure and logistics, lack of technology, insufficient skills, knowledge and management capacity of supply chain actors, and lack of access to markets. In addition, natural disasters play a role. Food waste refers to food appropriate for human consumption being discarded, whether or not after it is kept beyond its expiry date or left to spoil. Often this [wastage] is because food has spoiled but it can be for other reasons

such as oversupply due to markets or individual consumer shopping/eating habits.

FAO, 2013a

Food wastage can be divided further into an upstream and a downstream component. Upstream losses occur in the production phase, while downstream losses occur in the consumption phase (FAO, 2013a). It has been shown that food wastage is very dependent on the nature of the local conditions with a region or country. This regional attribute is also complicated by the fact that the source of food wastage (upstream vs downstream) depends on the overall income of the region (FAO, 2013a). For example, developed regions tend to have the greatest wastage downstream, while developing regions tend to have the greatest wastage upstream. The relationships between water and food outlined demonstrate the importance of decreasing food wastage. Reductions in food wastage will reduce the overall blue water footprint reported previously. The specific solutions deployed to reduce wastage and hence reduce the water footprint will vary not only by region, but also by regional income. A number of countries are implementing strategies to combat food waste. For example, in the USA, USEPA is conducting several studies on how to reduce food waste and use food waste as a value-added product (USEPA, 2016). The European Commission's new Circular Economy Package has food waste prevention as an important part (http://ec.europa.eu/food/safety/food_waste/eu_actions/index_en.htm).

The discussions above outline the additional complexities of the water/food nexus as compared to the water/energy nexus. Another consideration for the water/food nexus is not only food wastage but also activities that decrease the *quality* of the water supply. Regions may have sufficient water supply but if that supply is contaminated, it is not usable in the food supply chain unless decontamination procedures are deployed. The challenge is that activities that contaminate the water supply can range from industrial releases to the everyday use of pharmaceuticals and personal care products (PPCPs). These sources represent two extremes and are indicative of the complications of clean-up and management of water supplies.

Another unique aspect of the water/food nexus is that the means to mitigate risks related to water and food can be designed also to impact the water/energy nexus. One example relates to the management of food waste. Nearly 40% of the food produced within the USA is not consumed, but instead becomes food waste (Gunders, 2012). It has been shown that food waste can be collected and used as an input stream to anaerobic digesters (Nazaroff and Alvarez-Cohen, 2001; Smith, 2009). These digesters can be located at wastewater treatment facilities. The net result impacts both water and energy. The food waste is repurposed and used as a feed stock for the anaerobic digester instead of being sent to a landfill. The anaerobic digester produces biogas that is then used as an energy source within the wastewater treatment facility (Fulton, 2014; USEPA, 2016).

4.3.2.1 Water/Food Nexus Summary

The interdependencies of the water/food nexus become obvious when the results from the discussion above are summarised:

- Regional water resources directly influence the type of food production and how long it can be sustained; therefore regions with low water supplies should focus on regional food supplies that have low water needs.
- Good quality water is important for food production.
- Reductions in food wastage will dramatically decrease water consumption.
- Food waste could be used as a value-added product to generate energy without using additional water resources.

4.3.3 Water/Energy/Food Nexus: Summary and Next Steps

The water/energy/food nexus demonstrates the risks associated with climate change on a global basis. Risks, and therefore their

mitigation strategy, will vary based on the specific region of the globe. As indicated previously, regions will modify their electricity generation portfolio based on water considerations as well as CO_2 emission reduction considerations. Food security and resiliency issues will also vary with the specific region of the globe. The challenge with the water/food nexus is the need for not only *quantity* but also *quality* of water. These requirements illustrate why water management will be crucial in driving the economies of the future. The resulting interlinkage between water, food, energy, cities, and the environment motivates the suggestion of defining an "expanded water nexus" to emphasize water dependency (World Bank, 2016b).

Geopolitical events also help to create risks related to this nexus. They demonstrate the need to include resilience factors when examining potential solutions. It is important to start considering solutions that impact *all three components* (water, energy, food). Too often solutions are being pursued that reduce risks around one aspect (e.g., water/energy) but have a neutral or negative impact on the other aspect (e.g., water/food). It also is important to develop solutions that start with "low hanging fruit" approaches, such as efficiency, and then transition to more costly or complex solutions. In the food waste management world, this solution methodology is defined as the food waste pyramid. It suggests starting with *reducing* waste, then exploring *reusing, recycling or recovering*, followed only by the least environmentally friendly solution of *landfill* (FAO, 2013b). It means always starting with *efficiency* improvements that will inherently reduce overall demand.

This approach requires organizations that have the ability to benchmark current resources, estimate their level of resilience, and then understand how climate change, geopolitical events, and other factors can impact the resources. Organizations such as the Prairie Research Institute (PRI; www.prairie.illinois.edu) at the University of Illinois are engaged in this systematic analysis, which enables various scenarios to be examined. Typical activities conducted by PRI and that should be done globally include:

- Tracking weather, water, and soil data such as done by the PRI's Water and Atmospheric Resources Monitoring (WARM) program.
- Water planning.
- Water use and reuse.
- Disaster response scenarios.
- Energy efficiency.
- Alternative energy sources.
- Food wastage reduction and management.

The water/energy/food nexus provides a major challenge at a global scale, yet it must be addressed at a regional level with region-specific solutions. It requires coordination across utility and market sectors that have had limited coordination in the past. Failure to coordinate this effort will not only impact economic growth, but also could ignite civil unrest. As indicated by the World Bank (2016b) in their report: "...water management will be crucial in determining whether the world achieves the Sustainable Development Goals (SDGs) and aspirations for reducing poverty and enhancing shared prosperity."

Acknowledgments

Special thanks to Nancy L. Holm, Elizabeth L. Meschewsk, and Jim Dexter, Illinois Sustainable Technology Center, Prairie Research Institute, University of Illinois at Urbana-Champaign, for their contribution to the manuscript.

References

Al-Kharabshed, S. and YogiGoswami, D. (2003). Analysis of an innovative water desalination system using low-grade solar heat. *Desalination* 156, 323–332.

Ashbolt, N.J. (2004). Microbial contamination of drinking water and disease outcomes in developing regions. *Toxicology* 198, 229–238.

Ashbolt, N.J., Grabow, W.O., and Snozzi, M. (2001). Indicators of microbial water quality. In: Fewtrell, L. and Bartram, J. (eds), *Water Quality: Guidelines, Standards and Health*. London: World Health Organization and IWA Publishing, pp. 289–316.

Asperen van, I.A., Medema, G., Borgdorff, M.W., Sprenger, M.J., and Havelaar, A.H. (1998). Risk of gastroenteritis among triathletes in relation to faecal pollution of fresh waters. *Int J Epidemiol* 27, 309–315.

Backer, H. (1995). Field water disinfection. In: Auerbach, P. (ed.), *Wilderness Medicine*. St Louis, MO: Mosby, pp. 1060–1110.

Backer, H. (2002). Water disinfection for international and wilderness travelers. *Clin Infect Dis* 34, 355–364.

Backer, H. and Hollowell, J. (2000) Use of iodine for water disinfection: iodine toxicity and maximum recommended dose. *Environ Health Perspect* 108, 679–684.

Cabelli, V.J., Dufour, A.P., McCabe, L.J., and Levin, M. A. (1982). Swimming-associated gastroenteritis and water quality. *Am J Epidemiol* 115, 606–616.

Chalmers, R.M. (2012). Waterborne outbreaks of cryptosporidiosis. *Ann Ist Super Sanita* 48, 429–446.

Chaplin, B. (2014). Critical review of electrochemical advanced oxidation processes for water treatment applications. *Environ Sci Processes Impacts* 16, 1182–1203.

Council of the European Union (1998). Council directive on the quality on the water intended for human consumption (98/83/EC). Available at: http://eur-lex.europa.eu/legal-content/EN/TXT/?uri=CELEX:019 98L0083-20151027 (accessed November 20, 2017).

Courtenay, M., Sweeney, J., Zielinska, P, Brown Blake, S., and La Ragione, R. (2015). One

Health: An opportunity for an interprofessional approach to healthcare. *J Interprof Care* 29, 641–642.

Dyck, A., Exner, M., and Kramer, A. (2007) Experimental based experiences with the introduction of a water safety plan for a multi-located university clinic and its efficacy according to WHO recommendations. *BMC Public Health* 7, doi:10.1186/1471-2458-7-34.

Dziuban, M. (2011). Scarcity and Strategy in the GCC. Center for Strategic & International Studies. Available at: https://www.csis.org/analysis/scarcity-and-strategy-gcc (accessed November 20, 2017).

Economist Intelligence Unit (2010). The GCC in 2020: Resources for the future. *The Economist*. Available at: http://graphics.eiu.com/upload/eb/GCC_in_2020_Resources_WEB.pdf (accessed November 20, 2017).

Edberg, S.C., Rice, E.W., Karlin, R.J., and Allen, M.J. (2000). *Escherichia coli*: the best biological drinking water indicator for public health protection. *Symp Ser Soc Appl Microbiol* 29, 106S–116S.

Elhadj, E. (2014). Camels don't fly, deserts don't bloom: an assessment of Saudi Arabia's experiment in desert agriculture. Occasional Paper No. 48. Water Issues Study Group, SOAS/King's College London.

Eurostat (2016). Renewable energy statistics. Available at: http://ec.europa.eu/eurostat/statistics-explained/index.php/Renewable_energy_statistics (accessed December 18, 2017).

Faeth, P. and Sovacool, B.K. (2014). *Capturing Synergies between Water Conservation and Carbon Dioxide Emissions in the Power Sector*. Arlington, VA: CNA Analysis and Solutions.

FAO (Food and Agriculture Organization) (2013a). Food wastage footprint: Impacts on natural resources. FAO.

FAO (Food and Agriculture Organization) (2013b). Toolkit: reducing the food wastage footprint. FAO.

Franzen, C. and Muller, A. (1999). Cryptosporidia and microsporidia—waterborne diseases in the immunocompromised host. *Diagn Microbiol Infect Dis* 34, 245–262.

Fulton, A. (2014). Food Scraps to Fuel Vertical Farming's Rise in Chicago. The Salt. Available at: http://www.npr.org/sections/thesalt/2014/04/09/300620735/food-scraps-to-fuel-vertical-farmings-rise-in-chicago (accessed December 18, 2017).

Gall, A.M., Mariñas, B.J., Lu, Y., and Shisler, J.L. (2015). Waterborne viruses: a barrier to safe drinking water. *PLoS Pathog* 11(6): e1004867.

Goodyer, L. and Behrens, R.H. (2000). Safety of iodine based water sterilization for travelers. *J Travel Med* 7, 38.

Granit, J. (2010). Elaborating on the nexus between energy and water. *J Energy Security* [online]. Available at: http://www.ensec.org/index.php?option=com_content&view=article&id=238:elaborating-on-the-nexus-between-energy-and-water&catid=103:energysecurityissuecontent&Itemid=358 (accessed November 20, 2017).

Gunders, D. (2012). Wasted: how America is losing up to 40 percent of its food from farm to fork to landfill. Natural Resources Defense Council Issue Paper 12-06-B.

Gunnarsdottir, M.J., Gardarsson, S.M., Elliot, M., Sigmundsdottir, G., and Bartram, J. (2012). Benefits of Water Safety Plans: microbiology, compliance, and public health. *Environ Sci Technol* 46, 7782–7789.

Guzman-Herrador, B., Carlander, A., Ethelberg, S., et al. (2015). Waterborne outbreaks in the Nordic countries, 1998 to 2012. *Euro Surveill* 20. Available at: http://www.eurosurveillance.org/ViewArticle.aspx?ArticleId=21160 (accessed November 20, 2017).

Havelaar, A., Blumenthal, U., Strauss, M., Kay, D., and Bartram, J. (2001) Guidelines: the current position. In: Fewtrell, L. and Bartram, J. (eds), *Water Quality: Guidelines, Standards and Health*. London: World Health Organization and IWA Publishing, pp. 17–42.

Hoeger, S.J., Dietrich, D.R., and Hitzfeld, B.C. (2002). Effect of ozonation on the removal of cyanobacterial toxins during drinking water treatment. *Environ Health Perspect* 110, 1127–1132.

Hunter, P. and Fewtrell, L. (2001). Acceptable risk. In: Fewtrell, L. and Bartram, J. (eds), *Water Quality: Guidelines, Standards and Health*. London: World Health Organization and IWA Publishing, pp. 207–228.

Hunter, P., Andersson, Y., von Bonsdorff, C.H., et al. (2003). Surveillance and investigation of contamination incidents and waterborne outbreaks. In: Dufour, A., Snozzi, M., Koster, W., Bartram, J., Ronchi, E., and Fewtrell, L. (eds), *Assessing Microbial Safety of Drinking Water: Improving Approaches and Methods*. London: IWA Publishing, pp. 205–236.

Illinois State Water Survey (ISWS) (2015). Drought Trends in Illinois. Available at: http://www.sws.uiuc.edu/atmos/statecli/climate-change/ildrought.htm (accessed November 21, 2017).

International Atomic Energy Agency (2012). Efficient Water Management in Water Cooled Reactors. IAEA Nuclear Energy Series: No. NP-T-2.6. [Online]. Available: http://www-pub.iaea.org/MTCD/Publications/PDF/P1569_web.pdf (02 February 2018).

International Energy Agency (2012). Technology Roadmap: High-Efficiency, Low-Emissions Coal-Fired Power Generation. Available at: https://www.iea.org/publications/freepublications/publication/technology-roadmap-high-efficiency-low-emissions-coal-fired-power-generation.html (accessed November 21, 2017).

International Energy Agency (2013a). Technology Roadmap: Carbon Capture and Storage. Available at: https://www.iea.org/publications/freepublications/publication/technologyroadmapcarboncaptureandstorage.pdf (accessed November 21, 2017).

International Energy Agency. (2013b) Technology Roadmap: Wind Energy. Available at: https://www.iea.org/publications/freepublications/publication/Wind_2013_Roadmap.pdf (accessed November 21, 2017).

International Energy Agency (2014). Technology Roadmap: Solar Photovoltaic Energy. Available at: https://www.iea.org/publications/freepublications/publication/TechnologyRoadmapSolarPhotovoltaicEnergy_2014edition.pdf (accessed November 21, 2017).

International Energy Agency (2017). World Energy Outlook 2017. Available at: http://www.worldenergyoutlook.org/weo2017/ (accessed November 21, 2017).

International Energy Agency and Nuclear Energy Agency (2015) Technology Roadmap: Nuclear Energy. Available at: https://www.iea.org/media/freepublications/technologyroadmaps/TechnologyRoadmapNuclearEnergy.pdf (accessed November 21, 2017).

IWA (2004). *The Bonn Charter for Safe Drinking Water*. London: International Water Association.

Kenny, J.F., Barber, N.L., Hutson, S.S., Linsey, K.S., Lovelace, J.K., and Maupin, M.A. (2009). Thermoelectric power. In: *Estimated Use of Water in the United States in 2005*. Reston, VA: United States Geological Survey.

Koplin, D.W., Furlong, E.T., Meyer, M.T., et al. (2002). Pharmaceuticals, hormones, and other organic wastewater contaminants in U.S. streams, 1999–2000: A national reconnaissance. *Environ Sci Technol* 36, 1202–1211.

LeChevallier, M.W. and Au, K. (2004). *Water Treatment and Pathogen Control: Process Efficiency in Achieving Safe Drinking Water*. London: IWA Publishing.

Li, X., Hubacek, K., and Siu, Y.L. (2012). Wind power in China—dream or reality? *Energy* 37, 51–60.

Llewellyn, G.T., Dorman, F., Westland, J.L., et al. (2015). Evaluating a groundwater supply contamination incident attributed to Marcellus Shale gas development. *Proc Natl Acad Sci USA* 112(20), 6325–6330.

Loftus, L., Jin, G., Armstrong, S., et al. (2015) Fate of Pharmaceuticals and Personal Care Products in Irrigated Wastewater Effluent. Illinois Sustainable Technology Reports, TR-052.

Macler, B.A. and Regli, S. (1993) Use of microbial risk assessment in setting US drinking water standards. *Int J Food Microbiol* 18, 245–256.

McGuigan, K.G., Joyce, T.M., Conroy, R.M., Gillespie, J.B., and Elmore-Meegan, M. (1998) Solar disinfection of drinking water contained in transparent plastic bottles: characterizing the bacterial inactivation process. *J App. Microbiol* 84, 1138–1148.

Medema, G.J., Payment, P., Dufour, A., et al. (2003). Safe drinking water: An ongoing challenge. In: Dufour, A., Snozzi, M., Koster, W., Bartram, J., Ronchi, E., and Fewtrell, L. (eds), *Assessing Microbial Safety of Drinking Water: Improving Approaches and Methods.* London: IWA Publishing, pp. 11–45.

Meinhardt, P.L. (2005). Water and bioterrorism: preparing for the potential threat to U.S. water supplies and public health. *Annu Rev Public Health* 26, 213–237.

Meixner, T., Manning, A., Stonestrom, D., et al. (2016). Implications of projected climate change for groundwater recharge in the western United States. *J Hydrol* 534, 124–138.

Mohanty, A. and Chaturvedi, D. (2015). Relationship between electricity energy consumption and GDP: evidence from India. *Int J Econ Finance* 7(2), 186–202.

Mudaliar, M.M. (2012). Success of failure: Demonstrating the effectiveness of a Water Safety Plan. *Water Sci Technol* 12, 109–116.

Nazaroff W.W. and Alvarez-Cohen, L. (2001) *Environmental Engineering Science.* Wiley.

Rivera-Utrilla, J., Sánchez-Polo, M., Ferro-García, M., Prados-Joya, G., and Ocampo-Pérez, R. (2013). Pharmaceuticals as emerging contaminants and their removal from water. A review. *Chemosphere* 93, 1258–1287.

Rompre, A., Servais, P., Baudart, J., de Roubin, M.R., and Laurent, P. (2002). Detection and enumeration of coliforms in drinking water: current methods and emerging approaches. *J Microbiol Methods* 49, 31–54.

Rose, J.B. (2002). Water quality security. *Environ Sci Technol* 36, 246–250.

Schijven, J.F., Teunis, P.F., Rutjes, S.A., Bouwknegt, M., and de Roda Husman, A.M.

(2011). QMRAspot: a tool for quantitative microbial risk assessment from surface water to potable water. *Water Res* 45, 5564–5576.

Schönberg-Norio, D., Takkinen, J., Hänninen, M. L., et al. (2004). Swimming and *Campylobacter* infections. *Emerg Infect Dis* 10, 1474–1477.

Scott, T.M., Rose, J.B., Jenkins, T.M., Farrah, S.R., and Lukasik, J. (2002). Microbial source tracking: current methodology and future directions. *Appl Environ Microbiol* 68, 5796–5803.

Sfakianakis, J., Al Hugail, T.A., and Merzaban, D. (2010). Full steam ahead: Saudi power, water sectors occupy centre stage as demand soars. *Saudi Arabia Sector Analysis* March 14.

Smeets, P.W., Medema, G., and van Dijk, J. (2009). The Dutch secret: how to provide safe drinking water without chlorine in the Netherlands. *Drink Water Eng Sci* 2, 1–14.

Smeets, P.W., Rietveld, L.C., van Dijk, J.C., and Medema, G.J. (2010). Practical applications of quantitative microbial risk assessment (QMRA) for water safety plans. *Water Sci Technol* 61, 1561–1568.

Smith, J.E. (2009). State of the science on cogeneration of heat and power from anaerobic digestion of municipal biosolids. United States Environmental Protection Agency. Available at: https://cfpub.epa.gov/si/si_public_record_report.cfm?dirEntryId=212025 (accessed November 21, 2017).

Stanfield, G., LeChevallier, M., and Snozzi, M. (2003). Treatment efficiency. In: Dufour, A., Snozzi, M., Koster, W., Bartram, J., Ronchi, E., and Fewtrell, L. (eds), *Assessing Microbial Safety of Drinking Water: Improving Approaches and Methods.* London: IWA Publishing, pp. 159–178.

Stuart, J.M., Orr, H.J., Warburton, F.G., et al. (2003). Risk factors for sporadic giardiasis: a case-control study in southwestern England. *Emerg Infect Dis* 9, 229–233.

Szewzyk, U., Szewzyk, R., Manz, W., and Schleifer, K.H. (2000). Microbiological safety of drinking water. *Annu Rev Microbiol* 54, 81–127.

The Economist (2014). Coal: The fuel of the future, unfortunately. Available at: http://www.economist.com/news/business/21600987-cheap-ubiquitous-and-flexible-fuel-just-one-problem-fuel-future (accessed December 18, 2017).

United Nations (2002). The right to water. Committee on Economic, Social and Cultural Rights. Twenty-ninth Session, Agenda Item 3. General Comment No. 15. Available at: http://www2.ohchr.org/english/issues/water/docs/CESCR_GC_15.pdf (accessed November 21. 2017).

United Nations (2010). The human right to water and sanitation. Resolution adopted by the General Assembly on 28 July 2010. Sixty-fourth session, Agenda Item 48. A/RES/64/292. Available at: http://www.un.org/es/comun/docs/?symbol=A/RES/64/292&lang=E (accessed November 21, 2017).

United Nations (2015). The Millennium Development Goals. Report 2015. New York: United Nations.

United Nations World Water Assessment Programme (2015). The United Nations World Water Development Report 2015: Water for a Sustainable World. Paris: UNESCO.

USEIA (United States Energy Information Administration) (2013). U.S. economy and electricity demand growth are linked, but relationship is changing. *Today in Energy* March 22. Available at: http://www.eia.gov/todayinenergy/detail.cfm?id=10491 (accessed November 21, 2017).

USEIA (United States Energy Information Administration) (2016). Clean power plan for existing power plants. Available at: https://19january2017snapshot.epa.gov/cleanpowerplan/fact-sheet-overview-clean-power-plan_.html (accessed November 21, 2017).

USEPA (United States Environmental Protection Agency) (2016). Turning Food Waste into Energy at the East Bay Municipal Utility District (EBMUD). Available at: https://www3.epa.gov/region9/waste/features/foodtoenergy/index.html (accessed December 18, 2017).

Vaidyanathan, G. (2016). Fracking can contaminate drinking water. *Scientific American.* Available at: http://www.scientificamerican.com/article/fracking-can-contaminate-drinking-water/ (accessed December 18, 2017).

Vinten-Johansen, P., Brody, H., Paneth, N., Rachman, S., Rip, M., and Zuck, D. (2003). *Cholera, Chloroform, and the Science of Medicine: A Life of John Snow.* Oxford University Press.

WHO (2002). *The World Health Report 2002.* Geneva: World Health Organization.

WHO (2003). *Emerging Issues in Water and Infectious Disease.* Geneva: World Health Organization.

WHO (2011). *Guidelines for Drinking-water Quality*, 4th edn. Geneva: World Health Organization.

WHO (2012). *Pharmaceuticals in Drinking-Water.* Geneva: World Health Organization.

WHO (2014). Briefing Note. Antimicrobial Resistance: An Emerging Water, Sanitation and Hygiene Issue. Available at: http://www.who.int/water_sanitation_health/emerging/AMR_briefing_note.pdf?ua=1 (accessed November 21, 2017).

World Bank (2016a). World Development Indicators. Available at: https://openknowledge.worldbank.org/bitstream/handle/10986/23969/9781464806834.pdf (accessed November 21, 2017).

World Bank (2016b). High and Dry: Climate Change, Water, and the Economy. Washington, DC: International Bank for Reconstruction and Development/The World Bank. Available at: http://www.worldbank.org/en/topic/water/publication/high-and-dry-climate-change-water-and-the-economy (accessed November 21, 2017).

World Bank (2017). Water: Overview. The World Bank IBRD-IDA. Available at: http://

www.worldbank.org/en/topic/water/ overview (accessed November 21, 2017).

World Nuclear Association (2016). World Nuclear Performance Report 2016. Report No. 2016/001. World Nuclear Association.

Zheng, W., Zou, Y., Li, X., and Machesky, M. (2013). Fate of estrogen conjugate 17α-estrodiol-3-sulfate in dairy wastewater: comparison of aerobic and anaerobic degradation and metabolite formation. *J Hazard Mater* 258-259, 109–115.

Zheng, W., Wiles, K., Holm, N., Deppe, N., and Shipley, C. (2014). Uptake, translocation, and accumulation of pharmaceutical and hormone contaminants in vegetables. In: Kyung, M., Satchivi, N.M., and Kingston, C.K. (eds), *Retention, Uptake, and Translocation of Agrochemicals in Plants*. ACS Symposium Series. Washington, DC: American Chemical Society, pp. 167–181.

Zurfluh, K., Hächler, H., Nüesch-Inderbinen, M., and Stephan, R. (2013). Characteristics of extended-spectrum β-lactamase- and carbapenemase-producing *Enterobacteriaceae* Isolates from rivers and lakes in Switzerland. *Appl Environ Microbiol* 79, 3021–3026.

5

One Toxicology, One Health, One Planet

Daniel Hryhorczuk[1], Val R. Beasley[2], Robert H. Poppenga[3], and Timur Durrani[4]

[1] *University of Illinois at Chicago, Chicago, IL, USA*
[2] *The Pennsylvania State University, University Park, PA, USA*
[3] *University of California Davis, School of Veterinary Medicine, Davis, CA, USA*
[4] *University of California at San Francisco School of Medicine, San Francisco, CA, USA*

5.1 Introduction

5.1.1 History

In 1956, a 25-year-old woman in Kumamoto Prefecture, Japan, was noted to have difficulty with balance, numbness of hands and feet, diminished visual fields, abnormal speech, muscle weakness, tremor, abnormal eye movements, and impaired hearing. By 2001, she and 2264 other people had been diagnosed with methylmercury poisoning. The population of the region relied on Minamata Bay as a food source, and consumed contaminated fish or shellfish. The mercury came from a nearby factory that manufactured acetaldehyde and vinyl compounds and dumped their waste into the local bay. Reduced fish populations, uncoordinated and dying birds, and tremors, muscle spasms, unsteady and slow movement, seizures, and deaths in cats were noted before or concurrent with the same signs in humans. The lesions of methylmercury poisoning in cats were also similar to those of humans with "Minamata disease" (Eto, 1997). The Minamata Bay tragedy illustrated how an industrial pollutant can be biomagnified in an aquatic ecosystem from marine microorganisms up the food chain, and how the poisoned fish, predators, and scavengers that ate them should have served as sentinels of this outbreak of environmental illness before the effects were manifest in the human population. Had the animals been monitored, diagnosed, and protected, their suffering and deaths could have been vastly reduced and human illness may have been avoided altogether. Sadly, it took over a decade to recognize the source of this mass poisoning and, only in 2013 did the countries of the world address this global contaminant through a broad-based agreement – the Minamata International Treaty on Mercury.

Six years after the index case of Minamata disease, Rachel Carson described a mythical American town where birds were "silenced" and all life – from apple blossoms to fish to children – were poisoned by the organochlorine insecticide dichlorodiphenyltrichloroethane, also known as DDT. Her book *Silent Spring* (Figure 5.1) was thoroughly researched and supported by 68 pages of cited references, yet it was written in nonscientific terms and had broad appeal to the public (Carson et al., 1962). She described the effects that toxicants such as organochlorine and organophosphorus insecticides were having on the environment and on

Beyond One Health: From Recognition to Results, First Edition.
Edited by John A. Herrmann and Yvette J. Johnson-Walker.
© 2018 John Wiley & Sons, Inc. Published 2018 by John Wiley & Sons, Inc.

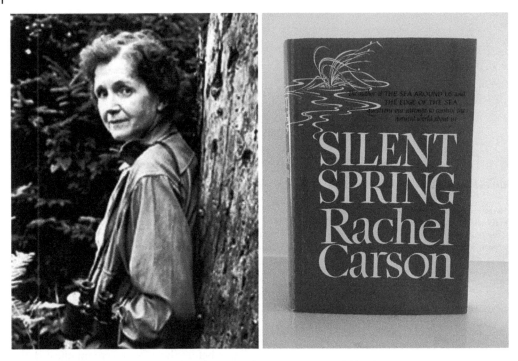

Figure 5.1 Rachel Carson and the jacket of her most famous and impactful book.

human health. Carson's book was controversial at the time of publication, particularly with chemical manufacturers and agricultural industries (Carson, 1962; Epstein, 2014). Even now, the risks and benefits of pesticides are debated. Carson noted, "It is not my contention that chemical insecticides must never be used. I do contend that we have put poisonous and biologically potent chemicals indiscriminately into the hands of persons largely or wholly ignorant of their potentials for harm." In today's world, we have more data about pesticides, but extraordinarily important research gaps remain.

Decades later, in 1991, Theo Colborn convened a meeting at the Wingspread Conference Center of the Johnson Foundation in Racine, Wisconsin, where experts compared overlapping impacts of synthetic chemicals on hormone signaling in wildlife and human populations. The conference and her 1996 book, co-authored by Dianne Dumanoski and John Peterson Myers, entitled *Our Stolen Future: Are We Threatening Our Fertility, Intelligence, and*

Survival? – A Scientific Detective Story (Figure 5.2), triggered concern among the public and expanded research effort in the scientific community. Colborn and co-workers referred to studies of abnormal sperm counts and testicular cancer in Danish men and reproductive abnormalities in alligators in Florida following exposure to high levels of dicofol, an organochlorine miticide chemically similar to DDT. But it was not only DDT and its related analogs that mimic natural hormones, amplifying or blocking their natural effects. Outcomes from exposures to these and many other endocrine disrupting chemicals (EDCs) retarded development of primary and secondary sex characteristics, and altered reproductive, immunological, and thyroid functions. Of particular concern were effects of chemicals on developing offspring, including those that may not fully manifest until later in their lives. This was illustrated by diethylstilbestrol (DES), thought of as a "wonder drug," to stop miscarriage a decade before the publication of Carson's book. Daughters of the mothers

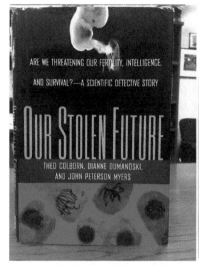 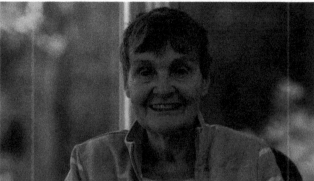

Figure 5.2 Theo Colborn and the jacket of *Our Stolen Future*. Photo by Brook Aitken. Book cover jacket used with permission of Penguin Publishing Group.

who took DES had reproductive tract abnormalities at birth and developed unique reproductive cancers as young women. Sons exposed to DES *in utero* had an increased risk for non-cancerous epididymal cysts (Niculescu, 1985).

At the end of a subsequent three-day Wingspread conference in 1998, Colborn and other scientists, ethicists, attorneys, and activists from the USA, Canada, and Europe articulated the group's consensus that "the release and use of toxic substances, the exploitation of resources, and physical alterations of the environment have had substantial unintended consequences affecting human health and the environment." They proposed that public health actions to protect human health and the environment are necessary even in the face of uncertainty. The "Precautionary Principle" states that "when an activity raises threats of harm to human health or the environment, precautionary measures should be taken even if some cause and effect relationships are not fully established scientifically." (SEHN, 1998; Hayes, 2005). Although Theo Colborn died in 2014 at age 87, her work on endocrine disruption continues with the website that she founded, The Endocrine Disruption Exchange (TEDX),

the Mission of which includes "to reduce or eliminate the production, use, accumulation, and dispersal of endocrine disruptors and other chemicals, which could cause harm to human and ecological health" (https://endocrinedisruption.org/). A subsequent section of this chapter addresses additional aspects of endocrine disruption.

5.1.2 Toxic Chemicals in Our Environment

Thousands of chemicals are produced and disseminated through manufacturing, pharmaceutical use, agriculture (nutrients, pesticides, and drugs), construction, cleaning and maintenance, commerce, transportation, energy generation, and other combustion processes.

Past regulation of chemicals used in the USA has proven to be insufficient to protect human and animal health. An example of shortcomings has been the Toxics Substances Control Act (TSCA), which was passed by the US Congress in 1976 and signed into law by President Gerald Ford. TSCA directed the Environmental Protection Agency (EPA) to regulate chemicals introduced and used in the USA (US Department of Health and

Human Services, 2006). However, with the passage of TSCA, many chemicals already in use were declared safe and not subject to the new regulation. In fact, by 2010, the EPA had required testing of less than 1% of the chemicals in commerce and had banned or restricted a total of nine (NCI, 2010). At the time of this writing, approximately 85 000 or more synthetic chemicals are approved for widespread use in the USA, and more than 600 new chemicals are being approved by the EPA each year (Trasande, 2016). Nevertheless, the EPA has ordered safety testing for only about 250 of the approved chemicals, and only nine have been banned or restricted. Examples of failed regulation are many. Officials lacked legal authority under TSCA to ban asbestos, which has caused lethal mesothelioma in over 107 000 people worldwide annually. The passage of TSCA, in effect, protected the manufacturers of 60 000 chemicals that were already in use from either having them banned or being required to undertake safety testing. Of importance is that TSCA gave the US Environmental Protection Agency little power to require proof of safety for newly manufactured chemicals as part of the review process.

Fortunately, in 2016 the US Congress passed the long-awaited TSCA Reform (the Frank R. Lautenberg Chemical Safety for the 21st Century Act) that addresses many of the deficiencies of the original TSCA Act. The new law 1) mandates safety reviews for large numbers of chemicals already in active commerce; 2) requires a safety finding for new chemicals before they can enter the market; 3) explicitly requires protection of vulnerable populations such as children and pregnant women; and 4) gives EPA enhanced authority to require testing of both new and existing chemicals (https://www.epa.gov/assessing-and-managing-chemicals-under-tsca).

The European Union (EU) took action at an earlier date to address the safety of chemicals already in the marketplace. The EU relies on the REACH Regulation, which draws its name from four processes, **R**egistration, **E**valuation, **A**uthorization, and restriction of **Ch**emicals, to protect human health and the environment. Implementation of REACH began in 2007, and its provisions are being phased in through 2018. The REACH Regulation places responsibility on industry to manage the risks from chemicals and to provide safety information on the substances. Manufacturers and importers are required to gather information on the properties of their chemical substances, which will allow their safe handling, and to register the information in a central database. The Regulation also calls for the progressive substitution of the most dangerous chemicals (referred to as "substances of very high concern") when suitable alternatives have been identified. According to the European Commission, one aim of REACH is to enhance innovation and competitiveness in the EU chemical industry (http://ec.europa.eu/environment/chemicals/reach/reach_en.htm).

The EU REACH regulations and the US TSCA Reform Act are but two examples of progressive legislation aimed at reducing risks imposed by chemicals in our environment. Globally, countries vary widely in their environmental protection even after adjusting for levels of income. These inter-country differences are associated with the quality of their environmental regulatory regimes. Other regulatory aspects of human, animal, and environmental toxicology are discussed in a subsequent section. While some may argue that more stringent regulations hamper economic competitiveness, global comparisons indicate that countries that have the most aggressive environmental policy regimes seem to be the most competitive and economically successful (Esty and Porter, 2005).

5.1.3 One Toxicology

The need for a One Health approach to toxicology is evident for several reasons. As illustrated by the Minamata Bay tragedy, humans and animals share a common environment (Buttke, 2011; Rumbeiha, 2012). Contamination of air, water, soil, and food by hazardous chemical pollutants can lead to toxic effects in multiple species. Bioconcentration of toxicants in our ecosystems and biomagnification up the food chain often result in the highest doses occurring at the highest trophic levels, that is, humans and other predators. Differences in susceptibility among species often allows for animal populations to serves as "sentinels" of toxicants in our common environment. Degradation of ecosystems by toxicants can also have indirect effects on human health, as in the case of declines in native small predator species that either consume free-living stages of parasites or vectors of parasitic or microbial diseases.

The term "One Toxicology" (Figure 5.3), has been suggested to encourage more efficient collaborative research, data and knowledge sharing, and stewardship actions among groups of toxicologists (Beasley, 2009). Biochemical systems are highly conserved such that toxic effects are often shared among multiple species. Molecular, comparative, preclinical, clinical, diagnostic, environmental, ecological, aquatic, and soil toxicology

need to inform one another as a matter of routine.

Human health has historically been protected through observations on domestic and wild as well as laboratory animals. The canary in the coal mine, of course, relied upon a captive animal to warn of hazards of methane (from geological formations) and carbon monoxide (from use of engines) in mines. Because of the high efficiency of avian respiration, effects on the canary were rapid, and when it showed signs of poisoning, it was time to grab the birdcage and head for fresh air.

To most readily benefit human, animal, plant, and ecosystem health in the broader world, toxicologists need to work in concert with other medical and nonmedical professionals, a variety of stakeholders and citizens at large. Toxicology is a basic, applied, and regulatory science. As in the case of methylmercury poisoning in Minamata Bay, effects on animals can often precede those noted in humans, but unless animals are observed antemortem and postmortem, a diagnosis is rendered, and toxicant exposure is

Figure 5.3 Toxicology in the context of One Health.

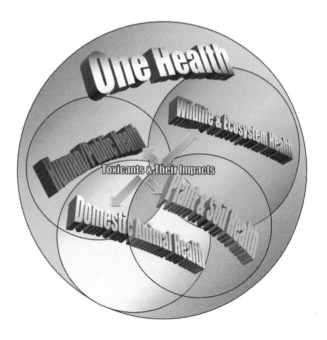

prevented, protection of other species will, at best, become just another lost opportunity. Accordingly, physicians, public health specialists, veterinary specialists, wildlife health professionals, plant specialists, ecologists, and different kinds of toxicologists should seek and create more opportunities to work together to prevent toxic injury to humans, animals, and plants. Surprisingly, the first session on One Health at a Society of Environmental Toxicology and Chemistry Annual Meeting took place only recently, in November 2015 (Aguirre et al., 2016). Fortunately, subsequent meetings of that group have continued to include One Health as a focus.

5.2 Key Concepts

5.2.1 Dose-Response Relationships

The father of modern toxicology, Paracelsus, is credited with the theory "The dose makes the poison." Figure 5.4 shows examples of various dose-response relationships. The classic toxicology dose-response relationships, whether positive or inverse, are *monotonic* and can be linear (Figure 5.4a) or nonlinear (Figure 5.4b). Most toxicants exhibit a *threshold* dose for a specific response, that is, the lowest dose at which a specific health effect is observed. A dose-response relationship that begins at (0,0), that is, no threshold, indicates that any dose of a toxicant has the potential to cause a response. These no threshold dose-response relationships most often occur when the response is stochastic, that is, the y axis measures the probability of a response occurring rather than the magnitude of a response. For example, many carcinogens exhibit stochastic dose-response relationships where even very small doses of the carcinogen have a probability, albeit small, of producing a carcinogenic response.

Figure 5.4c shows examples of *non-monotonic* dose-response relationships,

where the slope of the curve changes at least once from negative to positive, or vice versa. Such examples are seen with some endocrine disrupting chemicals. At low doses, some chemicals can induce breast cancer cells to multiply, but, as the dose increases, they may become overtly toxic, resulting in cell death (Vandenberg et al., 2012). Other non-monotonic dose curves include U-shaped, inverted U-shaped, and additional permutations. Non-monotonic dose curves have been associated with certain endocrine disruptors, and essential vitamins and trace elements including metals. Mechanistic studies have revealed the basis for a number of non-monotonic dose-response relationships (Welshons et al., 2003). For example, essential vitamins and minerals may have a U-shaped dose-response curve, which shows death at deficient levels for essential vitamins and trace elements, followed by homeostasis at adequate levels and, as doses increase, toxic responses of different types, including death. The beneficial effects of low doses of some chemicals, for example, vitamins, are referred to as hormetic effects (Luckey, 2006). Figure 5.4d shows a binary dose-response relationship, where one range of doses has no effect, and then a threshold is met, and all higher doses have the same effect. Understanding the shape of a dose-response relationship is clearly necessary if one wants to extrapolate a response from one dose to another.

5.2.2 Differences in Susceptibility

In some cases, humans and certain non-human species respond differently to chemical exposures. In general, any chemical that can cause cancer in humans can cause cancer in some other species of animals. However, because a chemical can cause cancer in one species or strain of animals does not mean that it will cause cancer in every other species or strain. Thus, some strains of laboratory mice, for example, may develop cancers from a given chemical that is innocuous to humans. This variability is explained by

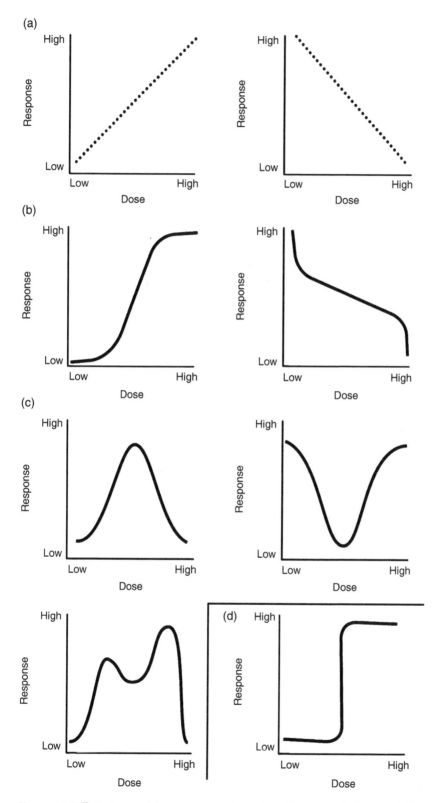

Figure 5.4 Different types of dose-response relationships. *Source:* Vandenberg et al., 2012. Reproduced with permission of Oxford University Press.

definable biological differences. For example, the exposure and accumulation of a toxic metabolite in tissues can vary among humans and animals. A well-known example is the use of the artificial sweetener, saccharin, which, when fed in large amounts, can accumulate and precipitate in the bladder of laboratory rats, leading to bladder cancer. This same precipitation does not occur in humans at doses consistent with dietary intake or even at high doses comparable to that consumed by laboratory rats (Cohen, 1998; Cohen et al., 2000). Another example is the difference in gene expression between animals, even among phylogenetically similar species such as rats, mice, guinea pigs, and hamsters. Rats, when given a diet containing aflatoxin B_1, a potent mycotoxin, at 15 parts per billion (ppb), develop liver tumors. Mice, however, when fed the same aflatoxin at 10 000 ppb, do not form tumors (Wogan et al., 1974). The difference can be explained in the detoxifying enzyme glutathione-*S*-transferase, which both species have, but the mouse version has a much higher rate of detoxification of aflatoxin compared to that of the rat (Eaton and Gallagher, 1994). Understanding differences among species and strains within species that can strongly influence disease outcomes is a key aspect of toxicology. Of importance, differences occur not only in regard to detoxification, but also in relation to processes of absorption, metabolic activation, which, by definition, makes a compound more toxic, and receptor affinity.

5.2.3 Periods of Increased Susceptibility

The timing of exposure to a toxicant in relationship to lifespan can be of critical importance in determining the severity or risk of an adverse response. Periods of increased susceptibility can include fetal as well as early childhood development. The biochemical coordination of cellular division and differentiation from fertilized ovum to highly coordinated interacting tissues, organs, and organ systems can be disrupted by xenobiotic chemicals and a host of other stressors.

Critical processes of development can be altered, resulting in lifelong and sometimes multigenerational health problems.

The study of birth defects, known as *teratology* – from the Greek, *teratos*, meaning monster – encompasses studies of biochemical mechanisms as well as clinical, pathologic, and epidemiologic investigations of alterations in form or function that arise during embryonic and fetal development. The embryonic period in humans is from the second through the eighth week of gestation. It encompasses organogenesis and thus is the most crucial period with regard to structural malformations. Figure 5.5 shows human fetal organ development throughout the embryonic period. During critical periods of susceptibility in embryonic and fetal development, toxic exposures can result in abnormalities. Because of the differing windows of susceptibility, the same dose of a chemical during different periods of development can have very different consequences. Thus, during development, not only does "Dose make the poison," but also "timing makes the poison" (Vogel, 2008). In addition to congenital malformations, other concerns for developmental and early life exposures are those that result in endocrine disruption with decreased fertility (Maffini et al., 2006), thyroid disorders (Diamanti-Kandarakis et al., 2009), or obesity (Heindel et al., 2015).

5.2.4 Receptors

In classical toxicology, a *receptor* is a target on or in a cell that interacts with natural or synthetic chemicals. There are many types and subtypes of receptors. Receptors are often initiating points for cascades of biological events that occur in response to endogenous and exogenous chemicals. Receptors may be selective for the natural endogenous chemical with which they interact. Interactions with receptors can involve either high- or low-affinity reactions. Some receptors are regarded as promiscuous, meaning that they react by being stimulated or inhibited after binding to a wide variety of compounds. The selectivity, affinity, and agonism or antagonism of a

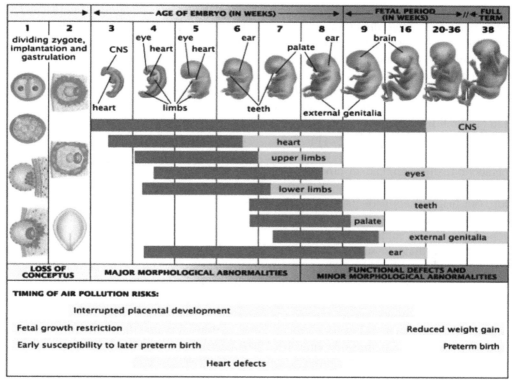

Note: Blue bars indicate time periods when major morphological abnormalities can occur, while light blue bars correspond to periods at risk for minor abnormalities and functional defects.

Figure 5.5 Developmental periods: pre-organogenesis, embryonic, and fetal.

receptor–chemical interaction serves as the basis for physiological and pharmacological responses of cells. *Selectivity* of a receptor describes the degree to which a compound acts on a given receptor relative to another receptor. *Affinity* describes the probability of the compound occupying a receptor at any given instant. *Agonism* at a receptor results in a physiological response, while *antagonism* blocks a response at the receptor.

5.2.5 Toxicokinetics and Toxicodynamics

Toxicokinetics, meaning "rate or movement" of toxic substances, is the study of the absorption, distribution, metabolism, and excretion of an exogenous chemical. *Absorption* describes the entry of the chemical into the organism, which would include inhalation (via breathing), transdermal (through the skin), ingestion (eating), or injection (into dif-

ferent body compartments including under the skin, into muscle/fat, or directly into the bloodstream). Limiting absorption, such as with activated charcoal for a range of ingested drugs or pesticides, can prevent or decrease the severity of toxic effects. *Distribution* describes the movement of the chemical from its initial absorption point throughout the body. Numerous properties can affect this. Chemicals that are fat soluble may be more likely to be transported to target tissues of the body such as the brain or to storage depots such as adipose tissue. In some clinical settings, intravenous administration of lipid emulsions is used to reduce concentrations of such substances at critical sites of action, thereby preventing or reducing toxicity. *Metabolism* describes the biochemical modification of exogenous chemicals. This modification, usually through enzymatic processes, can result in metabolites that are less, equally, or more potent, as compared to the parent chemical. An example of the latter is the herbicide paraquat. After direct ingestion by mammals, paraquat is metabolically activated in the lung and, with sufficient doses, pneumotoxicity is severe and often lethal. Conversely, with many chemicals, metabolic processes, especially in the liver, increase water solubility, making it easier to eliminate the chemical from the body. In some instances, administration of drugs that reduce metabolic toxification, and in others giving agents that promote metabolic detoxification, can help protect patients from further harm. *Elimination* is the final toxicokinetic step. Methods of elimination include via exhalation (breathing the substance out), urination (removal via the kidneys), or defecation (removal by the liver via the bile and through the gastrointestinal tract). When elimination is insufficient to avoid the buildup of a toxic chemical to a potentially harmful concentration in the body, appropriate therapy for some water-soluble chemicals includes enhancing elimination (e.g., via administration of intravenous fluids, potentially in concert with ion trapping of certain acidic or basic substances in the urine, or removal via hemodialysis). It is important to note that similar types of processes, including distribution, metabolism, and elimination also occur in the environment, reinforcing the concept that organisms and their ecosystems are not only biologically but also chemically interconnected.

Toxicodynamics focuses on what the poison does to the body. By definition, this interaction is injurious. Effects start at the molecular site, such as alteration of a receptor leading to blockade of an ion channel resulting in reduced activation of excitable tissues such as muscle or brain. The effects of other toxicants may be initiated by reactions with nuclear receptors that result in altered protein transcription, with multiple downstream consequences. In other cases, alterations may occur in DNA, inducing heritable changes in cells that result in degraded tissue function, carcinogenesis, or, if gametes are involved, multigenerational diseases. Yet other effects include changes in epigenetics, and in some instances, they too may lead to prolonged and even multigenerational problems. A variety of receptor interactions can result in organ failure, altered immune functions, and cancer.

5.3 Ecotoxicology and Human Exposures

5.3.1 Everyday Toxicology and Ecotoxicology: Contrasts, Complexities, and Challenges

Wild ecosystems, plants, and animals are critically important to a healthy human psyche and they provide essential ecosystem services that serve to protect animal and human health. But, wild places and wild organisms also have their own inherent value (van der Tuuk, 1999; de Groot et al., 2012; Curtin, 2009).

Domestic, laboratory, and wild animals are relied upon to warn against risks of toxic injury. From the canary in the coal mine to the household dog, and whether whale, wild bird, turtle, fish, arthropod, or mollusk, animals serve as sentinels of harmful and potentially lethal exposures to chemicals. For the animals to fill such roles, they need to be present, to be observed, and, when potential problems exist, to be examined (Burrell and Seibert, 1916; Reif, 2011; Reddy et al., 2001; Martineau, 2012; Holt and Miller, 2010). Additional information on environmental contaminants and their effects on terrestrial and aquatic wildlife is available in the primary literature and a number of books (e.g., Jorgensen, 2010; Newman, 2009; Walker et al., 2012).

Compared to human or veterinary clinical toxicology, ecotoxicology stands out due to: 1) vastly reduced control over the exposed individuals; 2) great complexity of exposures; 3) reduced knowledge about exposure histories; and 4) the everyday stressors of life in the wild (Newman and Clements, 2008). Clinicians in human and domestic animal medicine and those involved in agricultural plant health can readily examine individuals to determine their condition and assess their needs, but wildlife specialists and ecological toxicologists find and examine "their patients" often with considerable difficulty. Climatic and weather conditions (drought, storms, snow, ice, heat), and the time and expense of travel to sampling sites increases the challenges of making needed observations. Collecting permits from host governments may be necessary, transboundary issues must often be addressed, and property and privacy rights must be accommodated. In addition, the feasibility and risks associated with capture and restraint must be considered in light of potential harm or death in the organisms to be examined. Of course, risks to those involved in undertaking the examinations of specimens in and from the field must also be considered.

In ecotoxicology, the myriad chemicals introduced to the environment, in varying amounts – from such diverse sources as living organisms (biotoxins), geological deposits of metals, salts, or hydrocarbons (coal, petroleum, gas), mining and extraction activities, homes, businesses, industries, construction sites, agricultural settings, commercial forests,waste disposal, power plants, and vehicles of all types – produce an unending variety of exposures. Both individual toxicants and complex mixtures of toxicants directly interfere with life processes of resident microbial, plant, and animal communities, and they thereby alter the normal interplay among species.

Unfortunately, combined chemical exposures of humans, other animals, plants, and ecosystems and the effects of such exposures are rarely studied even in individual species, let alone in species assemblages or ecosystems. Consequently, ecotoxicologists are forced to rely on "educated guesses" as to risks of exposure until research can be completed. Such research ranges from modest short-term field investigations to modeling of massive data sets after sampling multiple similarly contaminated sites with comparisons to

multiple reference sites, or simply examining a wide variety of sites with different levels of contaminants present. Such field studies may give rise to hypotheses that can then tested with individual organisms in the lab or groups of organisms in microcosm or mesocosm studies (e.g., Rohr et al., 2008).

5.3.2 Toxicant Fate in the Environment

It has been estimated that there are between 8 and 16 million molecular species in the biosphere, and that up to 40 000 play major roles in the daily lives of human populations (Goméz et al., 2007). After release of a chemical into the environment, many processes influence exposure and toxicity. Environmental exposures vary as a function of release rates, dilution, spontaneous chemical reactions, binding phenomena, and metabolism by microbes, plants, and animals.

A windy area or a windy day may result in a great amount of dilution of a chemical volatilized from a field or suspended in dust, as well as of an airborne toxicant emitted by a vehicle, power plant, or factory. By contrast, stagnant air and thermal inversions may result in high ground-level exposures via inhalation, ocular, or dermal routes. Similarly, where runoff of a chemical enters a large lake or a large, rapidly moving stream, high concentrations may be fleeting even at the points of introduction, such that for many organisms, exposures do not exceed thresholds of toxicity. However, if the exposed environment is a small pool of water, and the chemical is not highly bound to soils and sediments, volatilized, or biodegraded, exposures may be high and prolonged. High levels of elements or compounds may overload the binding capacity of soils and sediments and the metabolic capacity of resident organisms (plants, bacteria, fungi, annelids, arthropods, mollusks, vertebrates) resulting in prolonged exposures and potential toxicity.

The chemical forms of certain elements and compounds in air, water, sediments, soils, plants, and animals can rapidly or slowly change as a consequence of abiotic and biotic reactions. Abiotic reactions include spontaneous hydrolysis, chemical reactions with elements and compounds also in the environment, UV-induced changes in the chemical structures of molecules, and binding to organic matrices and inorganic particles in soils. Each of these depends on what chemical is introduced to the area, the amounts released, the other chemicals that are already there, and local climate and weather conditions. Biotic reactions with chemicals include the uptake, alterations induced by, and elimination of elements and compounds by all forms of life (microbes, plants, and animals). Because of abiotic and biotic reactions, complex mixtures become more or less complex over time – even in the absence of deliberate human interventions. Such changes alter bioavailability and toxicity, increasing risks in some cases and decreasing risks in others.

Microbial metabolism is an important process in environmental fate that may result in complete elimination (termed mineralization) of a range of compounds. Knowledge of the physicochemical nature of compounds entering the environment and of pathways and organisms involved in their metabolism in a given area is used to predict: 1) the nature and duration of transfers of the parent chemical and its metabolites among organisms; 2) toxic impacts that may follow; and 3) the potential value of cleanup and bioremediation efforts. Bioremediation entails deliberate actions to increase the capacity of biological organisms in situ or in artificial systems to change contaminant structures or to trap and remove contaminants and thereby make the environment less toxic. Ecosystems change over time as a consequence of toxic chemicals. Areas contaminated for long time periods, whether because of long half-lives or frequent additions of the chemical(s), will favor persistence of tolerant individuals. In some instances, survivors will be those with reduced receptor sensitivity, but in others they will be those who can detoxify the pollutant. In many instances, organisms capable of detoxification, and especially those that can use the pollutant as a nutrient might be useful for environmental bioremediation (Nyman, 1999). Knowledge of interactions among chemicals with nonliving components and with living organisms in the environment, including those capable of detoxification, is also used in "green chemistry," which seeks to synthesize and deploy safer compounds to meet societal needs and demands (National Research Council, 2014).

UV-induced changes in chemical structures can increase or decrease toxicity. In many instances, aromatic molecules (e.g., aromatic hydrocarbons) become more reactive and thus exert greater toxicity after exposure to UV (Abdel-Shafy and Mansour, 2016). Halogenated compounds, when in the air, on the surface of soils or plants, or floating in microlayers on water bodies, may lose halogen atoms, which changes their fate in animals and may decrease or increase receptor activity and thus toxicity (e.g., Chen et al., 2015).

Binding to soils and sediments can largely immobilize many elements and compounds. The herbicide paraquat is a useful example of both UV-induced detoxification and binding to environmental matrices. In bright sunlight, unbound paraquat is photodegraded to less toxic compounds. In water, paraquat binds to plants or sediments, such that aqueous concentrations rapidly decline. Paraquat binds quite tightly to clay and other components of soils, and when bound to soils, it remains in its parent state for up to several years. Even though paraquat can be displaced from soils by such common ions as ammonium, potassium, sodium, and calcium, the available literature seems to indicate that toxicity to animals from soil-bound paraquat is not a major concern (Smith and Mayfield, 1978).

Chemicals introduced to the environment vary widely in mobility. Even heavy metals, which are often thought of as relatively immobile, may have quite different transport behaviors (Siegel, 2002). Coal-fired power plants and waste incinerators are important sources of atmospheric mercury. Mercury leaves power plants and waste incinerators as a vapor via smoke stacks as well as condensed on ash particles. In the environment, mercury can be present as elemental mercury, as mercury salts, and as a component of organic molecules. The fate of mercury in the environment (Figure 5.6) is influenced by temperature, soil moisture, and precipitation (Senior et al., 2000; Wallschläger et al., 1995; Song and Van Heyst, 2005; Wang et al., 2010). After methylation by sulfur-reducing bacteria in anaerobic sediments of aquatic ecosystems, methylmercury is biomagnified in aquatic foods and, in that form, it readily traverses both the placenta and the blood–brain barrier. Some of the effects of mercury on wildlife were discussed in the Introduction and others are discussed later.

The mobility of a given metal in soils and water, and uptake by plants and animals, will vary depending on pH, sorbent reactions with soils, soil organic and inorganic ligands, root extracts, nutrients, and redox reactions (Violante et al., 2010). Among classic concerns of heavy metal mobilization and toxicity are interactions among sulfides brought to the surface during mining where they react with atmospheric oxygen and water to form sulfuric acid, which dissolves metals and carries them into plants or water bodies (Yang et al., 2010). In water, the acid and the metals act both independently and together to harm aquatic life by impacting ion fluxes and damaging enzymes and other biochemical receptors, as best described in regard to the digestive (gut and liver), urinary (kidneys), immune, circulatory, and nervous systems. Moreover, when streams come together and more alkaline water buffers a more acidic stream, precipitation of metals, such as ubiquitous iron and aluminum, can smother the gills of both aquatic invertebrates and vertebrates (Rosseland et al., 1990; Youson and Neville, 1987; Stephens and Ingram, 2006).

Inorganic and organic molecules range from highly hydrophilic to extremely hydrophobic. Many hydrophobic molecules contain substantial numbers of halogen atoms (e.g., chlorine, bromine, and fluorine) in their structures, and they often lack atoms that can be readily ionized (hence they are not charged). Included in this regard are DDT and a number of other organochlorine insecticides; hexachlorobenzene, which was used as a fungicide; polychlorinated biphenyls (PCBs), which had many uses as electrical insulator fluids, in paints, coatings and carbonless carbon paper; polychlorinated dibenzofurans (PCDFs) and polychlorinated dibenzodioxins (PCDDs), which were byproducts of the chemical industry or produced from combustion of chlorine-containing materials; and polybrominated diphenyl ethers (PBDEs), which were more recently used in flame retardants. The bulky halogen atoms of such compounds interfere with metabolism. Due to their environmental stability and resistance to metabolism, such compounds are often referred to as persistent organic pollutants (POPs). They readily partition into lipid microlayers that float on water or that rest on or are incorporated into sediments. Animals that drink the water, and especially those that live at the surface or rely on the sediments, form the first links in food web exposures of predators. Fluorines are also among the halogens, but a number of polyfluorinated and perfluorinated organic compounds differ from the classical POPS in that they are both hydrophobic and oleophobic (Giesy and Kannan, 2002). Nevertheless, despite their differences in affinity for lipids and related differences in pathways of exchange among organisms, a number of the commercially important highly fluorinated compounds are biomagnified in aquatic food webs to an extent similar to DDT and PCBs (Haukås et al., 2007).

A temperature-related process that markedly influences the transport of semi-volatile organic compounds is the "grasshopper effect." Through this process, semi-volatile compounds evaporate in and are transported from warm areas (tropics, valleys, temperate zones in summer) to cooler areas (high elevations, over cold water bodies, temperate zones in winter, circumpolar environments)

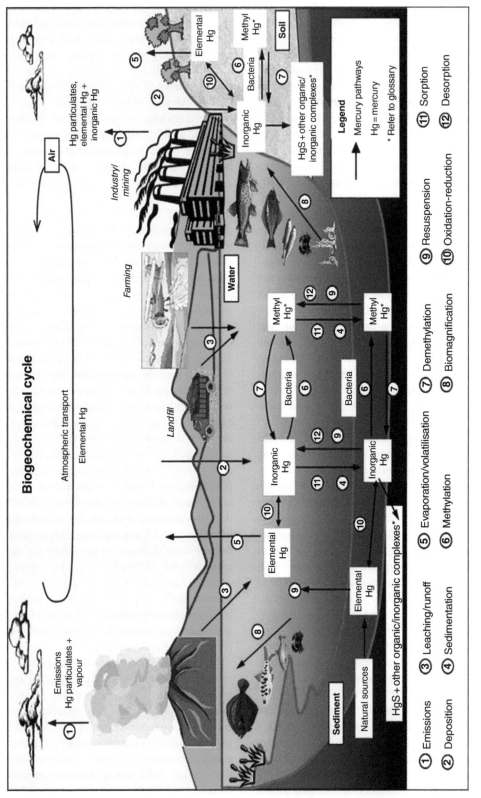

Figure 5.6 Mercury biogeochemical cycle. *Source:* New Zealand Ministry for the Environment, 2008.

with condensation, deposition with precipitation, and fractionation along the way (Gouin et al., 2004; Kirchner et al., 2009). The "grasshopper effect" and resistance to metabolism account for the high levels of POPs in Arctic polar bears and Antarctic birds, both of which feed at the apex of long and complex food webs (Cipro et al., 2013; Fox, 2001). Among the toxic effects of some such compounds are neurotoxicity, altered immunologic responses, and endocrine disruption.

Three similar sounding terms used in regard to concentrations of contaminants that arise in animals are bioconcentration, bioaccumulation, and biomagnification. In ecotoxicology, these three terms have quite different meanings. *Bioconcentration* refers to uptake of toxicants directly from water only (e.g., in a laboratory setting). *Bioaccumulation* accounts for the concentration in an animal that arises not only via the water through transport across respiratory epithelia (e.g., gills) and dermal absorption, but also via the diet. Finally, *biomagnification* becomes the most relevant term of the three in those cases in which the organism is exposed almost exclusively via the diet, and it becomes of major importance with a compound like methylmercury, which accumulates in the muscles of fish, or PCBs or organochlorine insecticides, which accumulate in adipose tissue. It can therefore become the process of greatest concern with POPs that work their way into aquatic top predators (Mackay and Fraser, 2000; Fraser et al., 2002; Sørmo et al., 2006; Férard and Blaise, 2013). Of course, coastal human communities may share the top predator position with marine mammals. The cooking process can substantially reduce contaminant exposures, but only if the lipids removed are not consumed. Public health agencies often issue fish advisories to limit or avoid eating certain types of fish and shellfish caught from specific water bodies due to chemical contamination. It can be important to weigh the cultural benefits of fishing and hunting as well as the nutritional value of consuming aquatic species (e.g., proteins, omega-3 fatty acids, vitamins) against the risks of the toxicants present (Moses et al., 2009).

5.3.3 Contrasts in Feasibility: Examinations and Interventions

When toxicological concerns arise, human, domestic animal, wildlife, or ecological practitioners and toxicologists generally strive to gather data on the individual(s) at risk, and on potential or confirmed chemical exposures, and they look for patterns that make sense (evidence of a toxic dose and effects that are consistent with those associated with the given agent). Unlike physicians whose roles focus on *Homo sapiens*, or domestic animal veterinarians who focus on companion or food-producing animals, a challenge to the wildlife veterinarian or ecotoxicologist, at least in many cases, is that multiple diverse species are exposed and of concern. Also, when threatened or endangered species are involved, sampling may necessarily rely on noninvasive methods, such as observations at a distance and studies of scats (feces), coupled with opportunistic examinations of individuals found dead, or sampling of surrogate species that share genetic characteristics, dietary habits, and the same or similar environments.

While exposures to complex mixtures of chemicals occur in every home, school, workplace, urban, rural, transitional, or wild environment, it is often the newly introduced substance that is of greatest concern in the patient presented to a physician or veterinarian for an acute toxicosis. When a clinical diagnosis of acute poisoning is made, such as to a highly toxic pesticide, the practitioners' goals of intervention typically include preventing further exposure to and absorption of the toxic agent, conserving/restoring physiological functions, protecting vital organs and, when possible, hastening elimination (Eddleston et al., 2008). Chronic toxicoses are also recognized and addressed by human and domestic animal medical professionals, as in the case of lead poisoning (Needleman, 2003; Morgan, 1994) (see case study in Box 5.1). When problems from chronic lead toxicosis

---

Box 5.1 Case study: lead

Lead has been used by humans for millennia due to its wide availability, ease of extraction and manipulation, and properties such as malleability (Tokar et al., 2013). However, recognition of its toxicity to humans and animals, even at very low concentrations, has led to restrictions on its use. For example, its removal from gasoline, paint, solder, and water supply lines has significantly reduced overall blood lead levels in the general population. Lead shot were phased out for use over wetlands in the USA in 1991, and increasingly strict regulation of lead in ammunition is occurring worldwide (Avery and Watson, 2009). However, lead remains a significant health concern due to its persistence in older homes and continued use in ammunition for upland game hunting and fishing tackle in much of the world. More recently, a major public health concern arose in relation to lead in Flint, Michigan, when leaching of lead from drinking water pipes followed a decision to rely on the highly corrosive water of the Flint River to supply the city (Tiemann, 2016). A recently recognized and unexpected source of lead to humans is through the consumption of eggs from backyard chickens exposed to old wood previously coated with lead-based paint. Backyard chicken flocks are becoming more popular across the USA, and the potential for lead exposure via contaminated eggs, especially of children, warrants education of the small poultry producers (Bautista et al., 2014).

Lead induces a wide range of adverse effects in humans that are dose- and exposure duration-dependent (Tokar et al., 2013). Toxic effects are diverse and include alterations of metal transport and energy metabolism, apoptosis, ion conduction, cell adhesion, inter- and intracellular signaling, enzymatic processes, protein maturation, and genetic regulation. Across multiple species, impacts are found in the form of dysfunction and lesions in the central nervous, gastrointestinal, renal, and hematopoietic systems. Children and young animals are more sensitive to the toxic effects of lead due to increased lead bioavailability compared to adults. In children, effects on neurodevelopment are of particular concern.

Numerous international studies have shown that increasing blood lead levels are inversely associated with IQ in children. The estimated IQ point decrements associated with an increase in blood lead from 2.4 to 10 μg/dL, 10 to 20 μg/dL, and 20 to 30 μg/dL were 3.9 (95% CI, 2.4–5.3), 1.9 (95% CI, 1.2–2.6), and 1.1 (95% CI, 0.7–1.5), respectively (Lanphear et al., 2005). Some believe that there is no safe level for lead exposure with regard to neurodevelopment. Subtle effects on neurodevelopment of animals have not been studied, but could be expected to occur. Unfortunately, the impact of such subtle effects on wildlife could conceivably affect long-term survival.

Acute lead encephalopathy in children can be manifested by such signs as lethargy, vomiting, irritability, anorexia, dizziness progressing to ataxia, coma, and death. In 2010, an outbreak of lead poisoning in Nigeria from unsafe processing of lead-containing ore resulted in the deaths of over 400 children up to 5 years of age (Bashir et al., 2014). In animals, predominant signs can vary depending on the species affected and the degree and duration of exposure.

Historically, in animals, the largest numbers of documented lead poisonings have involved waterfowl that ingested spent lead shot, cattle that ate lead from discarded vehicular batteries or motor oil contaminated from leaded gasoline, and pets exposed to older homes containing lead paint or lead paint residues. With the restrictions placed on lead in shot and removal of lead from gasoline and paint, the incidence of lead toxicosis in these species has declined. However, some wildlife species continue to be impacted by lead from sources such as lead ammunition and fishing tackle. The animal species most frequently reported to have lead poisoning in the USA at this time are avian scavengers such as California condors, and avian piscivores such as bald eagles and common loons. Intoxication of other wildlife is common, but the charismatic nature of the aforementioned species likely accounts for a disproportionate amount of attention given to them. In addition to lead, many piscivorous bird species such as bald

Box 5.1 (Continued)

eagles and loons are exposed to methylmercury, which is also neurotoxic. Unfortunately, little work has been done to assess the adverse effects from combined lead and mercury exposure.

Although lead concentrations in blood and tissues from exposed individuals have often been determined, the residue levels present in exposed bird species at the population level are generally unknown. It is clear, however, that lead intoxication has had a serious impact on the recovery of the California condor. The deaths of 135 released condors in California from October of 1992 through the end of 2009 were investigated by Rideout et al. (2012). A definitive cause of death was determined for 76 of 98 carcasses examined. Fifty-three deaths were attributed to an anthropogenic cause. Trash ingestion was the most important mortality factor for nestlings, and lead toxicosis was the leading cause of death among juvenile and adult birds (23/65). The authors concluded that, without effective adoption of mitigation measures, lead would remain the most important mortality factor undermining the sustainability of wild condor populations. Population models based upon condor demographic data indicate that the apparent recovery of the condor is entirely dependent upon the intensive, ongoing management efforts (Finkelstein et al., 2012).

The link between the use of leaded ammunition and condor mortality has been questioned (Starin, 2013). However, the evidence supporting an important role of lead poisoning in this species is overwhelming: it includes recovery of lead shotgun pellets and bullet fragments from GI tracts, tissue lead isotope ratios that match lead isotope ratios in lead ammunition, and exposures coinciding with hunting seasons and foraging activities in popular hunting areas. The cost of providing supplemental feeding, recapturing released birds, testing blood for lead, and treating lead-exposed birds is substantial.

In Arizona, a program to encourage hunters to voluntarily switch to non-lead ammunition and to remove gut piles from the field has had some success (Green et al., 2008). However, in California, restrictions on lead ammunition use

in the California condor range has had limited impacts, particularly in some natural areas used for condor release that were surrounded by private land (Kelly et al., 2014). As a result, California is currently the only state to have begun a process leading to a complete ban on the use of lead ammunition over a 5-year period, with the final stage of the phase-out scheduled for 2019.

People who consume a variety of game species shot with lead ammunition are clearly ingesting and absorbing the toxic metal (Iqbal et al., 2009; Green and Pain, 2012; Fachehoun et al., 2015; Arnemo et al., 2016). Figure 5.7 is a radiographic image of a bald eagle showing the presence of two radio-opaque lead bullet fragments in the gastrointestinal tract of the bird. In one study, people who consumed wild game had higher blood lead concentrations than those who did not consume wild game (Iqbal et al., 2009). In another study, it was estimated that 2.9%, 5.8%, and 7.7% of children who ate deer meat once, twice, or three times per week respectively would be exposed to a dose of lead associated with a 1 point IQ decrease.

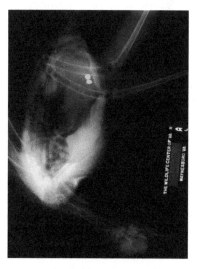

Figure 5.7 A radiographic image of a bald eagle showing the presence of two radio-opaque lead bullet fragments in the gastrointestinal tract of the bird. Courtesy of The Wildlife Center of Virginia and the Veterinary Department.

(Continued)

Box 5.1 (Continued)

(Fachehoun et al., 2015). The recent exhaustive review of Arnemo et al. (2016) cited several additional reports showing excessive intake of lead from game meat and excessive blood lead levels in consumers of the meat. Arnemo et al. (2016) concluded that existing reports on global use of lead ammunition and related risks of lead poisoning in humans are compelling, that comparatively nontoxic ammunition is widely available and affordable, and that the focus at this time should be on combating disinformation and pressing for legislation to permanently eliminate the risks to human health imposed by lead in ammunition used for hunting.

---

are encountered in humans or pet animals, goals for intervention may include preventing further exposure and absorption, promoting elimination, and close surveillance and intervention to counteract toxic manifestations. For children and domestic animals with severe lead poisoning, this may include changing the environment, lead remediation of housing, and chelation. Anticonvulsants may be used when needed for pets or children, and tutoring and counseling may be provided to lead-impaired children. While exceptions can be found[1], even the use of chelation alone is infrequently feasible for wildlife. For most acute or chronic toxicoses affecting free-ranging wildlife, interventions to prevent further exposure and absorption, close monitoring, and individually tailored treatments are difficult, impractical, or impossible. Prevention of toxic exposures in the wild may depend upon banning or restricting unsafe products such as lead ammunition for hunting and lead in fishing tackle, eliminating problem pesticides, implementing pollution controls on power plants, industries, and vehicles, and environmental cleanups that often take time (sometimes many years) and may cost many millions of dollars. Clearly, prevention of poisoning is rational for humans and domestic animals, but it is uniquely important for wild species.

5.3.4 Indirect Effects of Chemicals

Ecotoxicology differs from clinical and diagnostic toxicology because of the need to understand and address not only direct but also indirect effects of chemicals in the environment (Beasley and Levengood, 2012; Levengood and Beasley, 2007, 2012; Rohr et al., 2008; Newman and Clements, 2008). Greatly increased production of natural toxins and increased exposure to infectious pathogens are among the potential indirect effects of environmental contamination.

Nutrient additions from fertilizer applications, waste disposal, animal agriculture, and fossil fuel burning as well as climate change from emissions of carbon dioxide and methane tend to decrease the generation times of toxigenic cyanobacteria, diatoms, and dinoflagellates. Such changes may lead to important phycotoxin impacts on wildlife, domestic animals, and people (Beasley, 2011; Hilborn and Beasley, 2015). Examples of neurotoxic marine phycotoxins include:

- Domoic acid from marine diatoms – causes amnesic shellfish poisoning in people and neurological impairment and deaths of cetaceans, sea lions, otters, and water birds exposed via fish and shellfish (see case study in Box 5.2).

---

1 An exception to this is the case of California condors, which, through great expense, were rescued from extinction by removal of every wild individual alive to a captive setting. This was followed by captive breeding, release, monitoring, and periodic recapture, health monitoring, and chelation to address lead poisoning due to scavenging on lead-contaminated animals and "gut piles" left behind by hunters. Elimination of lead ammunition for hunting upland game is yet to be completed in environments relied upon by California condors (Finkelstein et al., 2012). An extraordinarily important One Health concern is that lead ammunition continues to be used in upland hunting in the USA and much of the world, even though it results in poisoning of human consumers of shot animals, as well as any carnivore or scavenger that ingests contaminated body parts (Arnemo et al., 2016). See Box 5.1.

Box 5.2 Case study: domoic acid

In 2015, one of the most extensive marine harmful algal blooms (HABs) ever encountered occurred along large stretches of the Pacific Coast of the USA. The bloom stretched from the central Californian coast north to Washington State, and the waters of several regions, including Monterey Bay and the central Oregon Coast, had some of the highest concentrations of the potent neurotoxin domoic acid (DA) detected to date (NOAA, 2015). DA is an amino acid belonging to the kainoid class of compounds.

DA is produced by a number of marine organisms. Along the west coast of the USA, marine diatoms belonging to *Pseudo-nitzschia* spp. are most commonly implicated in DA production. Under appropriate environmental conditions, the organisms undergo rapid growth (blooms) and produce the toxin. A definitive cause for the blooms and DA production has not been determined, making predictions of their occurrence difficult (Seubert et al., 2013). Anthropogenic eutrophication and climate change, drivers for the increased incidence of many HAB, are not the sole factors that account for the occurrence of *Pseudo-nitzschia* spp. Blooms and clearly conditions that give rise to upwelling along the coast are involved (http://oceandatacenter.ucsc.edu/home/news%20items/SG_narrative_FINAL.pdf).

DA accumulates in a wide array of marine species (Lefebvre et al., 2002). Fish as diverse as sanddabs, sardines, anchovies, and albacore tuna, mollusks such as mussels and clams, and crabs have been found to contain DA (Lefebvre et al., 2002). DA was first recognized as a phycotoxin in 1987, following an outbreak of toxic encephalopathy in humans from Canada after consumption of cultivated blue mussels (*Mytilus edulis*). The mussels originated from three river estuaries of Prince Edward Island (Perl et al., 1990). Acute illness was characterized by gastrointestinal and unusual neurologic symptoms. Severely affected patients exhibited unsteadiness, generalized weakness, confusion, and disorientation within 48 hours of consuming mussels. Five patients had seizures and 13 patients had altered states of consciousness ranging from agitation to coma. Over 100 individuals were affected, with 19 individuals requiring hospitalization (Jeffrey et al., 2004). Three patients died 11 to 24 days after consumption of the mussels. However, most patients recovered within 72 hours, although anterograde memory disorder and retrograde amnesia were noted in severely affected individuals even at 4 to 6 months after ingestion. The disease syndrome was called amnesic shellfish poisoning (ASP). In patients who died, neuronal necrosis or loss of astrocytes were noted in the CA1 and CA3 regions of the hippocampus and amygdaloid nucleus. Lesions were also evident in the thalamus of two individuals and the subfrontal cortex of three individuals.

The mechanism of toxic action of DA has been extensively studied both *in vitro* and *in vivo*. DA is structurally similar to glutamic and kainic acids. Kainic acid binds to a glutamate receptor subtype in the CNS called the kainate receptor. Kainate receptors are widely distributed in the mammalian brain but are especially concentrated in the CA1–3 regions of the hippocampus in rodents, the CA2 and CA3 regions in some nonhuman primates, and the CA3 region in humans. Receptor binding leads to stimulation of neuronal firing, influx of Ca^{2+} into neurons, failure to maintain ionic gradients and intracellular ion homeostasis, and cell death (Jeffrey et al., 2004).

Although *Pseudo-nitzschia* spp. have been recognized as part of the California marine microalgal community since the early 1900s, DA production by these species along the coast was not documented until 1991, when deaths in brown pelicans and Brandt's cormorants coincided with a DA-producing bloom of *Pseudo-nitzschia australis* (Work et al., 1993; Seubert et al., 2013). DA intoxication of wildlife species has been studied most extensively in California sea lions. In 1998, DA toxicosis was determined to be the cause of death of 48 sea lions stranded along the California coast during a *Pseudo-nitzschia australis* bloom (Scholin et al., 2000; Gulland et al., 2002). Similar outbreaks have occurred regularly since then.

(Continued)

Box 5.2 (Continued)

The neuropathology in affected animals has been extensively described (Buckmaster et al., 2014). Lesions noted in the hippocampus of sea lions with chronic DA toxicosis are similar to those of human patients with temporal lobe epilepsy (Figure 5.8). Spatial memory deficits could be predicted based upon the extent of lesion in the right dorsal hippocampus (Cook et al., 2015). DA exposure was also shown to disrupt hippocampal-thalamic brain networks, which could potentially impair spatial memory and affect survival in the wild. This has implications for the successful release of animals being rehabilitated after stranding due to DA exposure. Indeed, chronically affected sea lions re-strand at a rate much higher than that of sea lions rehabilitated and released for other reasons (71% vs ~0.5%, respectively; Goldstein et al., 2008).

Following the human outbreak of ASP in 1987, an action limit of 20 µg DA per gram of shellfish flesh was established in Canada and other parts of the world. No similar levels of concern have been developed for potentially affected wildlife species. Due to extensive monitoring for toxin levels in seafood, few people in North America have been exposed to highly toxic amounts of DA since the 1987 outbreak.

Because of the difficulty of predicting the occurrence of a DA-producing bloom, extensive monitoring programs have been implemented in many regions (Trainer and Hardy, 2015). The programs are designed to better detect and forecast HABs, and to ensure that commercial and recreational catches of seafood are safe for human consumption (NOAA, 2015).

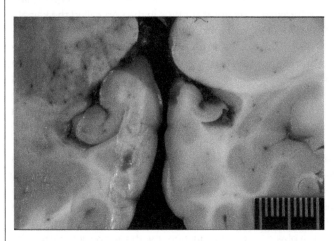

Figure 5.8 Lesions in the hippocampus of a domoic acid-poisoned sea lion (left) as compared to a normal sea lion (right). *Source:* Pathology Archives, UC Davis VMTH and the Marine Mammal Center.

- Brevetoxin from a dinoflagellate – causes nonsuppurative meningitis, respiratory tract irritation, hemolysis, immunosuppression, and may affect humans, manatees, dolphins, water birds, sea turtles, and fish exposed via the respiratory system and ingestion of contaminated food items.
- Saxitoxin from marine dinoflagellates and freshwater cyanobacteria – causes paralytic poisoning in humans and neurotoxicity in

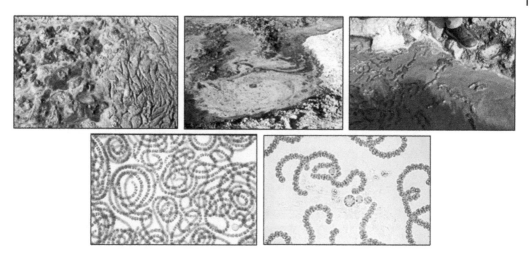

Figure 5.9 *Anabaena,* a commonly encountered toxigenic genus of cyanobacteria. Upper right, left, and middle: Photos of bloom materials in ponds where swine died after drinking the contaminated water. Lower left and right: Microscopic views of chains of *Anabaena* cells; the lower right image is of chains of *Anabaena* with nitrogen-fixing heterocyst (clear cell with two "dots") and spore (large cell).

marine mammals, water birds, sea turtles, and fishes, exposed through ingestion of shellfish and fish.

Cyanobacteria of the genus *Lyngbya* in estuarine or brackish water are producers of lyngbyatoxins, which can cause skin irritation and tumor promotion. In addition, cyanobacteria in freshwater may be ingested resulting in exposures to toxic amounts of the nicotinic agonist anatoxin-A, and the peripheral-acting cholinesterase inhibitor anatoxin-A(s); and either of these can cause lethal respiratory paralysis. While ruminants seem to be tolerant of anatoxin-A(s), other vertebrates should be considered at risk when drinking contaminated water. *Anabaena,* a genus often associated with production of anatoxins, is shown in Figure 5.9. *Microcystis* is shown in Figure 5.10. Ingestion of cyanobacteria, including strains of *Microcystis, Anabaena, Oscillatoria, Planktothrix, Nostoc,* and *Nodularia* or lysates of such organisms from nutrient-rich freshwater and coastal ecosystems, can produce hepatotoxicity due to microcystins or the structurally related nodularin. Also, the cyanobacterial toxin, cylindrospermopsin, from *Cylindrospermopsis,* is being found increasingly in warmer climates and, unlike the other phycotoxins above, is mainly a concern when it is free in the water; it can cause hepatotoxicity, nephrotoxicity, vomiting, bloody diarrhea, fever, headache, and genotoxicity following ingestion (Falconer and Humpage, 2005).

It should be no surprise that herbicides in aquatic environments are often toxic to plants or that they may cause direct toxicity in animals as well. However, indirect problems also arise because herbicides may damage or kill algae and macrophytes such that they no longer provide adequate dissolved oxygen for a host of invertebrates, fish, and amphibians. Also, after herbicide impact, the UV and nutrients that aquatic plants previously captured become available to other photosynthetic organisms. Herbicides may set the stage for blooms of toxigenic cyanobacteria as mentioned already (Lürling and Roessink, 2006), or alternatively, they may promote periphyton (slime algae)

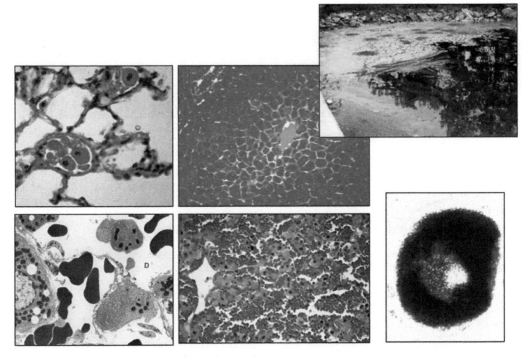

Figure 5.10 Top right: A wind-concentrated bloom of *Microcystis* along the shoreline of a pond in a heavily farmed area of central Illinois. Lower right: Microscopic view of thousands of cells of *Microcystis*. The colonies of cells are often surrounded by a clear coating. Upper middle: Histological section of liver showing early changes due to microcystin poisoning (initial separation of hepatocytes from one another). Lower middle: Histological section of liver showing massive separation of hepatocytes and intrahepatic hemorrhage. Upper left: hepatocytes lost from the damaged liver in capillaries of the lung. Lower left: Transmission electron photomicrograph of liver altered by microcystin poisoning, including damage to hepatocytes and endothelial cells, and red blood cells that have escaped from the damaged sinusoids.

growth, which supports more generations of snails and thus increased numbers of trematodes (trematodes reproduce asexually in snails) (Rohr et al., 2008).

Different trematodes infect invertebrate and vertebrate hosts, including wildlife, domestic animals, and humans. A recent study revealed that the combination of fertilizer, which stimulated growth of periphyton and thus snails, and the insecticide chlorpyrifos, which reduced arthropod predators that feed on snails, increased the infective load of *Schistosoma mansoni* cercariae in water. Of importance is that schistosomiasis undermines the health of hundreds of millions of people in the tropics, especially in Africa (Halstead et al., 2011). The life cycle and potential impacts of environmental change, including those induced by contaminants, are shown in Figure 5.11.

Herbicides and insecticides may reduce food items relied upon by seed-eating and carnivorous species, respectively (Boatman et al., 2004; Hallmann et al., 2014). While studies have demonstrated adverse effects on avian reproductive success, additional field research is needed to gauge the scale and importance of the impact of pesticide use in the food webs and nutrition of many more wild species. Likewise, studies are needed on the most effective ways to produce food without pesticide impacts to enable accelerated ecological recovery.

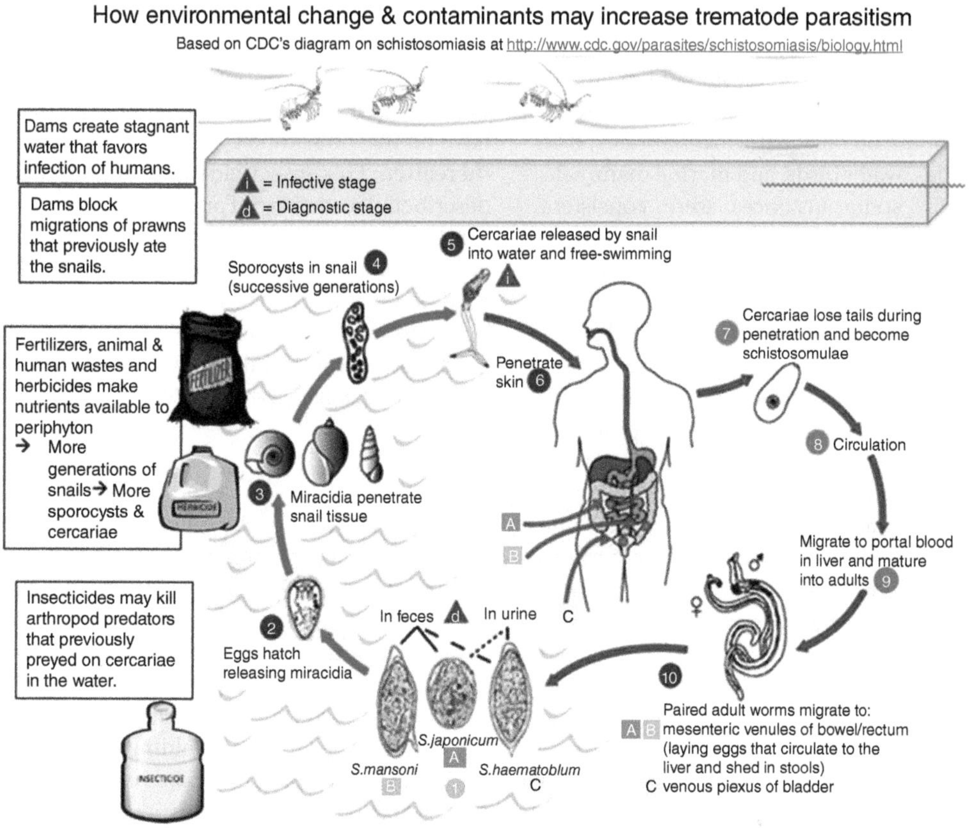

How environmental change & contaminants may increase trematode parasitism
Based on CDC's diagram on schistosomiasis at http://www.cdc.gov/parasites/schistosomiasis/biology.html

Figure 5.11 Life cycle of *Schistosoma mansoni* in humans and potential changes in the environment that may increase the extent of harm experienced. *Source:* Centers for Disease Control and Prevention (https://wwwnc.cdc.gov/parasites/schistosomiasis/biology.html).

5.3.5 Direct Immunotoxicity and Indirectly Mediated Immunosuppression

Toxicants in the environment may produce immunological dysfunction by various mechanisms:

1) Damaging epithelial barriers of the integument, respiratory system, or digestive tracts.
2) Impairing the production or functions of mononuclear or granulocytic white blood cells, and other cells of the body that are involved in immune system regulation and response.
3) Killing organisms that normally provide food for an animal and thus inducing malnutrition or starvation.
4) For aquatic animals that rely on dissolved oxygen, either killing phytoplankton or aquatic macrophytes that produce oxygen, or spurring the growth of phytoplankton blooms that ultimately die and are broken down by oxidative metabolism – causing hypoxic stress (Stämpfli and Anderson, 2009; Dietert and Luebke, 2012; Vos, 2007; Tanner et al., 2006).

Direct toxicity affecting a variety of other organs can also secondarily stress animals or concurrently affect the adrenals or hypothalamic-adrenal axis, resulting in chronic elevations of endogenous glucocorticoids, potentially causing immune suppression (Lall and Dan, 1999; Hopkins et al., 1997). One recent report described exposures and considered the relevant literature in regard to immunotoxicity and other effects following the Deepwater Horizon oil spill in the Gulf of Mexico (Barron, 2012). The author described effects of the oil on aquatic invertebrates, fish, sea turtles, water birds, and marine mammals, which in some instances were consistent with immunological dysfunction. Polyaromatic hydrocarbon-associated immunotoxicity has been comparatively well documented in laboratory mice (Holladay and Smialowicz, 2000; Abdel-Shafy and Mansour, 2016). Of importance is that people and other animals with immunological dysfunction may experience increased microbial and parasitic infections, reduced surveillance and elimination of precancerous or cancerous cells, and potential autoimmunity that may play a role in widespread gut, respiratory, joint, cardiovascular, and neurological diseases.

5.3.6 Neurotoxicity

The challenge of sorting out neurotoxicity through behavioral and pathology studies typically involves comprehensive studies of laboratory animals (Moser, 2011), and there should be reservations about extrapolations to other species, especially those with unique adaptations. Whether laboratory rodents are strong predictors of thresholds of neurotoxicity for unique and diverse animals, such as echolocating bats or marine mammals, cannot readily be tested. Bats present a special case, not only because of echolocation to find prey – such as insects – and to avoid crash injuries, but also because they may be exposed in areas of agricultural production and commercial forestry to neurotoxic neonicotinoid, pyrethroid, carbamate, organophosphorus, and organochlorine insecticides. Concerns include not only poisoning of the bats but also potential elimination of insects that provide their food (Wickramasinghe et al., 2003). If insecticide deployment eliminates insectivores, such as bats, arachnids, and predatory insects, agricultural producers and forest managers may experience greater losses to insect pests.

Similarly, health experts may witness increased impacts of arthropod pests and vectors on human and animal populations in urban settings as well. As a consequence, they may have an incentive to keep applying pesticides thereafter. This insecticide dependency was described decades ago. Fortunately, problems can be offset via cautious application of integrated pest management, use of genetically modified plants that target pest insects more than pest predators, and "organic" methods of production (Cowan and Gunby, 1996; Amman, 2005; Wickramasinghe et al., 2003).

5.3.7 Endocrine Disruption

Endocrine disruption by chemical contaminants in the environment can result from compounds that: 1) interfere with either synthesis or metabolism of hormones; 2) act as agonists or antagonists at subsets of nuclear hormone receptors; 3) alter epigenetic modifications; or 4) otherwise disturb protein transcription, translation, folding, or action. Endocrine receptors tend to be responsive to low concentrations of agonists and antagonists, and thus low-level exposures may be relevant to health. Hormonal effects may be increased or decreased at any life stage, but such changes may be extraordinarily important during development. Shared environments and food sources, as well as biomagnification via the food web, may be of considerable importance across a range of exposed species, but different groups of scientists and stakeholders vary in their level of concern regarding the importance of endocrine disruption, particularly in regard to potential effects on human beings (Marty et al., 2011; Vandenberg et al., 2013).

The insecticide DDT was used in the USA from the late 1940s until 1972, when most uses were banned. DDT is estrogenic, and DDE, its persistent metabolite and environmental product, is anti-androgenic. The compounds are known for effects on the shell gland in the reproductive tract of birds, resulting in eggshell thinning, such that eggs could not withstand the weight of the parent during incubation (Lincer, 1975). Such effects were associated with declines in fish-eating birds in the wild. Similar effects on the shell gland and eggshell thickness were reproduced in chickens given either DDT or the exogenous synthetic estrogen, ethynylestradiol (Holm et al., 2006). A number of other species of vertebrates are also sensitive to DDT and DDE. Alligators in Lake Apopka, Florida, that were exposed to DDT and had elevated DDE in their adipose tissue were found to have reduced testosterone concentrations as well as smaller phallus size (Guillette et al., 1996). In human babies, higher residues in breast milk of a combination of organochlorine insecticides, including DDT and DDE, were associated with a greater likelihood of cryptorchid testicles (Damgaard et al., 2006). Also, in a large study in South Africa comparing male babies from homes and villages sprayed with DDT to those not sprayed, there was a 33% greater chance of the DDT-exposed individuals having a urogenital birth defect, especially cryptorchidism and chordee (abnormal downward curvature of the penis) (Bornan et al., 2009). Other reviews have associated residential spraying of DDT with increased pre-term abortion, stillbirth, and shortened lactation (Damstra et al., 2004; Longnecker et al., 2005). Overall, wild animals have proven to be important sentinels for endocrine disruption in the case of DDT and DDE. Insecticides should be compared with one another and considered in light of feasible malaria protection in different locales. Of note is that, since 2006, the World Health Organization has recommended indoor residual spraying of homes with DDT in areas at high risk of malaria infection, including throughout Africa. Of course, risks of malaria can be offset through reduced exposures to mosquitoes, and hence the benefits of bed nets, screens, other comparatively benign insecticides, and additional mosquito control technologies.

Compounds that induce aromatase (synonymous with Cyp19A1) activity increase the conversion of androgens to estrogens, and the resultant feminization may affect a range of species (Sanderson et al., 2001; Hayes et al., 2010). Aromatase is induced by age, obesity, insulin, gonadotropins, and ethanol. Effects of the aromatase inducer, atrazine, a widely used herbicide in the USA, have been well demonstrated in frogs. In studies of a susceptible strain of African clawed frogs, atrazine caused complete transitions of some of the genetic males to functional females; the sex-reversed frogs bred with males; and they produced (as would be expected), all male offspring. Adverse reproductive effects of atrazine in fish, amphibians, reptiles, and mammals have been reviewed (Hayes et al., 2011). Additional studies of the reproductive toxicity of atrazine and other triazine herbicides, including their effects on endangered species are warranted.

Agents of a wide variety of compounds of varied chemical structure influence the hypothalamic-pituitary-gonadal axis, such that they should be considered for their potential to cause endocrine disruption. In this regard, genomics and computational biology are being employed to predict and account for observed effects (Ankley et al., 2009). Natural hormones in sewage effluents and wastes from large numbers of food-producing animals, humans, birth control products, phytoestrogens, pesticides, industrial compounds, accidentally synthesized contaminants, and household chemicals that may be persistent or only briefly present in the environment and the body may be important in the lives of terrestrial and aquatic species, depending upon their exposure scenarios.

In addition to chemically induced changes in reproductive endocrine physiology, effects on thyroid hormone production, degradation, receptor activity, and regulation are also important (Roelens et al., 2005; Mensching et al., 2012; Chow et al., 2015). One possible challenge in regard to studies that attempt to link residues in the body to hyperthyroidism is that the higher metabolism of affected individuals may deplete adipose tissues, mobilizing and increasing biodegradation and elimination of POPs, potentially including those responsible for the problem at the outset.

While there may be a strong and understandable tendency to focus on organic molecules in regard to endocrine disruption, concerns regarding environmental pollution with heavy metals are also relevant. Piscivorous birds and methylmercury illustrate the concern. Common loons (*Gavia immer*) are fish-eating birds that often nest at oligotrophic (low dissolved nutrient) lakes that have waters with low pH and little buffering capacity (Burgess et al., 2005). In one such locale, Kejimkukik National Park in Nova Scotia, 92% of the birds had blood mercury concentrations that exceeded 4 μg/g (wet wt). Such concentrations in the blood of birds have been associated with impaired reproduction, elevated corticosterone levels, asymmetrical plumage, and abnormal breeding behaviors (Burgess et al., 2005; Frederick and Jayasena, (2010). Because of concerns regarding declining numbers of fish-eating birds in southern Florida, a study was performed in which fish contaminated with methylmercury at concentrations equivalent to those in the environment were fed to captive white ibises. The ibises given the methylmercury-contaminated fish had a mean blood total mercury concentration of approximately 4 μg/g (wet wt), essentially the same as in the loons above. Mercury caused reduced courtship behaviors in the male ibises, homosexual pairings, and an overall 30% decline in egg production. A number of other heavy metals have also been shown to exert endocrine-disrupting effects (Iavicoli et al., 2009). Heavy metal-induced endocrine disruption warrants greater study, including in human populations.

In addition to ubiquitous organic chemicals and heavy metals, nitrite and nitrate can act, perhaps through endogenous conversion to nitric oxide, to cause endocrine disruption in a number of vertebrate species, including alligators and fish (Guillette and Edwards, 2005; Jannat et al., 2014). Nitrite and nitrate become elevated in the environment due to nitrogen oxides produced by internal combustion engines, protein degradation products in human and animal wastes, and ammonia and other ubiquitous lawn, garden, and agricultural fertilizers.

Hypoxia is an endocrine-disrupting stressor that affects fish through reduced pituitary and gonadal hormone concentrations as well as through reduced sex steroid receptors. Today's high nutrient concentrations in water give rise to high phytoplankton and macrophyte densities. When a limiting nutrient is depleted or due to seasonal changes, the dominant photosynthetic organisms begin to die and their metabolism by aerobic decomposers consumes oxygen, causing hypoxic areas that become "dead zones." Such areas are present in both small and very large lakes, streams, estuaries, and coastal zones the world over (Smith et al., 2006; Wu et al., 2003; Thomas et al., 2007). Considering the depletion of aquatic species and abstraction of freshwater from streams and aquifers for agriculture and other human uses, greater attention to nutrient contamination and related endocrine disruption in aquatic vertebrates is warranted. To restore normal fish reproduction and other ecological functions will depend upon closing the nutrient loop through wiser waste management combined with residential lawn, garden, and agricultural stewardship, and far greater reliance on renewable energy sources.

5.3.8 Reproductive and Developmental Toxicity

Sensitive coordination of reproductive behaviors and physiology, coupled with extraordinary cellular differentiation and growth during development, give rise to unique susceptibility to toxic insult. Exposures to toxic agents can therefore threaten populations in the wild. One example of a common problem is petroleum. Petroleum exposures of fish induced P450 enzymes and caused marked abnormalities in developing embryos, sufficient to raise serious concerns regarding population reductions in the wild (Dubansky et al., 2013). Developing embryos in birds' eggs are also extraordinarily sensitive to petroleum toxicity, and as little as 1–10 μL/egg was lethal during early incubation (Leighton, 1993). Devastating reproductive impacts in birds of herbicides as well as PCBs, PCB derivatives, chlorinated dibenzodioxins and dibenzo-furans, and other industrial chemicals are also of concern (Fry, 1995).

5.4 Toxicological Risk Assessment and One Health

5.4.1 Risk Assessment

Toxicological risk assessment is the quantitative or qualitative estimate of risk related to a recognized chemical hazard. The interdependence of human and planetary health would argue for an integrated risk assessment process that combines risk estimation for humans, biota, and natural resources. Yet the methodologies for human health and ecological risk assessments developed independently and remain largely disconnected. The basic steps in the process are similar. *Human health risk assessment* includes: 1) hazard identification; 2) dose-response assessment; 3) exposure assessment; and 4) risk characterization. Hazard identification examines whether a toxicant has the potential to cause harm in one or more species. For example, a given hazard identification might focus exclusively on humans. Dose-response assessment examines the quantitative relationship between exposure and effects. Exposure assessment examines the frequency, timing, and routes of exposure for a given toxicant. Risk characterization involves estimating the probability of an adverse effect, taking into account data on variation in exposures and responses to the chemical in question (https://www.epa.gov/risk). Protection of humans, however, will not necessarily result in the protection of nonhuman organisms and ecosystems. Indeed, we tend to protect one another far more effectively than we protect many other species.

The steps in *ecological risk assessment* include formulation of the problem, analysis,

and characterization of the risk. The ecological risk assessor defines an assessment endpoint to determine what ecological entity is important to protect (a species, community, ecosystem, or habitat) and conducts an analysis of the threat taking into account factors such as hazard quotients, bioavailability, and bioaccumulation in order to characterize the risk. Given the commonalities of mechanisms of action among human and ecological receptors, it would seem more efficient to estimate and manage toxicological risks holistically rather than separately. Recent attention in this direction is hopeful. *"Integrated risk assessment"* combines the processes of risk estimation for humans, biota, and natural resources (Reis et al., 2015). One Health approaches to integrated risk assessment are still under development but, given the interdependence of humans and their environment, closer interaction between the public health and ecosystem scientists is essential for the protection of our planet and the myriad species that it sustains.

5.4.2 Regulatory Toxicology

Regulatory toxicology encompasses the collection, processing, and evaluation of epidemiologic and experimental toxicology data to make scientifically sound decisions for the protection of health from harmful chemicals in our environment (Patel and Miller, 2012). In most cases, toxicological risk assessments have to rely on animal data. The extrapolation of an acceptable daily intake of a chemical from animals to humans can involve considerable uncertainty. Regulators typically divide the doses deemed to be safe from experimental toxicology studies in animals by uncertainty factors to estimate safe doses in humans (Steel, 2011). These uncertainty factors take into account: 1) interspecies extrapolation; 2) intraspecies variation; 3) extrapolation from subchronic to chronic toxicity; 4) extrapolation from a Lowest Observable Adverse Effect Level (LOAEL) to a No Observable Adverse Effect Level (NOAEL); and, when applicable, 5) a

Modifying Factor for residual uncertainties such as incomplete data.

The explosive growth in the chemical and pharmaceutical industry has created a large backlog for untested chemicals. It is estimated that the demand for testing will increase by fifteen-fold over the next decade (Rowlands et al., 2014). To meet this demand, chemical risk assessment is moving away from *in vivo* testing to testing *in vitro* (Tralau et al., 2015). In the USA, several regulatory agencies protect humans from toxicants. These include the Occupational Safety and Health Agency for workplace chemicals, the Food and Drug Administration for food and pharmaceuticals, and the United States Environmental Protection Agency (EPA) for chemicals in air, water, and soil. The Clean Air Act, the Clean Water Act, and the Comprehensive Environmental Response, Compensation, and Liability Act of 1980 (CERCLA, or Superfund) are important laws implemented by the EPA in concert with the states and the private sector that have reduced exposures and adverse impacts of chemicals on human, animal, and ecosystem health.

Regulatory ecotoxicology covers the protection of various species and ecosystems from toxicants, and authority is shared among governmental agencies. For example, the US Department of Interior, Fish and Wildlife Service, National Oceanographic and Atmospheric Administration, and National Marine Fisheries Service implement the development and enforcement of policies required for the Federal Endangered Species Act, Migratory Species Act, and other biological resource laws – and toxicants are among the stressors that must be considered. The US Food and Drug Administration, through its Center for Veterinary Medicine, regulates animal feed, and the US Department of Agriculture and the Public Health Service regulate humaneness for animal studies.

Previously mentioned in regard to regulatory toxicology were TSCA, TSCA reform, and REACH. Also mentioned was that companies are also contributing to pollution prevention by adopting a "green chemistry" approach.

In addition, corporate social responsibility initiatives are having some positive impacts (Institute of Medicine, 2007). To date, however, there has been little effort to adopt a One Health approach to regulatory toxicology. Future progress on One Health policymaking will likely depend on the advances in risk science, in particular on the success of efforts at integrated risk assessment.

5.4.3 One Health and One Toxicology on One Earth

While individual countries may have a robust regulatory framework for the assessment and management of toxicological risks, the reality of the global marketplace means that protection of borders is no longer a viable regulatory framework (Patel and Miller, 2012). Similarly, the trans-boundary movement of environmental toxicants can only be controlled through international regulatory frameworks. Toxicants such as POPs and mercury can migrate, bioaccumulate, and biomagnify in pristine areas of the planet thousands of miles from their points of emission.

The current global governance framework to address environmental health and sustainability evolved from a series of international meetings, reports, and commissions. Today there are several hundred international agreements aimed at protecting our global commons. In 1953, the World Health Assembly, which was the governing body of the World Health Organization (WHO), stated that the widening use of chemicals in food presented a new public health problem and charged WHO and the Food and Agricultural Organization (FAO) with the responsibility of undertaking relevant studies. This led to creation of the Codex Alimentarius in 1962, which seeks to harmonize food safety standards around the globe. The United Nations Conference on Human Health and Environment, held in Stockholm in 1972, moved national environmental concerns into the international political agenda and led to the establishment of the United Nations Environment Program (UNEP).

Among its many tasks, UNEP is working on the Strategic Approach to Chemicals Management. In 1987, the Brundtland Commission report on "Our Common Future" addressed the issue of sustainable development and influenced the Earth Summit in Rio de Janeiro in 1992 (Gudmundsson et al., 2016). The Global Environmental Facility (GEF), which was established as a separate institution from the World Bank following the Rio Summit, provides funding to developing nations to cover the incremental costs associated with transforming a project with national benefits into one with global environmental benefits.

Among the several international treaties aimed at addressing toxicants in our environment, the most successful has been the Montreal Protocol on Substances that Deplete the Ozone Layer (1987) (Winchester, 2009). Other treaties that specifically address toxicants include the Stockholm Convention on Persistent Organic Pollutants (1991), the Basel Convention on the Control of Transboundary Movements of Hazardous Wastes and Their Disposal (1992), and the Minamata Convention on Mercury (2013). A limitation of these treaties is that they need to be ratified by national governments even after they are signed. The Basel Convention, for example, has been ratified by only half of the countries needed to put it into force.

International bodies such as WHO, FAO, and UNEP can provide advice and guidance, but they lack the ability to enforce international agreements. Moreover, international environmental responsibilities, rather than being consolidated within UNEP, have been spread across multiple organizations, including other agencies within the UN system, the Bretton Woods institutions (e.g., the World Bank), the secretariats of Multilateral Environmental Agreements, and the World Trade Organization (WTO) (Ivanova and Roy, 2007). The WTO aims to promote trade by removing tariff and nontariff barriers. Although WTO permits measures to protect human, animal, or plant life or health,

other provisions make this exception difficult to sustain in practice. For example, a country can be required to prove that its laws and regulations represent alternatives that are least restrictive in regard to trade. The WTO Committee on Trade and Environment adjudicates issues of environment and sustainability as they pertain to the management of conditions for trade between states (Friel et al., 2015). Under these agreements, governments are facing some loss of sovereignty in policy-making that is pertinent to public health. The lack of an effective global governing framework to protect the global commons has resulted in a disaggregation of authority to multiple centers around the world. The political vacuum has been filled by nonstate actors such as non-governmental organizations and the private sector (Lee and Kamradt-Scott, 2014). This organizational multiplicity in the global environmental governance system has made it difficult to incorporate the One Health approach in these institutions (Lee and Brumme, 2012). Nevertheless, the interdependence of humans and the planet's ecosystems makes it imperative that we overcome an anthropocentric approach to global governance and realize that human health is ultimately dependent on the health of our planet. The recent (2015) adoption of the 2030 Agenda for Sustainable Development by the UN General Assembly offers opportunities to incorporate the One World, One Health approach into meaningful global action (Lueddeke, 2016).

5.5 Conclusions

The One Health approach views human health as inseparable from the health of the planet as a whole (King et al., 2008; Whitmee et al., 2015). Paradoxically, the advances in human health over the past several decades have coincided with vast degradation of our ecosystems. Humans have walled out climatic stress with climate-controlled buildings, protected and purified drinking water, and washed and cooked food. But, many domestic animals and all wild species do not live in our "protected bubble." As we have taken lands that were essential habitats, overharvested game, fish, and shellfish, and emitted toxic chemicals that undermine a variety of health forms we have created stressed and failing ecosystems that can no longer serve us or other species for the long term. Our species has traded off many of the planet's supportive processes by mortgaging the health of current and future generations of humans and nonhumans alike.

Wild ecosystems, plants, and animals provide essential ecosystem services and they have their own inherent value (van der Tuuk, 1999; de Groot et al., 2012; Curtin, 2009). A sustainable Earth relies upon vast biodiversity to regulate the atmosphere and climate, to produce soil, to purify the air and water, to pollinate and protect plants from pests and diseases, to protect animals from pests and diseases, and to confer natural beauty and a rational sense of well-being. Wiser applications of technologies including renewable energy, integrated pest management, selective use of genetically modified organisms in agriculture, pollution controls in industry and transportation, using native plants and avoiding pesticides in residential areas, careful nutrient management, and buffers as well as cover crops to protect water bodies from nutrients and pesticides, are urgent necessities now and will remain so in the future.

Toxic insult can be avoided through a deeper understanding of mechanisms of chemical action in living organisms, more comprehensive and efficient surveillance, faster and more reliable diagnoses, more effective interventions, and especially more astute prevention. Accordingly, molecular, clinical, diagnostic, environmental, ecological, and regulatory toxicologists all have parts to play in keeping humans and ecosystems alive, but for them to succeed in optimizing benefits for humans, plants, and animals, they must be nested in and rely upon other medical professionals, as well as the society at large.

References

Abdel-Shafy, H.I. and Mansour, M.S.M. (2016). A review on polycyclic aromatic hydrocarbons: source, environmental impact, effect on human health and remediation. *Egyptian Journal of Petroleum* 256, 107–123.

Aguirre, A.A., Beasley, V.R., Augspurger, T., Benson, W.H., Whaley, J., and Basu, N. (2016). One health – Transdisciplinary opportunities for SETAC leadership in integrating and improving the health of people, animals, and the environment. *Environmental Toxicology and Chemistry* 35(10), 2383–2391.

Amman, K. (2005). Effects of biotechnology on biodiversity: herbicide-tolerant and insect-resistant GM crops. *Trends in Biotechnology* 23, 388–394.

Ankley, G.T., Bencic, D.C., Breen, M.S., et al. (2009). Endocrine disrupting chemicals in fish: developing exposure indicators and predictive models based on mechanisms of action. *Aquatic Toxicology* 92, 168–178.

Arnemo, J.M., Andersen, O., Stokke, S., et al. (2016). Health and environmental risks from lead-based ammunition: science versus socio-politics. *EcoHealth* 13, 618–622.

Avery, D. and Watson, R.T. (2009). Regulation of lead-based ammunition around the world. In: Watson, R.T., Fuller, M.R., and Pokras, M. (eds), *Ingestion of Lead from Spent Ammunition: Implications for Wildlife and Humans*, 1st edn. Peregrine Fund, pp. 161–168.

Barron, M.G. (2012). Ecological impacts of the Deepwater Horizon oil spill: implications for immunotoxicity. *Toxicologic Pathology* 40, 315–320.

Bashir, M., Umar-Tsafe, N., Getso, K., et al. (2014). Assessment of blood lead levels among children aged < 5 years – Zamfara State, Nigeria, June-July 2012. *MMWR* 63(15), 325–327.

Bautista, A.C., Puschner, B., and Poppenga, R.H. (2014) Lead exposure from backyard chicken eggs: a public health risk? *Journal of Medical Toxicology* 10, 311–315.

Beasley, V. (2009). 'One Toxicology', 'Ecosystem Health', and 'One Health'. *Veterinaria Italiana* 45, 97–110.

Beasley, V.R. (2011) Pathophysiology and clinical manifestations of mycotoxin and phycotoxin poisonings. *Egyptian Journal of Natural Toxins* 8, 104–133.

Beasley, V.R. and Adkesson, A.M. (2012). Wildlife and ecosystem health. In: Norrgren, L. and Levengood, J.A. (eds), *Ecosystem Health and Sustainable Agriculture, Volume 3: Ecology and Animal Health*. Uppsala: Baltic University Press, pp. 13–26 and 329.

Beasley, V.R. and Levengood, J.M. (2012). Principles of ecotoxicology. In: Gupta, R.C. (ed.), *Veterinary Toxicology*. New York: Academic Press, pp. 83–855.

Boatman, N.G., Brickle, N.W., Justin, J.D., et al. (2004). Evidence for the indirect effects of pesticides on farmland birds. *Ibis* 146(s2), 131–143.

Bornan, R., de Jager, C., Worku, Z., Farias, P., and Reif, S. (2009. DDT and urogenital malformations in newborn boys in a malarial area. *BJU International* 106, 405–411.

Buckmaster, P.S., Wen, X., Toyada, I., Gulland, F.M., and Van Bonn, W. (2014). Hippocampal neuropathology of domoic acid-induced epilepsy in California sea lions (*Zalophus californianus*). *Journal of Comparative Neurology* 522, 1691–1706.

Burgess, N.M., Evers, D.C., and Kaplan, J.D. (2005). Mercury and other contaminants in common loons breeding in Atlantic Canada. *Ecotoxicology* 14, 241–252.

Burrell, G.A. and Seibert, F. (1916). Gases found in coal mines. In: Burrell, G.A. and Seibert, F. (eds), *Gases Found in Coal Mines* (Miner's Circular 14. Department of the Interior, Bureau of Mines). Washington, DC: Government Printing Office, pp. 5–23.

Buttke, D.E. (2011).Toxicology, environmental health, and the "One Health" concept. *Journal of Medical Toxicology* 7, 329–332.

Carson, R., Darling, L., and Darling, L. (1962). *Silent Spring*. Cambridge, MA: Houghton Mifflin/Riverside Press.

Chen, D., Hale, R.C., and Letcher, R.J. (2015). Photochemical and microbial transformation of emerging flame retardants: Cause for concern? *Environmental Toxicology and Chemistry* 34, 687–699.

Chow, K., Hearn, L.K., Zuber, M., Beatty, J.A., Mueller, J.F., and Barrs, V.R. (2015). Evaluation of polybrominated diphenyl ethers (PBDEs) in matched cat sera and house dust samples: investigation of a potential link between PBDEs and spontaneous feline hyperthyroidism. *Environmental Research* 136, 173–179.

Cipro, C.V.Z., Colabuono, F.I., Taniguchi, S., and Montone, R.C. (2013) Persistent organic pollutants in bird, fish, and invertebrate samples from King George Island, Antarctica. *Antarctic Science* 25, 545–552.

Cohen, S.M. (1998). Cell proliferation and carcinogenesis. *Drug Metabolism Reviews* 30(2), 339–357.

Cohen, S.M., Arnold, L.L., Cano, M., Ito, M., Garland, E.M., and Shaw, R.A. (2000). Calcium phosphate-containing precipitate and the carcinogenicity of sodium salts in rats. *Carcinogenesis* 21(4), 783–792.

Colborn, T., Dumanoski, D., and Myers, J.P. (1996). *Our Stolen Future : Are We Threatening Our Fertility, Intelligence, and Survival?: A Scientific Detective Story*. New York: Dutton.

Cook, P.F., Reichmuth, C., Rouse, A.A., et al. (2015). Algal toxin impairs sea lion memory and hippocampal connectivity, with implications for strandings. *Ecotoxicology* 350, 1545–1547.

Cowan, R. and Gunby, P. (1996). Sprayed to death: path dependence, lock-in and pest control strategies. *The Economic Journal* 106, 521–542.

Curtin, S. (2009). Wildlife tourism: the intangible, psychological benefits of human-wildlife encounters. *Animals in the Tourism and Leisure Experience* 12, 451–474.

Damgaard, I.N., Skakkebaek, N.E., Toppari, J., et al. (2006). Persistent pesticides in human breast milk and cryptorchidism. *Environmental Health Perspectives* 114, :1133–1138.

Damstra, T., Barlow, S., Bergman, A., Kavlock, R., and Van Der Kraak, G. (eds) (2004). Global Assessment of the State-of-the-Science of Endocrine Disruptors. International Programme on Chemical Safety. Geneva: World Health Organization. Available at: http://www.who.int/ipcs/publications/new_issues/endocrine_disruptors/en/ (accessed November 24, 2017).

de Groot, R., Brander, L., van der Ploeg, S., et al. (2012). Global estimates of the value of ecosystems and their services in monetary units. *Ecosystem Services* 1, 50–61.

Diamanti-Kandarakis, E., Bourguignon, J.P., Giudice, L.C., et al. (2009). Endocrine-disrupting chemicals: an Endocrine Society scientific statement. *Endocrine Reviews* 30(4), 293–342.

Dietert, R.R. and Luebke, R.W. (2012). *Immunotoxicity, Immune Dysfunction, and Chronic Disease.* New York: Springer.

Doss, M. (2013). Linear no-threshold model vs. radiation hormesis. *Dose Response* 11, 480–497.

Dubansky, B., Whitehead, A., Miller, J.T., Rice, C.D., and Galvez, F. (2013). Multitissue molecular, genomic, and developmental effects of the Deepwater Horizon oil spill on resident Gulf killifish (*Fundulus grandis*). *Environmental Science & Technology* 47, 5074–5082.

Eaton, D.L. and Gallagher, E.P. (1994). Mechanisms of aflatoxin carcinogenesis. *Annual Review of Pharmacology and Toxicology* 34, 135–172.

Eddleston, M., Buckley, N.A., Eyer, P., and Dawson, A.H. (2008). Management of acute organophosphorus pesticide poisoning. *Lancet* 371, 597–607.

Epstein, L. (2014). Fifty years since Silent Spring. *Annual Review of Phytopathology* 52, 377–402.

Esty, D.C. and Porter, M.E. (2005). National Environmental Performance: An Empirical Analysis of Policy Results and Determinants. Faculty Scholarship Series, Paper 430. Available at: http://digitalcommons.law.yale.edu/fss_papers/430 (accessed November 27, 2017).

Eto, K. (1997). Pathology of Minamata disease. *Toxicologic Pathology* 25(6), 614–623.

Fachehoun, R.C., Lévesque, B., Dumas, P., St Louis, A., Dubé, M., and Ayotte, P. (2015). Lead exposure through consumption of big game meat in Quebec, Canada: risk assessment and perception. *Food Additives & Contaminants: Part A* 32, 1501–1511.

Falconer, I.R. and Humpage, A.R. (2005). Health risk assessment of cyanobacterial (blue-green algal) toxins in drinking water. *International Journal of Environmental Research and Public Health* 2, 43–50.

Férard, J-F. and Blaise, C. (eds) (2013). *Encyclopedia of Aquatic Ecotoxicology.* Dordrecht: Springer.

Finkelstein, M.E., Doak, D.F., George, D., et al. (2012). Lead poisoning and the deceptive recovery of the critically endangered California condor. *Proceedings of the National Academy of Sciences of the USA* 109, 11449–11454.

Fox, G.A. (2001). Effects of endocrine disrupting chemicals on wildlife in Canada: past, present, and future. *Water Quality Research Journal Canada* 36, 233–251.

Fraser, A.J., Burkow, I.C., Wolkers, H., and Mackay, D. (2002). Modeling biomagnification and metabolism of contaminants in harp seals of the Barents Sea. *Environmental Toxicology and Chemistry* 21, 55–61.

Friel, S., Hattersley, L., and Townsend, R. (2015). Trade policy and public health. *Annual Review of Public Health* 36, 325–344.

Frederick, P. and Jayasena, N. (2010). Altered pairing behaviour and reproductive success in white ibises exposed to environmentally relevant concentrations of methylmercury.

Proceedings of the Royal Society B 278, 1851–1857.

Fry, D.M. (1995). Reproductive effects in birds exposed to pesticides and industrial chemicals. *Environmental Health Perspectives* 103(Suppl. 7), 165–171.

Giesy, J.P. and Kannan, K. (2002). Perfluorinated surfactants in the environment. *Environmental Science & Technology* 36, 147A–152A.

Goldstein, T., Mazet, J.A.K., Zabka, T.S., et al. (2008). Novel symptomatology and changing epidemiology of domoic acid toxicosis in California sea lions (*Zalophus californianus*): an increasing risk to marine mammal health. *Proceedings of the Royal Society B* 275, 267–276.

Goméz, M.J., Pazos, F., Guijarro, F.J., de Lorenzo, V., and Valencia, A. (2007). The environmental fate of organic pollutants through the global microbial metabolism. *Molecular Systems Biology* 3; Art. No. 114: doi:10.1038/msb4100156.

Gouin, T., Mackay, D., Jones, K.C., Harner, T., and Meijer, S.N. (2004). Evidence for the "grasshopper" effect and fractionation during long-range atmospheric transport of organic contaminants. *Environmental Pollution* 128, 139–148.

Green, R.E. and Pain, D.J. (2012). Potential health risks to adults and children in the UK from exposure to dietary lead in gamebirds shot with lead ammunition. *Food and Chemical Toxicology* 50, 4180–4190.

Green, R.E., Grainger Hunt, W., Parish, C.N., and Newton, I. (2008). Effectiveness of action to reduce exposure of free-ranging California condors in Arizona and Utah to lead from spent ammunition. *PloS One* 3, e4022.

Gudmundsson, H., Hall, R.P., Marsden, G., Zietsman, J. (2016). Sustainable development. In: *Sustainable Transportation, Indicators, Frameworks, and Performance Management*. Springer, Ppp. 15–49.

Guillette, L.J. Jr and Edwards, T.M. (2005). Is nitrate an ecologically relevant endocrine disruptor in vertebrates? *Integrative & Comparative Biology* 45, 19–27.

Guillette, L.J. Jr, Pickford, D.B., Crain, D.A., Rooney, A.A., and Percival, H.F. (1996). Reduction in penis size and plasma testosterone concentrations in juvenile alligators living in a contaminated environment. *General and Comparative Endocrinology* 101, 32–42.

Gulland, F.M.D., Haulena, M., Fauquier, D., et al. (2002) Domoic acid toxicity in California sea lions (*Zalophus californianus*): clinical signs, treatment and survival. *Veterinary Record* 150, 475–480.

Hallmann, C.A., Foppen, R.P.B., van Turnhout, C.A.M., de Kroon, H., and Jongejans, E. (2014). Declines in insectivorous birds are associated with high neonicotinoid concentrations. *Nature* 511, 341–343.

Halstead, N., Johnson, S.A., McMahon, T.A., and Rohr, J.R. (2011). Agrochemicals increase risk of human schistosomiasis. Conference Paper. *96th Ecological Society of America Convention*.

Haukås, M., Berger, U., Hop, H., Bulliksen, B., and Gabrielson, G.W. (2007). Bioaccumulation of per- and polyfluorinated alkyl substances (PFAS) in selected species from the Barents sea food web. *Environmental Pollution* 148, 360–371.

Hayes, A.N. (2005). The precautionary principle. *Archives of Industrial Hygiene and Toxicology* 56(2), 161–166.

Hayes, T.B., Khoury, V., Narayan, A., et al. (2010). Atrazine induces complete feminization and chemical castration in male African clawed frogs (*Xenopus laevis*). *Proceedings of the National Academy of Sciences of the USA* 107, 4612–4616.

Hayes, T.B., Anderson, L.L., Beasley, V.R., et al. (2011). Demasculinization and feminization of male gonads by atrazine: consistent across vertebrate classes. *Journal of Steroid Biochemistry and Molecular Biology* 127, 64–73.

Heindel, J.J., Newbold, R., and Schug, T.T. (2015). Endocrine disruptors and obesity. *Nature Reviews Endocrinology* 11(11), 653–661.

Hilborn, E.D. and Beasley, V.R. (2015). One Health and cyanobacteria in freshwater systems: animal illnesses and deaths as sentinel events for human health risk. *Toxins* 7, 1374–1395.

Holladay, S.D. and Smialowicz, R.J. (2000). Development of the murine and human immune system: differential effects of immunotoxicants depend on time of exposure. *Environmental Health Perspectives* 108, 463–473.

Holm, L., Blomqvist, A., Brandt, I., Brunström, B., Ridderstråle, Y., and Berg, C. (2006). Embryonic exposure to *o,p'*-DDT causes eggshell thinning and altered shell gland carbonic anhydrase expression in the domestic hen. *Environmental Toxicology and Chemistry* 25, 2787–2793.

Holt, E.A. and Miller, S.W. (2010). Bioindicators: using organisms to measure environmental impacts. *Nature Educational Knowledge* 3, 8.

Hopkins, W.A., Mendonça, M.T., and Congdon, J.D. (1997). Increased circulating levels of testosterone and corticosterone in southern toads, *Bufo terrestris*, exposed to coal combustion waste. *General and Comparative Endocrinology* 108, 237–246.

Iavicoli, I., Fontana, L., and Bergamaschi, A. (2009). The effects of metals as endocrine disruptors. *Journal of Environmental Health B, Critical Reviews* 12, 206–223.

Institute of Medicine (2007). Global Environmental Health in the 21st Century. From Governmental Regulation to Corporate Social Responsibility. Available at: http://www.nap.edu/catalog/11833.html (accessed November 27, 2017).

Iqbal, S., Blumenthal, W., Kennedy, C., et al. (2009). Hunting with lead: association between blood lead levels and wild game consumption. *Environmental Research* 109, 952–959

Ivanova, M. and Roy, J. (2007). The architecture of global environmental governance: pros and cons of multiplicity. Center for UN Reform Education. Available at: http://www.centerforunreform. org/?q=node/234 (accessed November 27, 2017).

Jannat, M., Fatimah, R., and Kishida, M. (2014). Nitrate (NO_3^-) and nitrite (NO_2^-) are endocrine disruptors to downregulate expression of tyrosine hydroxylase and motor behavior through conversion to nitric oxide in early development of zebrafish. *Biochemical and Biophysical Research Communications* 452, 608–613.

Jeffrey, B., Barlow, T., Moizer, K., Paul, S., and Boyle, C. (2004). Amnesic shellfish poison. *Food and Chemical Toxicology* 42, 545–557.

Johnson, C.K., Kelly, T.R., and Rideoout, T.A. (2013). Lead in ammunition: a persistent threat to health and conservation. *EcoHealth* 10, 455–464.

Jorgensen, E. (2010), *Ecotoxicology*, 1st edn. Amsterdam: Academic Press.

Kelly, T.R., Grantham, J, George, D., et al. (2014). Spatiotemporal patterns and risk factors for lead exposure in endangered California condors during 15 years of reintroduction. *Conservation Biology* 28, 1721–1730.

King, L.J., Anderson, L.R., Blackmore, C.G., et al. (2008). Executive summary of the AVMA One Health Initiative Task Force report. *JAVMA* 233(2), 259.

Kirchner, M., Faus-Kessler, T., Jakobi, G., et al. (2009). Vertical distribution of organochlorine pesticides in humus along Alpine altitudinal profiles in relation to ambiental parameters. *Environmental Pollution* 157, 3238–3247.

Lall,, S.B. and Dan, G. (1999). Role of corticosteroids in cadmium induced immunotoxicity. *Drug and Chemical Toxicology* 22, 401–409.

Lanphear, B.P., Hornung, T., Khoury, J., et al. (2005). Low-level environmental lead exposure and children's intellectual function: an international pooled analysis. *Environmental Health Perspectives* 113(7), 894–899.

Lee, K. and Brumme, Z.L.(2013). Operationalizing the One Health approach: the global governance challenge. *Health Policy and Planning* 28, 778–785.

Lee, K. and Kamradt-Scott, A. (2014). The multiple meanings of global health governance: a call for conceptual clarity. *Globalization and Health* 12, 28.

Lefebvre, K.A., Bargu, S., Kieckhefer, T., and Silver, M.W. (2002). From sanddabs to blue whales: the pervasiveness of domoic acid. *Toxicon* 40, 971–977.

Leighton, F.A. (1993). The toxicity of petroleum oils to birds. *Environmental Reviews* 1, 92–103.

Levengood, J.M. and Beasley, V.R. (2007). Principles of ecotoxicology. In: Gupta, R.C. (ed.), *Veterinary Toxicology*. New York: Elsevier, pp. 689–708.

Levengood, J.M. and Beasley, V.R. (2012). Ecotoxicology. In: Aguirre, A.A., Ostfeld, R.S., and Daszak, P. (eds), *Conservation Medicine: Applied Cases of Ecological Health*. New York: Oxford University Press, pp. 345–358.

Lincer, J.L. (1975). DDE-induced eggshell-thinning in the American kestrel: A comparison of the field situation and laboratory results. *Journal of Applied Ecology* 12, 781–793.

Longnecker, M.P., Klebanoff, M.A., Dunson, D.B., Guo, X., Zhou, H., and Brock, J.W. (2005). Maternal serum level of the DDT metabolite DDE in relation to fetal loss in previous pregnancies. *Environmental Research* 97, 127–133.

Luckey, T.D. (2006). Radiation hormesis: the good, the bad, and the ugly. *Dose Response* 4(3), 169–190.

Lueddeke, G. (2016). Achieving the UN-2030 Sustainable Development Goals through the 'One World, One Health' concept. *Oxford Public Health Magazine* 4, 36–40.

Lürling, M. and Roessink, M. (2006). On the way to cyanobacterial blooms: impact of the herbicide metribuzin on the competition between a green alga (*Scenedesmus*) and a cyanobacterium (*Microcystis*). *Chemosphere* 65, 618–626.

Mackay, D. and Fraser, A. (2000). Bioaccumulation of persistent organic chemicals: mechanisms and models. *Environmental Pollution* 110, 375–391.

Maffini, M.V., Rubin, B.S., Sonnenschein, C., and Soto, A.M. (2006). Endocrine disruptors and reproductive health: the case of bisphenol-A. *Molecular and Cellular Endocrinology* 254-255, 179–186.

Martineau, D. (2012) Contaminants and health of beluga whales of the Saint Lawrence Estuary. In: Norrgren, L. and Levengood, J.M. (eds), *Ecosystem Health and Sustainable Agriculture 2: Ecology and Animal Health*. Uppsala: Baltic University Press, pp. 139–148 and 342–346.

Marty, M.S., Carney, E.W., and Rowlands, J.C. (2011). Endocrine disruption: historical perspectives and its impact on the future of toxicology testing. *Toxicological Sciences* 120, S93–S108.

Mensching, D.A., Slater, M., Scott, J.W., Ferguson, D.C., and Beasley, V.R. (2012). The feline thyroid gland: a model for endocrine disruption by polybrominated biphenyl ethers (PBDEs)? *Journal of Toxicology and Environmental Health A* 75, 201–212.

Morgan, R.V. (1994). Lead poisoning in small companion animals: an update (1987-1992). *Veterinary and Human Toxicology* 36, 18–22.

Moser, V.C. (2011). Functional assays for neurotoxicity testing. *Toxicologic Pathology* 39, 36–45.

Moses, S.K., Whiting, A.V., Bratton, G.R., Taylor, R.J., and O'Hara, T.M. (2009). Inorganic nutrients and contaminants in subsistence species of Alaska: linking wildlife and human health. *International Journal of Circumpolar Health* 68, 53–74.

National Cancer Institute (2010). Reducing Environmental Cancer Risk: What We Can Do Now. 2008–2009 Annual Report, President's Cancer Panel. Available at: http://deainfo.nci.nih.gov/advisory/pcp/annualReports/pcp08-09rpt/PCP_Report_08-09_508.pdf (accessed November 27. 2017).

National Research Council (2014). *A Framework to Guide Selection of Chemical Alternatives*. Washington, DC: National Academies Press.

Needleman, H. (2003). Lead poisoning. *Annual Review of Medicine* 55, 209–222.

Newman, M.C. (2009). *Fundamentals of Ecotoxicology*, 3rd edn. Boca Raton, FL: CRC Press.

Newman, M.C. and Clements, W.H. (2008). *Ecotoxicology: A Comprehensive Treatment.* Boca Raton, FL: CRC Press.

New Zealand Ministry for the Environment (2009). Mercury Inventory for New Zealand: 2008. Publication CR 76. Available at: http://www.mfe.govt.nz/publications/waste/mercury-inventory-new-zealand-2008 (accessed November 27. 2017).

Niculescu, A.M. (1985). Effects of in utero exposure to DES on male progeny. *Journal of Obstetric, Gynecologic and Neonatal Nursing* 14(6), 468–470.

NOAA (2015). NOAA fisheries mobilizes to gauge unprecedented West Coast toxic algal bloom. National Oceanic and Atmospheric Administration. Available at: http://www.westcoast.fisheries.noaa.gov/mediacenter/6.15.2015_final_algal_bloom_pr.pdf (accessed 27 November, 2017).

Nyman, J.A. (1999). Effect of crude oil and chemical additives on metabolic activity of mixed microbial populations in fresh marsh soils. *Microbial Ecology* 37, 152–162.

Patel, M. and Miller, A. (2012). Impact of regulatory science on global public health. *Kaohsiung Journal of Medical Sciences* 28, S5–S9.

Perl, T.M., Bédard, L., Kosatsky, T., Hockin, J.C., Todd, E.C., and Remis, R.S. (1990). An outbreak of toxic encephalopathy caused by eating mussels contaminated with domoic acid. *New England Journal of Medicine* 322, 1775–1780.

Reddy, M.L., Dierauf, L.A., and Gulland, F.M.D. (2001). Marine mammals as sentinels of ocean health. In: Direauf, L. and Gulland, F.M.D. (eds), *CRC Handbook of Marine Mammal Medicine: Health, Disease, and Rehabilitation*, 2nd edn. Boca Raton, FL: CRC Press, pp. 3–13.

Reif, J.S. (2011). Animal sentinels for environmental and public health. *Public Health Report* 126(Suppl. 1), 50–57.

Reis, S., Morris, G., Fleming, L.E., et al. (2015). Integrating health and environmental impact analysis. *Public Health* 129, 1383–1389.

Rideout, B.A., Stalis, I., Papendick, R., et al. (2012). Patterns of mortality in free-ranging California condors (*Gymnogyps californianus*). *Journal of Wildlife Diseases* 48, 95–112.

Roelens, S.A., Aerts, B.V., Clerens, S., et al. (2005). Neurotoxicity of polychlorinated biphenyls (PCBs) by disturbance of thyroid hormone-regulated genes. *Annals of the New York Academy of Sciences* 1040, 454–456.

Rohr, J.R., Schotthoefer, A,M., Raffel, T.R., et al. (2008). Agrochemicals increase trematode infections in a declining amphibian species. *Nature* 455, 1235–1239.

Rosseland, B.O., Eldhuset, T.D., and Staurnes, M. (1990). Environmental effects of aluminum. *Environmental Geochemistry and Health* 12, 17–27.

Rowlands, J.C., Sander, M., and Bus, J.S. (2014). FutureTox: Building the road for 21st century toxicology and risk assessment practices. *Toxicological Sciences* 137(2), 269–277.

Rumbeiha, W.K. (2012). Toxicology and "One Health": Opportunities for multidisciplinary collaborations. *Journal of Medical Toxicology* 8(2), 91–93.

Sanderson, J.T., Letcher, R.J., Heneweer, M., Giesy, J.P., and van den berg, M. (2001). Effects of chloro-s-triazine herbicides and metabolites on aromatase activity in various human cell lines and on vitellogenin production in male carp hepatocytes. *Environmental Health Perspectives* 109, 1027–1031.

Scholin, C.A., Gulland, F., Doucette, G.J., et al. (2000). Mortality of sea lions along the central California coast linked to toxic diatom bloom. *Nature* 403, 80–84.

Scott, B.R., Walker, D.M., Tesfaigzi, Y., Schollnberger, H., and Walker, V. (2003). Mechanistic basis for nonlinear dose-response relationships for low-dose radiation-induced stochastic effects. *Nonlinearity in Biology, Toxicology and Medicine* 1(1), 93–122.

SEHN (Science & Environmental Health Network) (1998). Wingspread Conference on the Precautionary Principle. Available at: http://sehn.org/wingspread-conference-on-the-precautionary-principle/ (accessed November 27, 2017).

Senior, C.L., Sarofim, A.F., Zeng, T., Helble, J.J., and Mamani-Paco, R. (2000). Gas-phase transformations of mercury in coal-fired power plants. *Fuel Processing Technology* 63, 197–213.

Seubert, E.L., Gellene, A.G., Howard. M.D., et al. (2013). Seasonal and annual dynamics of harmful algae and algal toxins revealed through weekly monitoring at two coastal ocean sites off of southern California, USA. *Environmental Science and Pollution Research* 20, 6878–6895.

Siegel, F.R. (2002). Heavy metals mobility/immobility in environmental media. In: Siegel, F.R. (ed.), *Environmental Geochemistry of Potentially Toxic Metals*. Berlin/Heidelberg: Springer-Verlag, pp. 45–59.

Smith, E.A. and Mayfield, C.I. (1978). Paraquat: determination, degradation and mobility in soil. *Water, Air and Soil Pollution* 9, 439–452.

Smith, V.H., Joye, S.B., and Howarth, R.W. (2006). Eutrophication of freshwater and marine ecosystems. *Limnology and Oceanography* 51, 351–355.

Song, X. and Van Heyst, B. (2005). Volatilization of mercury from soils in response to simulated precipitation. *Atmospheric Environment* 39, 7494–7505.

Sørmo, E.G., Salmer, M.P., Jenssen, B.M., et al. (2006). Biomagnification of polybrominated diphenyl ether and hexabromocyclododecane flame retardants in the polar bear food chain in Svalbard, Norway. *Environmental Toxicology and Chemistry* 25, 2502–2511.

Stämpfli, M.R. and Anderson, G.P. (2009). How cigarette smoke skews immune responses to promote infection, lung disease and cancer. *Nature Reviews, Immunology* 9, 377–384.

Starin, D. (2013) Condors and carcasses. Natural History. Available at: http://www.naturalhistorymag.com/perspectives/082655/condors-and-carcasses (accessed November 27, 2017).

Steel, D. (2011). Extrapolation, uncertainty factors, and the precautionary principle. *Studies in History and Philosophy of Biological and Biomedical Sciences* 42, 356–364.

Stephens, F.J. and Ingram, M. (2006). Two cases of fish mortality in low pH, aluminium rich water. *Journal of Fish Diseases* 29, 765–770.

Tanner, C.A., Burnett, L.E., and Burnett, K.G. (2006). The effects of hypoxia on phenoloxidase activity in the Atlantic blue crab (*Callinectes sapidus*). *Comparative Biochemistry and Physiology, Part A* 144, 218–223.

Thomas, P.T., Rahman, M.S., Khan, I.A., and Kummer, J.A. (2007). Widespread endocrine disruption and reproductive impairment in an estuarine fish population exposed to seasonal hypoxia. *Proceedings of the Royal Society B* 274, 2693–2701.

Tiemann, M. (2016). Lead in Flint, Michigan's Drinking Water: Federal Regulatory Role. Congressional Research Service. Available at: http://fas.org/sgp/crs/misc/IN10446.pdf (accessed November 24, 2017).

Tokar, E.J., Boyd, W.A., Freedman, J.H., and Waalkes, M.P. (2013). Toxic effects of metals. In: Kaassen, C.D. (ed.), *Casarett and Doull's Toxicology. The Basic Science of Poisons*, 8th edn. New York: McGraw-Hill Education, pp. 981–1030.

Trainer, V.L. and Hardy, F.J. (2015). Integrative monitoring of marine and freshwater harmful algae in Washington State for public health protection. *Toxins* 7, 1206–1234.

Tralau, T., Oelgeschlager, M., Gurtler, R., et al. (2015). Regulatory toxicology in the twenty-first century: challenges, perspectives, and possible solutions. *Archives of Toxicology* 89, 823–850.

Trasande, L. (2016). Updating the Toxic Substances Control Act to protect human health. *JAMA* 315(15), 1565–1566.

US Department of Health and Human Services (2006). Toxicological profile for cyanide. Public Health Service – Agency for Toxic

Substances and Disease Registry. Available at: https://www.atsdr.cdc.gov/toxprofiles/tp8.pdf (accessed December 20, 2017).

Vandenberg, L.N., Colborn, T., Hayes, T.B., et al. (2012). Hormones and endocrine-disrupting chemicals: low-dose effects and nonmonotonic dose responses. *Endocrine Reviews* 33(3), 378–455.

Vandenberg, L.N., Colborn, T., Hayes, T.B., et al. (2013). Regulatory decisions on endocrine disrupting chemicals should be based on principles of endocrinology. *Reproductive Toxicology* 38, 1–15.

van der Tuuk, E. (1999). Intrinsic value and the struggle against anthropocentrism. In: Dol, M., van Vlissingen, M.F., Kasanmoentalib, S., Visser, T., and Zward H. (eds), *Recognizing the Intrinsic Value of Animals, Beyond Animal Welfare*. Assen: Van Gorcum, pp. 29–37.

Violante, A., Cozzolino, V., Perelomov, L., Caporale, A.G., and Pigna, M. (2010). Mobility and bioavailability of heavy metals and metalloids in soil environments. *Journal of Soil Science and Plant Nutrition* 10, 268–292.

Vogel, S.A. (2008). From 'The dose makes the poison' to 'The timing makes the poison': Conceptualizing risk in the synthetic Age. *Environmental History* 13(4), 667–673.

Vos, J.G. (2007). Immune suppression as related to toxicology. *Journal of Immunotoxicology* 4, 175–200.

Walker, C.H., Sibly, R.M., Hopkin, S.P., and Peakall, D.B. (2012). *Principles of Ecotoxicology*, 4th edn. Boca Raton, FL: CRC Press.

Wallschläger, D., Hintelmann, H., Evans, R.D., and Wilken, R-D. (1995). Volatilization of dimethylmercury and elemental mercury from river Elbe floodplain soils. *Water, Air, and Soil Pollution* 80, 1325–1329.

Wang, S.X., Zhang, L., Li, G.H., et al. (2010). Mercury emission and speciation of coal-fired power plants in China. *Atmospheric Chemistry and Physics* 10, 1183–1192.

Welshons, W.V., Thayer, K.A., Judy, B.M., Taylor, J.A., Curran, E.M., and vom Saal, F.S. (2003). Large effects from small exposures. I. Mechanisms for endocrine-disrupting chemicals with estrogenic activity. *Environmental Health Perspectives* 111(8), 994–1006.

Whitmee, S., Haines, A., Beyrer, C., et al. (2015). Safeguarding human health in the Anthropocene epoch: report of the Rockefeller Foundation-*Lancet* Commission on planetary health. *Lancet* 386, 1973–2028.

Wickramasinghe, L.P., Harris, S., Jones, G., and Vaughan, N. (2003). Bat activity and species richness on organic and conventional farms; impact of agricultural intensification. *Journal of Applied Ecology* 40, 984–993.

Winchester, N.B. (2009). Emerging global environmental governance. *Indiana Journal of Global Legal Studies* 16(1), Article 2.

Wogan, G.N., Paglialunga, S., and Newberne, P.M. (1974). Carcinogenic effects of low dietary levels of aflatoxin B1 in rats. *Food and Cosmetics Toxicology* 12(5-6), 681–685.

Work, T.M., Barr, B., Beale, A.M., Fritz, L., Quilliam, M.A., and Wright, J.L.C. (1993). Epidemiology of domoic acid poisoning in brown pelicans (*Peleacanus occidentalis*) and Brandt's cormorants (*Phalacrocorax penicillatus*) in California. *Journal of Zoo and Wildlife Medicine* 24, 54–62.

Wu, R.S.S., Zhou, B.S., Randall, D.J., Woo, N.Y.S., and Lam, P.K.S. (2003). Aquatic hypoxia is an endocrine disruptor and impairs fish reproduction. *Environmental Science and Technology* 37, 1137–1141.

Yang, S-X., Liao, B., Li, J-T., Guo, T., and Shu, W-S. (2010). Acidification, heavy metal mobility and nutrient accumulation in the soil-plant system of a revegetated acid mine wasteland. *Chemosphere* 80, 852–859.

Youson, J.H. and Neville, C.M. (1987). Deposition of aluminum in the gill epithelium of rainbow trout (*Salmo gairdneri* Richardson) subjected to sublethal concentrations of the metal. *Canadian Journal of Zoology* 65, 647–656.

6

Biodiversity and Health

Dominic A. Travis[1], Jonathan D. Alpern[1], Matteo Convertino[1], Meggan Craft[1], Thomas R. Gillespie[2], Shaun Kennedy[1], Cheryl Robertson[1], Christopher A. Shaffer[3], and William Stauffer[1]

[1] University of Minnesota, Minneapolis, MN, USA
[2] Emory University & Rollins School of Public Health, Math and Science Center, GA, USA
[3] Grand Valley State University, Allendale, MI, USA

6.1   Introduction

Health is not merely the absence of disease or infirmity, but a state of complete physical, mental, and social well-being (WHO, 2006). Although historically viewed largely within an organismal context, there has been increased recognition of the complexity of health and its connection to, or dependence upon, the natural world. Recently, integrative approaches have gained traction, defining health as "a state of equilibrium between human [and/or animals] and the physical, biological, and social environment compatible with full functional activity. A sustainable state in which humans and other living creatures can coexist indefinitely in equilibrium." (White et al., 2013).

Addressing complex health problems has been a slow, expensive, and often failure-prone process due to an almost exclusive dependence on a reductionist approach. For instance, disease modeling has traditionally been used to simplify or reduce complex problems to a manageable size. Unfortunately, simple models of complex realities rarely improve our understanding or ability to predict future outcomes. Several

paradigms – "One Health," "Ecosystem Health," and "Planetary Health" – have recently provided platforms to embrace complexity through new methods and approaches. The "discipline" of Ecosystem Health (sometimes termed "Ecosystem Approaches to Health") is grounded in a systems-based methodology and interdisciplinary, or interprofessional, science. "Ecosystem Health recognizes the inherent interdependence of the health of humans, animals and ecosystems and explores the perspectives, theories and methodologies emerging at the interface between ecological and health sciences" (Wilcox et al., 2004); it has a deep record in peer-reviewed publications highlighting the approach and methodologies used (Rapport, 2003).

According to the One Health Commission, "One Health" is the collaborative effort of multiple health science professions, together with their related disciplines and institutions – working locally, nationally, and globally – to attain optimal health for people, domestic animals, wildlife, plants, and our environment (Zinsstag et al., 2011). In essence, this movement provides guidance on "the way" for interdisciplinary science to achieve the intended results above. It provides much of the current backbone for collaborative science under the Global Health Security Agenda (GHSA), a partnership of over 50 nations, international organizations, and non-governmental stakeholders launched in 2014, to help build collective capacity toward a world safe and secure from infectious disease threats (https://www.ghsagenda.org). However, there is still great need for the development and validation of methodologies used for this approach (Häsler et al., 2014; Hueston et al., 2013).

Biological diversity (or *biodiversity*) has been defined as "the variability among living organisms from all sources including, terrestrial, marine and other aquatic ecosystems and the ecological complexes of which they are part; this includes diversity within species, between species and of ecosystems." (United Nations, 2014). The term is complex in that it can be discussed on many scales (molecular and genetic, microbial, taxonomic, and ecological), including those representing global processes in the biosphere: lithosphere (physical environment), hydrosphere (aquatic), and more recently human society (so-called sociosphere). The human societal connection is reflected by the popularization of the term "Anthropocene" (Box 6.1).

Biodiversity is difficult to quantify since only a small portion of life on Earth has been catalogued. Thus, estimates usually include predictive modeling. Mora et al. published a relatively recent model that predicts ~ 8.7 million (± 1.3 million SE) eukaryotic species globally, of which ~ 2.2 million (± 0.18 million SE) are marine. "In spite of 250 years of taxonomic classification and over 1.2 million species catalogued in a central database, our results suggest that some 86% of existing species on Earth and 91% of species in the ocean still await description" (Mora et al., 2011).

Humans and animals are part of the biodiversity of our planet genetically and taxonomically. However, our choices and actions are sculpting ecosystems across the globe, influencing biodiversity perhaps more than at any other time in history. We, in turn, are greatly influenced by the diversity of life around us (Whitmee et al., 2015; Myers et al., 2013; Myers and Patz, 2009). At a completely different scale, humans and animals themselves serve as ecosystems for diverse microbial communities. For instance, we now know that symbiotic microbial communities present in our gastrointestinal system influence – and are influenced by – our nutrition, as well as playing a role in regulating immune, cardiovascular, and reproductive function.

Box 6.1 The Anthropocene

The Anthropocene is an "unofficial" term used to characterize the current geological period, wherein human activities have a powerful effect on the global environment. Recently, scientists have been looking for evidence to support making the Anthropocene "official." Any formal recognition of an Anthropocene epoch in the geological time scale hinges on whether humans have changed the Earth system sufficiently to produce a stratigraphic signature in sediments and ice that is distinct from that of the Holocene epoch. Waters et al. (2016) believe they have found enough evidence to support formal recognition: "We review anthropogenic markers of functional changes in the Earth system through the stratigraphic record. The appearance of manufactured materials in sediments, including aluminum, plastics, and concrete, coincides with global spikes in fallout radionuclides and particulates from fossil fuel combustion. Carbon, nitrogen, and phosphorus cycles have been substantially modified over the past century. Rates of sea-level rise and the extent of human perturbation of the climate system exceed Late Holocene changes. Biotic changes include species invasions worldwide and accelerating rates of extinction. These combined signals render the Anthropocene stratigraphically distinct from the Holocene and earlier epochs."

Box 6.2 Global microbiome projects

In the past 10 years, advances in genomics and computational science have allowed for sequencing of full genomes from humans and many other taxa. This breakthrough quickly led to an expansion of these ideas connecting multidisciplinary teams of experts on a global scale. The Earth Microbiome Project (EMP) was launched in August 2010, with the ambitious aim of constructing a global catalogue of the uncultured microbial diversity of this planet. The primary vision of the Earth Microbiome Project was to process the microbial diversity and functional potential from approximately 200 000 environmental samples (Gilbert et al., 2014). The Human Microbiome Project (HMP) is designed to understand the microbial components of our genetic and metabolic landscape, and how they contribute to our normal physiology and disease predisposition. It is a global

and interdisciplinary project that promises to break down the artificial barriers between medical and environmental microbiology (Turnbaugh et al., 2007). Central to this interface, the Primate Microbiome Project was established to develop a systematic map of variation in microbiome structure and function across all primates and to relate this to primate health, evolution, behavior, and conservation. The primate gastrointestinal tract is home to trillions of bacteria that play major roles in digestion and metabolism, immune system development, and pathogen resistance, among other important aspects of host health and behavior. A recent finding suggests that captivity and loss of dietary fiber in nonhuman primates are associated with loss of native gut microbiota and convergence toward the modern human microbiome (Clayton et al., 2016).

Thus, microbial biodiversity directly impacts human and animal homeostasis and health at the human/animal organismal level (Gilbert et al., 2014) (Box 6.2).

6.2 Connectivity

Biodiversity provides building blocks for systems that underpin ecosystem functioning, and in turn support animals and humans. As a group, this is termed "ecosystem services" (Figure 6.1). Ecosystems provide four categories of services: provisioning (e.g., food), regulating (e.g., water quality regulation and pollination), cultural (e.g., recreation), and supporting (e.g., nutrient cycling) (Harrison et al., 2014).

So, when ecosystems function correctly, they provide direct benefits to humans and animals such as clean air and water, food, and products for shelter, religious/cultural practices, health, and medicine. Diverse ecosystems support human food systems, from soil quality and richness to pollination services, that provide natural food products and pest

control through direct consumption (bats) or competition. Globally, diverse ecosystems support many human and animal life support systems through the cycling of carbon or nutrients that underpin a stable climate. Most fundamentally, biodiverse ecosystems provide a kind of insurance account against both natural and man-made disasters (Soliveres et al., 2016; UNEP et al., 2015) (Box 6.3).

6.2.1 Biodiversity as an Indicator of Health

There are natural and anthropogenic processes that drive the dynamics of biodiversity. Many drivers of biodiversity change include human activities and choices such as habitat conversion, natural resource overexploitation, pollution, invasive species introduction, and climate change. These choices often result in suboptimal benefits to ecosystem services, yet cause damage to ecosystems (Sala et al., 1997). Biodiversity loss may in turn affect human/animal health directly or indirectly. Direct consequences such as overexploitation or the introduction of

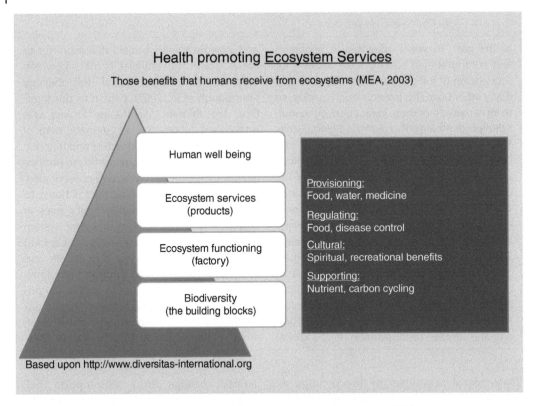

Figure 6.1 Ecosystem services. Adapted from Millennium Ecosystem Assessment, 2005.

invasive species may result in the loss of natural products upon which we depend (e.g., wild protein or medicinal plants) (Grifo et al., 1997). Another important example includes the extremely high use of antibiotics and/or other pharmaceuticals resulting in resistance or accidental effects on off-target species upon entering the environment, usually via human disposal, excretion, or secretion. These biological effects may affect the health and survival of off-target species directly, while indirectly affecting the sustainability of populations, food webs, or ecological niches that support human and animal health.

Despite the fact that most of these changes occur at a local level, they are often interdependent and create a cascade of organized effects at the global level. Without careful consideration of the sustainability of natural resources that provide direct services to humans and animals, these resources may quickly disappear with cascading effects on human and animal health and well-being (Harrison et al., 2014). Thus, decisions made in our daily lives influence biodiversity and, directly or indirectly, our own health.

Potentially more insidious are indirect drivers of biodiversity loss such as large-scale land use policy resulting in habitat loss, pollution, and climate change. War, civil strife, refugee crises, and other socioecological outcomes are indeed linked as well. Such linkages have been recognized by international organizations such as the World Risk Forum (Winickoff et al., 2005). These drivers act as long-term stressors on the building blocks of the biodiversity pyramid, decreasing resilience of systems and leading to degradation of ecosystem function and linked services over time, until a potential systemic collapse occurs. Of particular importance in these situations is the presence of multiple stressors that may have synergistic effects (identifiable by systems analysts as a functional

---

Box 6.3 Pollination services

Animal pollination, usually via insects, birds, or bats, influences the reproductive success of 87% of flowering plants worldwide. Over 1500 crops require insect pollination, and 3–8% of global crop production depends on insect pollination. In temperate regions, most animal pollination is provided by honeybees (*Apis mellifera*), bumblebees (*Bombus* spp.), solitary bees, wasps, and hoverflies; while in the tropics, butterflies, moths, birds, and bats become important (Klein et al., 2007). While most of this occurs via wild insects, a growing proportion are managed, as with the honeybee in the temperate regions of the world. Since pollination is an ecosystem service, which humans depend on through its link to world food production, it has become an often-cited example of how ecosystem services are economically valuable. Recent estimates suggest that crop pollination by insects underpins £430 million of crop production in the UK, with an equivalent figure of $361 billion worldwide. However, there is considerable doubt over the precision, reliability, usefulness, and interpretation of such figures. The ecosystem service values derived from

pollinators depend to a large extent on the condition and extent of the stock of pollinators, which is part of an area's natural capital (Hanley et al., 2015). A list of pressures that affect pollinators, and thus pollination services, includes:

- Landscape change in agricultural landscapes decreasing food sources for wild bees.
- Growing use of pesticides such as neonicotinoids with lethal and nonlethal effects on both wild and managed bees.
- Introduction of alien species, which may displace native flowers (food sources – although this can work in both directions) or directly outcompete native/local bees.
- Pathogens and parasites (bacterial, viral, protozoan, and fungal diseases), the best known of which is the mite *Varroa destructor*, accidentally introduced to Europe and the Americas from Asia.
- Climate change, which has been linked with changes in species range (adaptability) due to such factors as growing mismatches between insect emergence and floral bloom and changing drop choices (Spivak et al., 2011; European Commission, 2015).

---

network), increasing the scale of the problem and/or decreasing the time to degradation. The concept is laid out in Figure 6.2, and these relationships are fully explored in the proceedings of two major works: The Lancet Commission on Planetary Health (Whitmee et al., 2015) and the State of Knowledge Review of the World Health Organization (WHO) and the Secretariat for Convention of Biological Diversity (WHO and SCBD, 2015).

If these relationships are true, to what extent is biodiversity an "indicator" of human, animal, or ecosystem health? There is still a lot of research to be done as multiple biodiversity metrics exist and the universal patterns between these metrics and population health have not yet been mapped and analyzed systemically. It is clear that maintaining a certain level of biodiversity is necessary for proper

ecosystem functioning and the provisions of ecosystem services to humanity, and that this is a complex relationship across and between multiple trophic levels (Soliveres et al., 2016). Harrison et al. (2014) found over 530 studies with positive linkages between different biodiversity attributes and 11 ecosystem services. So, biodiversity loss could result in compromised ecosystem function, which, in turn indirectly influences human health. However, direct linkages between biodiversity health/preservation and human/animal health are less clear and have been less explored quantitatively (Ford et al., 2015). For instance, the fact that undisturbed ecosystems are often – but not always – "epidemic hotspots" for emerging and non-emerging infectious diseases of both humans and animals, clouds the linkages between biodiversity and health

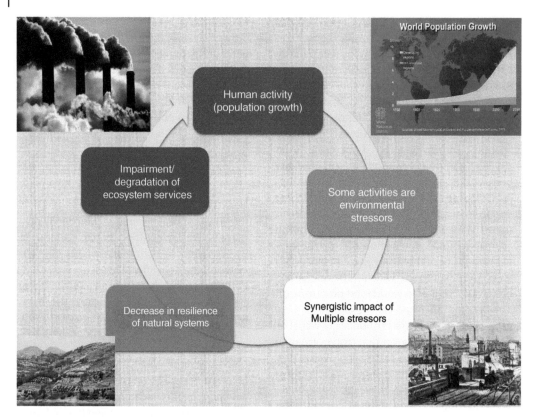

Figure 6.2 Synergistic effects of ecosystem stressors.

in this area. Therefore, better defining these biodiversity-health relationships is one of the top priorities in global and ecological health sciences (Millennium Ecosystem Assessment, 2005) (Box 6.4).

6.2.2 Social Factors

Human culture, society, and decision making has a profound influence on the drivers of biodiversity sustainability and its connection to health. It is no secret that population growth is one of the key drivers of the human-animal-environment relationship at local, regional, and global scales (Foley et al., 2011). However, the principles of epidemiology show us that population health is greatly influenced by social, economic, and environmental factors, whether they be by circumstance or choice. Economic and political instability, density of human (i.e., rural vs

urban) and animal habitats (farming systems), as well as gender, culture, and age all factor into this relationship. Vulnerable people tend to be more dependent on natural resources and services, for instance, and many cultures have long-standing gender roles that partition risk accordingly. At a larger scale, governance and policy directly supports or undermines the sustainability of biodiversity and the systems it supports. Even in highly stable countries and cultural situations, the priorities of different leadership administrations drive both short- and long-term relationships between biodiversity and health.

One of the most glaring shortcomings of the One Health paradigm is the relative lack of social science inclusion and engagement. Social sciences can contribute to our understanding of how combined changes in environmental, animal, and human health affect

---

Box 6.4 Relating biodiversity and health

Exploring the hypothesis that loss of biodiversity results in adverse human health consequences through the use of several indicators on a global scale, Huynen et al. selected indicators of human health (life expectancy, disability adjusted life expectancy, infant mortality rate, and percentage low-birth-weight babies), biodiversity (percentage threatened species, current forest as a percentage of original forest, percentage of land highly disturbed by man), and socioeconomic development (health expenditure as percentage of GNP, percentage 1-year olds immunized, illiteracy rate, GNP per capita, and development grade) on a country level. After controlling for relevant socioeconomic confounders, several measures of habitat loss and/or disturbance had no relationship with health indicators. Unexpectedly, there was a positive association between the logarithm of the percentage of threatened species, human life expectancy, and disability adjusted life expectancy. Thus, there was no empirical proof of a negative association between loss of biodiversity and human health at the global scale. There were several assumptions and data comparison issues that complicated the model and limited interpretation (Huynen et al., 2004). Additionally, results from studies of this kind are always dependent on the scale and resolution available from the data, so a comprehensive scale-invariance study of biodiversity-health patterns is required.

---

human psychosocial outcomes and of the cyclical relationship between humans and their environment. For example, it is becoming clear that climate change will result in changes in temperature and water availability all over the world. This will influence the movement and health of wild animals and will also influence the ways in which humans care for domestic animals. It will yield changes to human migration and well-being including food security and the frequency of human conflicts (Lapinski et al., 2015).

Social scientists have often been critical of traditional approaches to biodiversity conservation and human development, questioning "top-down," protectionist strategies on both ethical and practical grounds (Wilshusen et al., 2002). This has resulted in an unfortunate and sometimes profound rift between many conservationists in the natural sciences and many critics of conservation policy from the social sciences (Campbell, 2005). Yet bridging this gap is essential for simultaneously sustaining biodiversity and human welfare. Theoretical perspectives like *political ecology*, with its emphasis on elucidating the relationship between larger political forces and local environmental pressures, have considerably improved our ability to understand human–environmental interactions (Adams and Hutton, 2007). As a result, many social scientists have called for a more "people-oriented" approach to conservation, stressing the need for understanding the diverse worldviews of local people and the unequal power relations that often drive environmental conflict. Methodologically, the rich contextual data provided by ethnographic research allow for an understanding of the complex cultural drivers of human resource use and cross-cultural variation in ecosystem services. More complete integration of theoretical and methodological approaches from the social sciences into the One Health paradigm is critical for designing effective interventions to mitigate the loss of biodiversity and improve human health.

6.3 Grand Challenges, Development Goals, Global Health Security, and Ecosystem Health

In September 2000, 147 heads of state met at the United Nations (UN) headquarters to plan a course of action on the most pressing problems of humanity and the environment. The UN Millennium Declaration, which came out of that meeting, committed member nations to reduce extreme poverty and set out a series of time-bound targets that became known as the Millennium Development Goals (MDG). The Goals, with an ultimate target date of 2015, spanned a large range of topics, including poverty, infectious disease, education, and gender equality (United Nations 2015a) (Table 6.1). Several MGDs (nos. 4–6) are directly aimed at health and prevention/control of infectious diseases, many of which occur at the interface of humans, domestic animals, and wildlife. In recognition that health is inextricably linked to the sustainability of natural resources, MDG 7, "Ensure environmental sustainability," recognizes several human activity-related challenges to the environment by listing four target areas:

- "integrate the principles of sustainable development into country policies and programmes and reverse the loss of environmental resources;
- reduce the rate of biodiversity loss by 2010;
- reduce by half the proportion of people without sustainable access to safe drinking water and basic sanitation;
- achieve significant improvement in lives of at least 100 million slum dwellers by 2020."

In 2003, the Gates Foundation announced a $200 million medical research initiative, the Grand Challenges (GC) in Global Health, based upon on the assumption that with enough funding, contemporary science could remove some of the obstacles to more rapid progress against diseases that disproportionately affect the developing world (Varmus et al., 2003). From this time, the MDG and GC language and goals have been largely intertwined, even though the Gates initiative (GC) was meant to be largely complementary to the MDG program. There has been progress to be sure; but more importantly, lessons learned have stimulated an entire new round of thinking aimed at approaching these goals/challenges from a nontraditional perspective, which includes ecological approaches to health.

One of the widely acknowledged shortcomings of the MDG and GC targets was the lack of cross-sectoral integration among social, economic, and environmental goals, targets, and priorities (Haines et al., 2012). Opposing trends have been reported among the key indicators for the MDGs, with many negative trends for environmental indicators, including biodiversity, where anthropocentric progress was being made (UNEP et al., 2015). Since many of the grand challenges of our time are a product of the interconnectedness between humans, animals, and ecosystems, this broader focus requires new approaches and methods for solving problems of greater complexity at a larger scale. For instance, how can we decouple human-animal health threats such as emerging zoonotic diseases from the cofactors of climate change, food and water insecurity, extreme poverty, and land use/conversion?

The Grand Challenge movement combined with the lessons learned from the MDG program, as well as several others, has reinforced the need for a transdisciplinary approach to addressing the world's most pressing complex problems. At the same time, there has been broad global support for approaches such as "One Health" and "Ecosystem Health," among others, and they are quickly becoming codified in the language of international development, global health, and natural resource conservation and sustainability. This is reflected in the new set of Sustainable Development Goals, "a universal call to action to end poverty, protect the planet and ensure that all people enjoy peace and prosperity." These 17 goals build upon the successes of the MDGs, while including new areas such as climate change, economic inequality, innovation, sustainable consumption, peace, and justice, among other priorities (Table 6.1). The goals are interconnected – often the key to success on one will involve tackling issues more commonly associated with another (Clark, 2015; UN Development Programme, 2016).

Table 6.1 Millennium and Sustainable Development Goals compared.

Themes of Millennium Development Goals	Themes of Sustainable Development Goals	
Poverty and hunger	No poverty	Industry, innovation and infrastructure
Primary education	Zero hunger	
Gender equality and women's empowerment	Good health and well-being	Reduced inequalities
	Quality education	Sustainable cities and communities
Child mortality	Gender equality	Responsible consumption and production
Maternal health	Clean water and sanitation	
Infectious disease (HIV, malaria, etc.)	Affordable and clean energy	Climate action
Environmental sustainability	Decent work and economic growth	Life below water
Global development partnerships		Life on land
		Peace, justice and strong institutions
		Partnerships for goals

6.3.1 The Case of Agriculture, Food Security, and Biodiversity

The advancement of agriculture since the 1950s has been driven substantially by improved agricultural knowledge, technology, and improved crop and animal genetics. This has dramatically increased food production, which in turn has reduced food insecurity and increased economic development. Considering just cereal grains, UN Food and Agriculture Organization (FAO) estimates of production rose from 1.35 billion tons in 1961 to 2.82 billion tons in 2014. On a percentage basis, meat and poultry production has grown even more, from 8.9 million tons in 1961 to 112.9 million tons in 2014 (FAO, 2017). As a result, food insecurity has decreased, but it has not been eliminated. While the food insecure population has fallen by 15% from 930 million in 2000–2002 to 795 million in 2014–2016, this is still well above the Millennium Development Goal (FAO et al., 2015). By 2050 WHO estimates that the world population will grow to 9.2 billion, an increase of 2.4 billion. At the same time, as economic development continues, the diets of those in the developing world are expected to shift to greater consumption of meat and dairy products. Livestock already utilize one-quarter of the available global arable land and consume one-third of all grain grown; increased meat and dairy consumption will likely only increase that. The combination of anticipated population growth by 2050 with consumer demand shifting to more resource-intensive food sources in much of the world, drives the FAO forecast that 60% more food will be needed in 2050 (Alexandratos and Bruinsma, 2012).

These land use choices and subsequent rapid growth have come with dramatic consequences. Much of the increase in crop production resulted from improved genetic technologies, which have resulted in the use of more monoculture grains that can be intensively farmed efficiently. Intensive farming often requires increased use of chemical inputs such as fertilizers and pesticides, which have direct or indirect environmental and health impacts. Some negative impacts are projected far from the source, as evidenced by hypoxic areas such as the Gulf of Mexico "dead zone," caused by fertilizer run-off into rivers and streams in the central plains and upper Midwest that feed the Mississippi River. In 2016 the National Oceanic and Atmospheric Administration estimated the "dead zone" as over 6800 square miles of ocean where aquatic species would be negatively affected.

Decreased crop diversity can result in poor soil fertility, requiring additional chemical inputs to maintain production, which, in turn, increase the negative impacts of chemical use. Plant diseases and pest risk also increase with decreased biological diversity. Diverse agriculture systems tend in general to be more resilient to disruptions or insults, resulting in food systems that can better prevent food insecurity. Similar risks are faced in the animal agriculture sector (Frison et al., 2011).

The increase in the land dedicated to agriculture, and the inevitable use of synthetic fertilizers and chemicals, have had negative impacts for flora and fauna, in general, but more specifically on organisms that are important to the health of agriculture, such as pollinators. Pollinators are required for the majority of crops, and, in many cases, the crops dependent on pollinators are central to diets on a caloric and micronutrient level, making them a key link from biodiversity loss to human health (Spivak et al., 2011). Importantly, while harvested honeybees are commonly used for pollination services in intensive farming systems, they are less effective at boosting overall production compared to wild pollinators. Thus, the negative impacts of agriculture on pollinators actually pose both direct and indirect risks to agriculture production and human health (Garibaldi et al., 2013).

Finally, land use choices that result in human encroachment into previously undisturbed – or at least less disturbed – areas of wildlife habitat have been directly responsible for several emerging infectious disease outbreaks in humans. Salient examples include spillover from bats to domestic animals and then humans, such as with the emergence of Nipah virus from bats to pork producers and from bats to palm wine/sap to humans in Southeast Asia, as well as Hendra virus being released from bats to horses to humans in Australia (Plowright et al., 2014).

Meeting the anticipated food demand of the future will require advancements on a range of fronts, especially given the long-term benefits of at least reducing, if not reversing, the negative impacts of decreased biodiversity on wildlife and the sustainability of crops and animal agriculture. The pressure on increased primary food production can be reduced by more efficient systems from farm to consumer. This importantly includes food waste, ranging from crops that never make it to market due to poor infrastructure, food that is diverted due to economic and trade policy, and food that is wasted at processing and consumption. The overall impact of food waste is estimated at nearly one-third of total food produced, including 45% of fruits, vegetables, roots, and tubers. Trade and economic policies, including limited access to credit in the developing world, impose other challenges.

If progress can be made on improved agriculture practices such as crop and animal selection, crop rotation, crop and animal management practices that decrease the need for additional chemical inputs, and food waste, then the actual demand on feeding the world in 2050 can be reduced. Agricultural research that results in more productive practices, crops, and livestock can also help achieve the food production goals with less impact on the environment and ecosystem services. Reducing food waste and more efficient production of food are both needed if hunger is going to be reduced and the diversity of agriculture and the environment are to be sustained.

6.3.2 The Case of Wildlife Trade, Bushmeat, and Biodiversity

The legal global trade in wildlife and wildlife products involves the movement of billions of plants and animals comprising an economic value estimated at US$300 billion per annum. The illegal aspect of wildlife trade is estimated to be a $5–20 billion dollar industry, comparable to the international trade of narcotics and weapons. There are no adequate estimates of the full scale of wildlife traded throughout the world given its diversity, scope, and partial underground existence (Smith et al., 2017) (Box 6.5). Bushmeat (nutritional products sourced from free-ranging, noncaptive animals) represents one type of wildlife commodity that is either

---

Box 6.5 The scale of US wildlife imports

A summary of 14 years (2000–2013) of the most comprehensive data available (USFWS LEMIS system), shows that the USA imported over 11 billion individual specimens and an additional 977 million kilograms of wildlife during that time. The majority of shipments contained mammals (27%), while the majority of specimens imported were shells (57%) and tropical fish (25%). Most imports were facilitated by the aquatic and pet industry, resulting in one-third of all shipments containing live animals. The importer-reported origin of wildlife was 77.7% wild-caught and 17.7% captive-reared. Indonesia was the leading exporter of legal shipments, while Mexico was the leading source reported for illegal shipments. At the specimen level, China was the leading exporter of legal and illegal wildlife imports. The number of annual declared shipments doubled during the period examined, illustrating continually increasing demand, which reinforces the need to scale up capacity for border inspections, risk management protocols, and disease surveillance (Smith et al., 2017).

---

directly consumed or sold at local or regional markets, and sometimes transported long distances. Local offtake from the forest depends upon cultural preferences and norms, food insecurity, economics, availability/abundance, and local or international law. Thus, it is very hard to estimate global wild animal consumption or its impact on global food security.

However, around the world, people consume a huge diversity of wild-sourced terrestrial and aquatic animals, as well as plants and fungi. Wildlife from aquatic and terrestrial ecosystems is not just a source of protein, but also provides critical fat calories and micronutrients for many people (Sarti et al., 2015). For instance, fish provide more than 3 billion people with important sources of protein, vitamins, and minerals (Godfray et al., 2010). As we know, wildlife populations are in worldwide decline as a result of habitat destruction, overexploitation, pollution, and invasive species. Global declines will likely present major challenges in low-income and resource-restricted areas. It is possible that conservation strategies could provide significant public health dividends (Millennium Ecosystem Assessment, 2005).

The collection and trade of wild foods indirectly contributes to health and well-being by providing income for household needs, particularly in less developed countries. Aggregating across numerous local level studies, estimates of the annual value of the bushmeat trade alone in west and central Africa range between US$42 and 205 million (at 2000 values). This scale of economy poses important subsistence benefits. Hunting, butchering, consumption, global trade, and/or contact in markets with other species can also present risks of transmission and spread of infectious diseases (Millennium Ecosystem Assessment, 2005). A study conducted by the Centers for Disease Control and Prevention (CDC) and US Fish and Wildlife Services found evidence of herpesviruses (cytomegalovirus and lymphocryptovirus) and simian foamy virus within confiscated bushmeat samples at US ports of entry (Smith et al., 2012). The association between bushmeat and Ebola virus disease has also been established. Bushmeat often contains bats, which is the proposed animal reservoir for Ebola virus (Leroy et al., 2005) and many other known human pathogens. Despite bushmeat importation into the USA being prohibited, the practice is widespread among immigrants originating from countries where bushmeat consumption and trade is a common practice (Bair-Brake et al., 2014). Yet many of the social drivers of bushmeat trade remain poorly understood (Box 6.6).

Although nutritional acquisition is an obvious and important part of this discussion, there are other sociocultural drivers of the bushmeat trade. In many areas of the world, bushmeat hunting is an essential

---

Box 6.6 The bushmeat trade

Bushmeat consumption and importation into the USA by West African immigrant communities was of heightened concern during the recent Ebola virus disease epidemic. Yet, the knowledge, attitudes, practices, and economics (KAPE) driving bushmeat importation and consumption are poorly understood. There exist few examples of science-based community engagement to understand cultural drivers of this practice (Bair-Brake et al., 2014). Hence, intervention and mitigation strategies currently mainly rely on strict regulation through border protection, which has limited effect. A more comprehensive approach, including understanding the KAPE and community-derived interventions or mitigation techniques, should be sought through direct cultural engagement. In Minneapolis, Minnesota, a key community of West Africans (Liberians) were engaged through focus groups that were facilitated in collaboration with a community-based partner. The social drivers of local (US) bushmeat consumption included maintaining a cultural connection to home (most common), desirable taste, and belief in health benefits. In addition, consumption of bushmeat abroad while visiting friends and relatives in West Africa was a common practice. Participants acquired bushmeat in Minnesota from contacts who smuggled it in airline luggage (with detailed descriptions on how they successfully got past immigration officials), or through mailed packages as well as from (purchased) local ethnic groceries. Confusion about regulations surrounding bushmeat importation were common, and the idea that consuming bushmeat could transmit disease was a contentious topic. Many thought that the preparation or cooking processes mitigated most risk. This study confirmed bushmeat importation into the USA is common among West Africans living in Minnesota, and positive attitudes toward bushmeat may be a driver for continued demand in first-generation immigrant populations. Moving forward, opportunities exist to improve community education regarding the risks of bushmeat consumption, engage the community in intervention or mitigation projects to decrease risk, clarify import regulations, and help promote safer behavioral practices while traveling abroad (Walz et al., 2017).

---

social and symbolic practice that is strongly linked to cultural identity, material culture, mythology, and personhood. For example, among many Amazonian societies, humanity is defined in reference to nonhuman animal "persons" and hunting is an important realm for societies to negotiate and assert their own humanity (Rival, 2002; Cormier, 2003). Hunted animals feature prominently in the myths of symbiotic humans around the world, and primate parts are often used for folk medicine and ritual objects (de Melo et al., 2014). These beliefs and practices, in turn, influence the harvesting behavior of hunters in ways that may not be predicted by solely economic models of human behavior (Remis and Robinson, 2012). Further, these factors can make unsuccessful interventions that propose alternative livelihoods and/or protein sources. Understanding the complex

sociocultural context underlying bushmeat hunting is thus critical for informing successful conservation and health policy.

Creative solutions are being formulated for these issues. For example, participatory monitoring and management programs are becoming an increasingly common approach to biodiversity conservation and sustainability across the world (Danielsen et al., 2009). These programs are designed to empower local stakeholders by engaging communities in the collection and analysis of environmental data and the implementation of conservation policy. While these strategies pose a number of challenges (e.g., logistical issues, the need for shared conservation goals among diverse groups of people, governance issues) they offer tremendous potential for sustainable management in many areas. They provide a number of sustainability benefits over

---

Box 6.7 Co-management of Waiwai bushmeat hunting

Participatory monitoring and management (or "co-management") programs have become an important strategy for enhancing sustainable resource use in Amazonia, a region where more than 50% of protected areas are under indigenous control. In these areas, indigenous groups seek to maintain traditional subsistence strategies while simultaneously conserving biodiversity. For many Amazonians, bushmeat hunting is integral to food security and is a fundamental social and symbolic practice. Unfortunately, increased population density, changes in hunting technology, and the cumulative effects of habitat degradation and hunting pressure are imperiling wildlife populations and increasing the risk of zoonotic disease emergence. In the 625 000 hectare Konashen Community Owned Conservation Area in Guyana, researchers are working with indigenous Waiwai forager-horticulturalists for co-management of bushmeat hunting and health (Shaffer et al., 2017; M. Milstein et al., unpublished). This co-management program seeks to combine theoretical and methodological approaches from conservation biology, anthropology, and ecosystems health for people-oriented conservation. The partnership involves training indigenous parabiologists to collect data on their own harvesting practices, conduct line transect surveys, and conduct gross necropsies on hunted animals. Hunters collect data on offtake and hunting locations through self-monitoring forms and a participatory geographic information system (GIS). These data are used to assess long-term sustainability for the harvesting of vulnerable species and manage offtake accordingly. Indigenous parabiologists also conduct hunter-based disease surveillance, identifying gross pathologies in hunted animals and sampling tissues for histopathological and parasitological analysis. In addition, ethnographic research is being conducted to identify the cultural drivers of bushmeat hunting, indigenous perceptions of disease, cultural practices that may mitigate or enhance the potential for zoonotic transmission, and to determine community goals for sustainability and implement culturally appropriate interventions. The long-term goals of this program are to provide the capacity building necessary for the Waiwai to sustainably manage their own resource use and health.

---

externally driven conservation programs, including low cost, increased data gathering, more rapid interventions, and, perhaps most importantly, increasing the local relevance of policy by empowering local people to make management decisions. Successful co-management programs have been applied for ecotourism, fisheries management, bushmeat hunting, swidden agriculture, REDD (Reducing Emissions from Deforestation and forest Degradation) schemes, and water quality, among others (Box 6.7).

6.3.3 The Case of Infectious Diseases and Biodiversity

The health of humans, domestic animals, and wildlife are inextricably linked, especially through infectious diseases. Spillover of infectious diseases at "interfaces" (between humans and wildlife, wildlife and domestic animals, and domestic animals and humans) is receiving increasing attention from public health, conservation, and economic perspectives. For example, over 60% of infectious diseases in humans can be transmitted between humans and animals (i.e., zoonotic), and of those infectious diseases deemed to be emerging, 75% are zoonotic (Taylor et al., 2001). Emerging infectious diseases of wildlife appear to be especially problematic as they threaten both human health and biodiversity (Daszak et al., 2000). Infectious disease has been implicated as a contributing driver of global species extinctions (Smith et al., 2006, 2009) and can threaten economies through diseases in livestock (Cleaveland et al., 2001; Rist et al., 2015). The drivers of infectious disease emergence events are likely anthropogenic and driven by, among other things, land-use change (Patz et al., 2004). In the future, we expect to see a continued increase in anthropogenic perturbations, leading to emerging infectious disease events, especially in areas that are considered hotspots of wildlife biodiversity (Jones et al., 2008).

The relationship between biodiversity and disease is not as straightforward as it might appear and has been the subject of much scientific debate. It has been posited that biodiversity loss increases disease transmission risk (Keesing et al., 2010). The proposed negative association between biodiversity and disease risk, also called the "dilution effect hypothesis," is appealing because it suggests that protecting biodiversity is a win-win for both the environment and society (Ostfeld and Keesing, 2000; Wood et al., 2014). One proposed mechanism for the dilution effect is that with biodiversity loss comes the loss of competitors, thereby increasing the abundance of those hosts who are most able to become infected and effectively transmit disease (i.e., competent reservoir hosts). An alternative mechanism for the dilution effect hypothesis is that biodiversity loss might disproportionately affect the less competent reservoir hosts, thereby leaving the competent reservoir hosts to thrive. The most competent reservoir hosts for multi-host diseases are often widespread, abundant, and resilient species (Han et al., 2015). The dilution effect hypothesis has been supported with a few well-documented case studies of vector-borne, host-pathogen systems (e.g., Lyme disease, West Nile virus, hantavirus pulmonary syndrome), as well as a recent meta-analysis that found that disease prevalence is often higher in less diverse systems, holding true for plants, animals, and humans, experimental and comparative settings, and micro and macroparasites (Civitello et al., 2015).

However, it seems that a loss in biodiversity does not always lead to an increase in disease transmission risk, which brings into question the generalizability of the dilution effect as a general principle. Of course, areas of naturally high biodiversity may also serve as a source of new pathogens emerging out of these rich areas (Keesing et al., 2010; Young et al., 2013). A meta-analysis of six parasites found no consistent directionality in the biodiversity-disease relationship (Salkeld et al., 2013). Another recent review suggests that biodiversity likely has little effect on most human diseases, and when it does, biodiversity actually increases infectious disease risk, creating a positive relationship between biodiversity and disease (Wood et al., 2014). If this were true, public health officials would promote the reduction of biodiversity in undisturbed landscapes near human settlements (e.g., draining wetlands, culling wildlife, clear cutting brush and forests), or if biodiversity was to be preserved, public health efforts should be increased instead of decreased in these biodiverse areas (Wood et al., 2014) (Box 6.8).

Although there is a growing body of literature, more rigorous studies need to be done to clarify the directionality of the biodiversity-disease relationship, or figure out the conditions by which there is a positive or negative relationship.

6.3.4 The Case of Climate Change, Conflict, and Human and Animal Migration

The forced migration of families and communities is a complex phenomenon, driven by armed conflict, climate change, and the allocation of scarce, nonrenewable natural resources. War is no longer the only driver of displacement in the world. In 2014, climate-related disasters, rather than wars, accounted for the forced displacement of 32.4 million people worldwide, with the numbers steadily increasing (UNHCR, 2014). The UN Security Council identifies climate change as a "threat multiplier" in many of today's conflicts, from Darfur to Somalia to Iraq and Syria (United Nations 2015b). Climate-driven migration, as in armed conflict alone, is often a gendered experience, disproportionally affecting

---

Box 6.8 Understanding disease dynamics and habitat change

In recognition of the need for a more rigorous approach to this theme, a working group of the National Center for Ecological Analysis and Synthesis (NCEAS)and the National Socio-Environmental Synthesis Center (SESYNC) optimized an allometrically scaled multi-host model with empirical data from diverse natural systems undergoing habitat reduction, and thus declining biodiversity. The study found that greater biodiversity can lead to a decrease (dilution effect) or increase (amplification effect) in infection prevalence depending on the pathogen transmission mode and how host competence scales with body size. Dilution effects were detected for most frequency-transmitted pathogens; but amplification effects were detected for most density-dependent pathogens (Faust et al., 2017a). This group also developed a general model for the transmission of pathogens from species in intact habitat (core species) undergoing landscape-level conversion to predict the risk of spillover into species outside of core habitat (matrix species). Interestingly, this model suggests the risk of spillover is a nonlinear function of land conversion, with the highest probability of emergence at intermediate levels of conversion (Faust et al., 2017b).

---

women. As in displacement from armed conflict, women are left responsible for finding and providing food, and maintaining family cohesion and safety during the pre-flight and flight experience (Robertson and Hoffman, 2014; Robertson et al., 2016).

While contributing minimally to human-induced climate change, Africa is geographically among the most vulnerable to its effects and generally lacks adequate capacity to mitigate the impact of environmental degradation (Kolmannskog, 2010). Published discourse on climate change and forced migration reflects an interdisciplinary consensus that the impact of climate change on the human experience requires urgent intervention (Assan and Rosenfeld, 2012; Cohen et al., 2013; UNHCR, 2014). Food insecurity, pre- and post-migration conflict, shifts in urbanization patterns, and human rights abuses are among the threats resulting from the displacement of communities in search of habitable land (Barrios et al., 2006; Assan and Rosenfeld, 2012; Cohen et al., 2013; UNHCR, 2014). Within this context, climate change has not created new challenges, but has magnified existing disparity among the world's most vulnerable (Raleigh, 2011; Kjellstrom and McMichael, 2013; UNHCR, 2016). For example, in South Sudan 340 000 individuals were internally displaced during 2012 as a result of rainy season floods (UNHCR, 2014). Already in South Sudan, existing internal and cross-border displacement has impacted a significant proportion of the population as a result of recent conflict (IDMC, 2013; UNHCR, 2014). Regardless of the circumstance of mobility, interventions and policies supporting the protection and resilience of mobile communities are necessary, particularly as global climate patterns become increasingly less predictable (Kolmannskog, 2010; Cohen et al., 2013; UNHCR, 2016) (Box 6.9).

Less prominent in the literature is the discussion of ways that communities engage in strategies to support the cultural, physical, and psychosocial health of their members in the face of climate-related displacement (Bersaglio et al., 2015; Cohen et al., 2013). Yet, the set internal processes of self-determination, identity preservation, and healing will be critical to manage and strengthen communities in the face of the destabilizing effects of climate change, and, ultimately, to minimize intercommunity conflict in the coming decades (Opiyo et al., 2015; Piguet et al., 2011; Kjellstrom and McMichael, 2013). Published discourse on climate change and forced migration reflects an interdisciplinary consensus that the impact of climate change on the human experience requires urgent intervention (Assan and Rosenfeld, 2012; Cohen et al., 2013; UNHCR, 2014). We hypothesize

---

Box 6.9 The human experience of forced displacement

In 2016, Robertson and East African research partners used ethnographic methods – archival data collection, participant observation, in-depth unstructured interviews – in northern Kenya to better understand the human experience of climate, conflict, and forced displacement in pastoralist communities. Preliminary analyses suggest a complex story of drought, violence, livelihood loss, migration, decentralized government, emerging extractive industries, population pressures, ethnic and refugee tensions, hunger, opportunity, and of course, resilience. As this text is written, famine has been declared in six countries – four of which are enmeshed in armed conflicts deeply intertwined with drought and depleted resources.

---

that the community experience of culture shifts, disruption, and violence is similar to those in war zones, but this is not known. Community interventions that have been designed to address trauma and improve coping in war-affected communities may be relevant.

6.4 Conclusions and a Way Forward

Health is our most basic human right and therefore one of the most important indicators of sustainable development. At the same time, the conservation and sustainable use of biodiversity is imperative for the continued functioning of ecosystems at all scales, and for the delivery of ecosystem services that are essential for human health. There are many opportunities for synergistic approaches that promote both biodiversity conservation and the health of humans. However, in some cases there must be trade-offs among these objectives (WHO and SCBD, 2015). Many organizations, such as the World Health Organization and the Convention on Biological Diversity, have been cooperating to promote greater awareness about, and action on, the interlinkages between human health and biodiversity (Romanelli et al., 2014). The post-2015 United Nations Sustainable Development Goal Agenda provides a unique opportunity to advance the parallel goals of improving human health and protecting biodiversity

(Whitmee et al., 2015). Ongoing evaluation of synergistic and antagonistic effects of complementary sustainable development goals and targets is needed. This includes sustainable development goals and targets addressing health, food and freshwater security, climate change, and biodiversity loss (WHO and SCBD, 2015).

Measuring health at an individual or population level is seldom easy; measuring integrated ecosystem health in a dynamic world is a much greater challenge. It requires the use of standardized methods, indicators and metrics that can be implemented across disciplines. Numerous paradigms or frameworks are emerging to address this issue. The One Health Paradigm is providing "the way" for teams to come together, collaborate, and communicate; while the Ecosystem Health Paradigm provides participatory tools for design and implementation – as well as teaching – ecological methods for assessing health. However, the real solution may be embedded in the roots of "Complexity Science."

6.4.1 The Application of Complexity Science and Technology Tools to Optimize Health and Environmental Outcomes

Technological advancements have a role to play in understanding and "solving" the biodiversity-health "equation." New computational technologies can support predictions of ecosystem health and resilience trajectories over space and time, which in turn allow for the development of optimized solutions or strategies for the sustainability of species and/or ecosystem services that support health. Complexity science, anchored in statistical physics and coupled with applied engineering, strives to advance technologies that drive our synthetic understanding of the real world. Complexity science, when applied to ecological problems, has vastly improved our understanding of universal ecosystem dynamics, and has helped define limits to their resilience in the face of a multitude of threats and pressures. However, little has been done to validate "universal indicators" across a variety of ecosystem types and, unfortunately, single driver/single effect approaches are much more common to date.

Without a much-needed systemic definition of health, it is difficult to validate universal indicators needed to study complexity. However, syndemic theory has highlighted a successful pathway using an approach similar to macroecology for assessing multiple indicators in scenarios where trade-offs between ecosystem services are expected (Lim et al., 2016; Singer et al., 2017). This is important because the health of biodiversity and humans are not necessarily synchronized functions: in many cases the maximization of biodiversity leading to "species health" requires trade-offs for human health. For instance, in the Amazon, a combination of deforestation and the construction of hydropower plants has led to increased loss of species and a higher incidence of infectious diseases, while increasing food security and reliable local power; both are consequences of ecosystem alteration. However, in other ecosystem types such as wetlands (e.g., the Florida Everglades), both infectious disease incidence and species loss have negative trends as a result of an optimized hydro-control infrastructure. In the Everglades the number of native species has been very stable over time while the incidence of infectious diseases has declined. Any future reconstruction of these wetlands toward the original drainage configuration would likely lead to a dramatic resurgence of infectious diseases due to increased habitat for mosquito breeding and increasing human population density in this region of the USA.

In defining an optimal solution for the maintenance of multiple ecosystem services (i.e., a function that maximizes biodiversity and energy production, while minimizing infectious disease incidence) conventional "recipes," such as single-factor deterrence strategies, or simplified models, are often insufficient. Many common modeling and management approaches do not provide a good picture of the actual system behavior; the complex and often counterintuitive behavior of socioecological systems and their macro-level collective dynamics can be better understood by means of complexity science (Park et al., 2013; Helbing et al., 2014). Complexity science – in particular information, network, and decision sciences – can indeed capture the complexity of complex ecosystems, and models can be embedded into applied technologies for real use in the field. Certainly complexity science cannot solve all problems, but it is useful for understanding ecosystem dynamics and for ecosystem management.

Sustainable ecosystem design and management must include the anticipation of undesirable cascades of events that lead to loss of resilience. Grand challenges in ecosystem health are not one-dimensional problems of ecology, sociology, veterinary medicine, public health, or engineering, but are complex, collective issues where all disciplines and stakeholders need to collaborate for the common good. To this end, complexity science – by characterizing relationships between universal patterns of system stressors and health outcomes – can help to save animal and human lives while preserving the environment. Thus, these technologies may also be invaluable science-based policy tools for stakeholder engagement when assessing the suitability of potential solutions and management options (Convertino et al., 2013, 2014).

References

Adams, W.M. and Hutton, J. (2007). People, parks and poverty: political ecology and biodiversity conservation. *Conservation and Society* 5(2), 147–183.

Alexandratos, N. and Bruinsma, J. (2012). World Agriculture Towards 2030/2050: The 2012 Revision. Rome: UN Food and Agriculture Organization. Available at: http://www.fao.org/fileadmin/templates/esa/Global_persepctives/world_ag_2030_50_2012_rev.pdf (accessed November 29, 2017).

Assan, J.K. and Rosenfeld, T. (2012). Environmentally induced migration, vulnerability and human security: consensus, controversies and conceptual gaps for policy analysis. *Journal of International Development* 24(8), 1046–1057.

Bair-Brake, H., Bell, T., Higgins, A., et al. (2014). Is that a rodent in your luggage? A mixed method approach to describe bushmeat importation into the United States. *Zoonoses and Public Health* 61(2); doi:10.1111/zph.12050.

Barrios, S., Bertinelli, L., and Strobl, E. (2006). Climatic change and rural-urban migration: the case of sub-Saharan Africa. *Journal of Urban Economics* 60(3), 357–371.

Bersaglio, B., Devlin, J., and Yap, N. (2015). Contextualising emergency responses to famine among Turkana pastoralists in Kenya. *Development in Practice* 25(5), 688–702.

Campbell, L.M. (2005). Overcoming obstacles to interdisciplinary research. *Conservation Biology* 19(2), 574–577.

Civitello, D.J., Cohen, J., Fatima, H., et al. (2015). Biodiversity Inhibits Parasites: Broad Evidence for the Dilution Effect. *Proceedings of the National Academy of Sciences of the USA* 112(28), 8667–8671.

Clark, H. (2015). Governance for planetary health and sustainable development. *The Lancet* 386(10007), e39–41.

Clayton, J.B, Vangay, P., Huang, H., et al. (2016). Captivity humanizes the primate microbiome. *Proceedings of the National Academy of Sciences of the USA* 113(37), 10376–10381.

Cleaveland, S., Laurenson, M.K., and Taylor, L.H. (2001). Diseases of humans and their domestic mammals: pathogen characteristics, host range and the risk of emergence. *Philosophical Transactions of the Royal Society of London. Series B, Biological Sciences* 356(1411), 991–999.

Cohen, I.S., Spring, Ú.O., Padilla, G.D., et al. (2013). Forced migration, climate change, mitigation and adaptive policies in Mexico: some functional relationships. *International Migration* 51(4), 53–72.

Convertino, M., Foran, C.M., Keisler, J.M., et al. (2013). Enhanced adaptive management: integrating decision analysis, scenario analysis and environmental modeling for the Everglades. *Scientific Reports* 3, Art. No. 2922; doi:10.1038/srep02922.

Convertino, M., Liu, Y., and Hwang, H. (2014). Optimal surveillance network design: a value of information model. *Complex Adaptive Systems Modeling* 2(1), 6; doi:10.1186/s40294-014-0006-8.

Cormier, L.A. (2003). Animism, cannibalism, and pet-keeping among the Guajá of Eastern Amazonia. *Tipití: Journal of the Society for the Anthropology of Lowland South America* 1(1), 81–96.

Danielsen, F., Burgess, N.D., Balmford, A., et al. (2009). Local participation in natural resource monitoring: a characterization of approaches. *Conservation Biology* 23(1), 31–42.

Daszak, P., Cunningham, A.A., and Hyatt, A.D. (2000). Emerging infectious diseases of wildlife – threats to biodiversity and human health. *Science* 287(5452), 443–449.

de Melo, R.S., da Silva, O.C., Souto, A., Alves, R.R.N., and Schiel, N. (2014). The role of mammals in local communities living in conservation areas in the northeast of Brazil: an ethnozoological approach. *Tropical Conservation Science* 7(3), 423–439.

European Commission (2015). Decline in bees and wasps linked to land-use changes. Science for Environment Policy. Available at: http://step-project.net/img/uplf/decline_in_bees_wasps_linked_to_agriculture_urban_land_use_changes_424na2_en.pdf (accessed November 29, 2017).

FAO (2017). FAOSTAT. Food and Agriculture Organization of the United Nations. Available at: http://www.fao.org/faostat/en/#data (accessed November 29, 2017).

FAO, IFAD, and WFP (2015). The State of Food Insecurity in the World. Rome: Food and Agriculture Organization of the United Nations, International Fund for Agricultural Development, and World Food Programme. Available at: http://www.fao.org/3/a-i4646e.pdf (accessed November 29, 2017).

Faust C., Dobson, A.P., Gottdenker, N., et al. (2017a). Null expectations for disease dynamics in shrinking habitat: dilution or amplification? *Philosophical Transactions of the Royal Society B Biological Sciences* 372(1722); doi: 10.1098/rstb.2016.017.

Faust, C., Dobson, A.P., Gottdenker, N., et al. (2017b). Null expectations for disease dynamics in shrinking habitat: dilution or amplification? *Philosophical Transactions of the Royal Society B Biological Sciences* 372 doi: 10.1098/rstb.2016.0173

Foley, J.A., Ramankutty, N., Brauman, K.A., et al. (2011). Solutions for a cultivated planet. *Nature* 478(7369), 337–342.

Ford, A.E.S., Graham, H., and White, P.C.L. (2015). Integrating human and ecosystem health through ecosystem services frameworks. *EcoHealth* 12(4), 660–671.

Frison, E.A., Cherfas, J., and Hodgkin, T. (2011). Agricultural biodiversity is essential for a sustainable improvement in food and nutrition security. *Sustainability* 3(12), 238–253.

Garibaldi, L.A., Steffan-Dewenter, I., Winfree, R., et al. (2013). Wild pollinators enhance fruit set of crops regardless of honey bee abundance. *Science* 339(6127), 1608–1611.

Gilbert, J.A., Jansson, J.K., Knight, R., et al. (2014). The Earth Microbiome project: successes and aspirations. *BMC Biology* 12(1), 69.

Godfray, H.C.J., Beddington, J.R., Crute, I.R., et al. (2010). Food security: the challenge of feeding 9 billion people. *Science* 327(5967), 812–818.

Grifo, F. and Rosenthal, J. (1997). Chapter 1: Introduction. In: Grifo, F. and Rosenthal, J. (eds), *Biodiversity and Human Health*. Island Press.

Haines, A., Alleyne, G., Kickbusch, I., and Dora, C. (2012). From the Earth Summit to Rio + 20: integration of health and sustainable development. *The Lancet* 379, 2189–2197.

Han, B.A., Schmidt, J.P., Bowden, S.E., and Drake, J.M. (2015). Rodent reservoirs of future zoonotic diseases. *Proceedings of the National Academy of Sciences of the USA* 112(22), 7039–7044.

Hanley, N., Breeze, T.D., Ellis, C., and Goulson, D. (2015). Measuring the economic value of pollination services: principles, evidence and knowledge gaps. *Ecosystem Services* 14, 124–132.

Harrison, P.A., Berry, P.M., Simpson, G., et al. (2014). Linkages between biodiversity attributes and ecosystem services: a systematic review. *Ecosystem Services* 9, 191–203.

Häsler, B.L., Cornelsen, L., Rushton, J., and Shankar, B. (2014). A review of the metrics for One Health benefits. Leverhulme Centre for Integrative Research on Agriculture and Health. Available at: http://www.lcirah.ac.uk/node/141 (accessed November 29, 2017).

Helbing, D., Brockmann, D., Chadefaux, T., et al. (2014). Saving human lives: what complexity science and information systems can contribute. *Journal of Statistical Physics* 158(3), 735–781.

Hueston, W., Appert, J., Denny, T., King, L., Umber, J., and Valeri, L. (2013). Assessing global adoption of One Health approaches. *EcoHealth* 10(3), 228–233.

Huynen, M.M.T.E., Martens, P., and De Groot, R.S. (2004). Linkages between biodiversity loss and human health: a global indicator analysis. *International Journal of Environmental Health Research* 14(1), 13–30.

IDMC (2013). Global Estimates 2012. People Displaced by Disasters. Oslo: Internal Displacement Monitoring Centre. Available at: http://www.internal-displacement.org/assets/publications/2013/2012-global-estimates-corporate-en.pdf (accessed November 29, 2017).

Jones, K.E., Patel, N.G., Levy, M.A., et al. (2008). Global trends in emerging infectious diseases. *Nature* 451(7181), 990–993.

Keesing, F., Belden, L.K., Daszak, P., et al. (2010). Impacts of biodiversity on the emergence and transmission of infectious diseases. *Nature* 468(7324), 647–652.

Kjellstrom, T. and McMichael, A.J. (2013). Climate change threats to population health and well-being: the imperative of protective solutions that will last. *Global Health Action* 6(1), 1–9.

Klein, A.-M., Vaissière, B.E., Cane, J.H., et al. (2007). Importance of pollinators in changing landscapes for world crops. *Proceedings of the Royal Society B: Biological Sciences* 274(1608), 303–313.

Kolmannskog, V. (2010). Climate change, human mobility, and protection: initial evidence from Africa. *Refugee Survey Quarterly* 29(3), 103–119.

Lapinski, M.K., Funk, J.A., and Moccia, L.T. (2015). Recommendations for the role of social science research in One Health. *Social Science & Medicine (1982)* 129, 51–60.

Leroy, E.M., Kumulungui, B., Pourrut, X., et al. (2005). Fruit bats as reservoirs of Ebola virus. *Nature* 438(7068), 575–576.

Lim, S.S., Allen, K., Bhutta, Z.A., et al. (2016). Measuring the health-related sustainable development goals in 188 countries: a baseline analysis from the Global Burden of Disease Study 2015. *The Lancet* 388(10053), 1813–1850.

Millennium Ecosystem Assessment (2005). *Ecosystems and Human Well-Being: Biodiversity Synthesis*. Washington, DC: World Resources Institute.

Mora, C., Tittensor, D.P., Adl, S. et al. (2011). How many species are there on earth and in the ocean? *PLoS Biology* 9(8), e1001127.

Myers, S.S. and Patz, J.A. (2009). Emerging threats to human health from global environmental change. *Annual Review of Environment and Resources* 34, 223–252.

Myers, S.S., Gaffikin, L., Golden, C.D. et al. (2013). Human health impacts of ecosystem alteration. *Proceedings of the National Academy of Sciences of the USA* 110(47), 18753–18760.

Opiyo, F., Wasonga, O., Nyangito, M., Schilling, J., and Munang, R. (2015). Drought adaptation and coping strategies among the Turkana pastoralists of northern Kenya. *International Journal of Disaster Risk Science* 6(3), 295–309.

Ostfeld, R.S. and Keesing, F. (2000). Biodiversity series: the function of biodiversity in the ecology of vector-borne zoonotic diseases. *Canadian Journal of Zoology* 78, 2061–2078.

Park, J., Seager, T.P., Rao, P.S.C., Convertino, M., and Linkov, I. (2013). Integrating risk and resilience approaches to catastrophe management in engineering systems. *Risk Analysis* doi:10.1111/j.1539-6924.2012.01885.x.

Patz, J.A., Daszak, P., Tabor, G.M. et al. (2004). Unhealthy landscapes: policy recommendations on land use change and infectious disease emergence. *Environmental Health Perspectives* 112(10), 1092–1098.

Piguet, E., Pécoud, A., and de Guchteneire, P. (2011). Migration and climate change: an overview. *Refugee Survey Quarterly* 30(3), 1–23.

Plowright, R.K., Eby, P., Hudson, P.J., et al. (2015). Ecological dynamics of emerging bat virus spillover. *Proceedings of the Royal Society B: Biological Sciences* 282; doi: 10.1098/rspb.2014.2124.

Raleigh, C. (2011). The search for safety: the effects of conflict, poverty and ecological influences on migration in the developing world. *Global Environmental Change* 21 (Suppl. 1), S82–93.

Rapport, D.J., Lasley, W.L., Rolston, D.E., et al. (eds) (2003). *Managing for Healthy Ecosystems*. Lewis Publishers.

Remis, M.J. and Jost Robinson, C.A. (2012). Reductions in primate abundance and diversity in a multiuse protected area: synergistic impacts of hunting and logging in a Congo Basin forest. *American Journal of Primatology* 74(74); doi:10.1002/ajp.22012.

Rist, C.L., Ngonghala, C.N., Garchitorena, A., et al. (2015). Modeling the burden of poultry disease on the rural poor in Madagascar. *One Health* 1, 60–65.

Rival, L.M. (2002). *Trekking Through History: The Huaorani of Amazonian Ecuador*. New York: Columbia University Press.

Robertson, C.L. and Hoffman, S.J. (2014). Conflict and forced displacement. *Nursing Research* 63(5), 307–308.

Robertson, C.L., Savik, K., Mathiason-Moore, M., Mohamed, A., and Hoffman, S. (2016). Modeling psychological functioning in refugees. *Journal of the American Psychiatric Nurses Association* 22(3), 225.

Romanelli, C., Cooper, H.D., and de Souza Dias, B.F. (2014). The integration of biodiversity into One Health. *Revue Scientifique et Technique (International Office of Epizootics)* 33(2),487–496.

Salkeld, D.J., Padgett, K.A., and Holland Jones, J. (2013). A meta-analysis suggesting that the relationship between biodiversity and risk of zoonotic pathogen transmission is idiosyncratic. *Ecology Letters* 16(5), 679–86.

Sarti, F.M., Adams, C., Morsello, C., et al. (2015). Beyond protein intake: bushmeat as source of micronutrients in the Amazon. *Ecology and Society* 20(4), 22.

Shaffer, C.A., Milstein, M.S., Yukuma, C., Marawanaru, E., and Suse, P. (2017). Sustainability and comanagement of subsistence hunting in an indigenous reserve in Guyana. *Conservation Biology*. doi:10.1111/cobi.12891.

Singer, M., Bulled, N., Ostrach, B., and Mendenhall, E. (2017). Syndemics and the biosocial conception of health. *The Lancet* 389(10072), 941–50.

Smith, K.F., Sax, D.F., and Lafferty, K.D. (2006). Evidence for the role of infectious disease in species extinction and endangerment. *Conservation Biology* 20(5), 1349–1357.

Smith, K.F., Acevedo-Whitehouse, K., and Pedersen, A.B. (2009). The role of infectious diseases in biological conservation. *Animal Conservation* 12(1), 1–12.

Smith, K.M., Anthony, S.J., Switzer, W.M., et al. (2012). Zoonotic viruses associated with illegally imported wildlife products. *PloS One* 7(1), e29505.

Smith, K.M., White, A., Asmussen, M., et al. (2017). Summarizing US wildlife trade with an eye toward assessing the risk of infectious disease introduction. *EcoHealth* 14, 29–39.

Soliveres, S., van der Plas, F., Manning, P., et al. (2016). Biodiversity at multiple trophic levels is needed for ecosystem multifunctionality. *Nature* 536(7617), 456–459.

Spivak, M., Mader, E., Vaughan, M., and Euliss, N.H. (2011). The plight of the bees. *Environmental Science & Technology* 45(1), 34–38.

Taylor, L.H., Latham, S.M., and Woolhouse, M.E. (2001). Risk factors for human disease emergence. *Philosophical Transactions of the Royal Society of London B: Biological Sciences* 356(1411), 983–89.

Turnbaugh, P.J., Ley, R.E., Hamady, M., Fraser-Liggett, C.M., Knight, R., and Gordon, J.I. (2007). The Human Microbiome Project. *Nature* 449(7164), 804–810.

UN Development Programme (2016). UNDP Policy and Programme Brief: UNDP Support to the Implementation of the 2030 Agenda for Sustainable Development. New York: United Nations Development Programme. Available at: http://www.undp.org/content/dam/undp/library/SDGs/SDG Implementation and UNDP_Policy_and_Programme_Brief.pdf (accessed November 29, 2017).

UNEP, CBD, and WHO (2015). *Connecting Global Priorities: Biodiversity and Human Health: A State of Knowledge Review*. United Nations Environment Programme,

Convention on Biological Diversity, World Health Organization. Available at: https://www.cbd.int/health/stateofknowledge/(accessed November 29, 2017).

UNHCR (2014). 2014 Country Operations Profile – South Sudan. Geneva: United Nations High Commissioner for Refugees. Available at: http://www.unhcr.org/pages/4e43cb466.html (accessed November 29, 2017).

UNHCR (2016). Challenges relating to climate change induced displacement. Remarks by Mr José Riera. International Conference "Millions of People without Protection: Climate Change Induced Displacement in Developing Countries". United Nations High Commissioner for Refugees. Available at: http://www.unhcr.org/5151bf239.html (accessed November 29, 2017).

United Nations (2014). *Global Biodiversity Outlook. Secretariat of the Convention on Biological Diversity.* Vol. 25. doi:10.2143/KAR.25.0.504988.

United Nations (2015a). The Millennium Development Goals Report 2015. New York: United Nations. Available at: http://www.un.org/millenniumgoals/2015_MDG_Report/pdf/MDG 2015 rev (July 1).pdf (accessed November 29, 2017).

United Nations (2015b). UN Security Council Meeting on Climate Change as a Threat Multiplier for Global Security. The Center for Climate and Security. Available at: https://climateandsecurity.org/2015/07/08/un-security-council-meeting-on-climate-change-as-a-threat-multiplier-for-global-security/(accessed November 29, 2017).

Varmus, H., Klausner, R., Zerhouni, E., Acharya, T., Daar, A.S., and Singer, P.A. (2003). Grand challenges in global health. *Science* 302(5644), 398–399.

Walz, E., Wilson, D., Wanduragala. D., et al. (2017). Drivers of bushmeat consumption and importation among Liberians living in Minnesota, USA. *J Emerg Inf Dis* 23(12). doi: https://doi.org/10.3201/eid2312.170563.

Waters, C.N., Zalasiewicz, J., Summerhayes, C., et al. (2016). The Anthropocene is functionally and stratigraphically distinct from the Holocene. *Science* 351(6269); doi: 10.1126/science.aad2622.

White, F., Stallones, L., and Last, J.M. (eds) (2013). *Global Public Health: Ecological Foundations.* Oxford: Oxford University Press.

Whitmee, S., Haines, A., Beyrer, C., et al. (2015). Safeguarding human health in the Anthropocene epoch: report of the Rockefeller Foundation-Lancet Commission on Planetary Health. *The Lancet* 6736(15), 1973–2028.

WHO (2006). *Constitution of the World Health Organization.* Geneva: World Health Organization, pp. 1–18.

WHO and SCBD (2015). Connecting Global Priorities: Biodiversity and Human Health: A State of Knowledge Review. Geneva: World Health Organization and Secretariat of the Convention on Biological Diversity. Available at: https://cgspace.cgiar.org/bitstream/handle/10568/67397/SOK-biodiversity-en.pdf?sequence=1&isAllowed=y (accessed November 29, 2017).

Wilcox, B.A., Alonso Aguirre, A., Daszak, P., et al. (2004). EcoHealth: A transdisciplinary imperative for a sustainable future. *EcoHealth* 1(1), 3–5.

Wilshusen, P.R., Brechin, S.R., Fortwangler, C.L., and West, P.C. (2002). Reinventing a square wheel: critique of a resurgent "protection paradigm" in international biodiversity conservation. *Society and Natural Resources* 15, 17–40.

Winickoff, D., Jasanoff, S., Busch, L., and Grove-White, R. (2005). Adjudicating the GM food wars: science, risk, and democracy in World Trade law. *Yale Journal of International Law* 30(1), Article 3. Available at: http://digitalcommons.law.yale.edu/cgi/viewcontent.cgi?article=1246&context=yjil (accessed November 29, 2017).

Wood, C.L., Lafferty, K.D., Deleo, G., Young, H.S., Hudson, P.J., and Kuris, A.M. (2014).

Does biodiversity protect humans against infectious disease? *Ecology* 95(4), 817–832.

Young, H., Griffin, R.H., Wood, C.L., and Nunn, C.L. (2013). Does habitat disturbance increase infectious disease risk for primates? *Ecology Letters* 16(5), 656–663.

Zinsstag, J., Schelling, E., Waltner-Toews, D., and Tanner, M. (2011). From 'One Medicine' to 'One Health' and systemic approaches to health and well-being. *Preventive Veterinary Medicine* 101(3), 148–156. 3.

7

Emerging Infectious Diseases: Old Nemesis, New Challenges

Ronald C. Hershow[1] and Kenneth E. Nusbaum[2]

[1] *University of Illinois at Chicago, Chicago, IL, USA*
[2] *Auburn University, Auburn, AL, USA*

7.1 Introduction

The human population has confronted infectious disease emergences throughout recorded history. For much of that time, there was little or no understanding of infectious disease etiology and transmission. The nineteenth century witnessed the advent of germ theory and the assignment of specific causative organisms to individual infectious diseases through the application of Koch's postulates (Gradmann, 2014). This led to an explosion of knowledge about infectious diseases and to growing optimism about the eventual control and elimination of these diseases. The sense of confidence was fostered by the development and widespread use of vaccines and, more recently, antimicrobials. The global eradication of smallpox in 1976 was perceived as a watershed moment that seemingly suggested that infectious diseases were in full retreat (Henderson, 2011). That sentiment was short lived, however. In the same year that the eradication of smallpox was triumphantly announced, Ebola virus disease (EVD) outbreaks were first reported from Sudan and Zaire (WHO, 1978). Concurrently, the discovery of the bacterial cause of Legionnaire's disease, in Philadelphia, USA, indicated that it was not only developing countries that could be affected by novel pathogens, but rich countries as well (CDC, 2017).

In 1981, the first cases of what was later named the acquired immunodeficiency syndrome (AIDS) were reported in the *Morbidity and Mortality Weekly Report* (CDC, 1996). The discovery of the causative agent, the human immunodeficiency virus (HIV), which jumped from apes to humans in western Africa, heralded a sustained, global pandemic that, by 2010, was the leading cause of disability adjusted life years for 30–44-year-old persons worldwide and the fifth leading cause of death for persons of all ages (Ortblad et al., 2013). These and other infectious disease emergences during the last four decades have led to a growing awareness of the importance of emerging infectious diseases and refocused research on animal origins of human diseases, especially those originating from spillover from wildlife sources.

Outbreaks of infectious and contagious diseases have garnered great public attention, sometimes disproportionate to their effect on morbidity (illness) and mortality (death). The economic disruption they cause may be out of balance with their direct impact on human health. A case in point is the 2003 severe acute respiratory syndrome (SARS) pandemic, caused by a coronavirus

Beyond One Health: From Recognition to Results, First Edition.
Edited by John A. Herrmann and Yvette J. Johnson-Walker.
© 2018 John Wiley & Sons, Inc. Published 2018 by John Wiley & Sons, Inc.

(SARS-CoV), which emerged initially in November 2002 in six municipalities of Guangdong province, China. After the pandemic ended in July 2003, the World Health Organization (WHO) reported 8098 probable cases affecting 29 countries and regions with 774 deaths (case-fatality rate 9.6%) (WHO, 2003). Although the macroeconomic effects of this pandemic are debated, several studies have estimated a global impact of US$30 to 100 billion (Keogh-Brown and Smith, 2008). This translates to approximately US$3.7 to 12.3 million per case. The costs were mainly attributable to detrimental effect on travel and tourism but analyses have identified a broader range of affected economic sectors (Smith, 2006). As a result of the great public concern associated with the SARS epidemic, and the subsequent socioeconomic impacts engendered by recent emerging outbreaks, public health leaders and the 24-hour news media may be criticized for immoderate risk communication to the public. Elements of science, and a modern media focused on viewership, color our understanding of these diseases, and the media, in particular, may be a source of sound information and calm reassurance or it may send panic throughout the population. However, because of the unpredictable and unknown nature of emerging infectious diseases, it may be difficult to avoid outbreak management based on worst-case scenarios. A delicate balance often exists between an aggressive yet careful and thoughtful outbreak response and mitigation strategy, which may lead to public anxiety, and a too conservative approach, which may prolong the outbreak and lead to excess morbidity and mortality. The key is risk communication in a manner that is easily understood by the public (Abraham, 2009).

Despite the significance of infectious disease emergences in human history, it wasn't until 1992 that the Institute of Medicine, now called the National Academy of Medicine, of the National Academies of Sciences formally defined emerging infectious diseases and identified six key drivers associated with

infectious disease emergence. Disease emergence, re-emergence, and persistence is associated with:

- Human behaviors, culture, economics, technology, trade, and transport.
- Human–animal interface through agriculture, incursions into wildlife areas, and exposure to companion animals.
- Human–environment interface in the built and natural environments.
- Animal behavior, range, biodiversity loss, response to climate change.
- Environmental temperature, humidity, and other responses to climatic change.
- Animal–environment interface and how changes in habitat range (altitude and latitude) affect individual immunity and pathogen-host dynamics (Institutes of Medicine, 2009).

Fineberg and Wilson (2010) described three additional determinants that encompass the six delineated above: 1) social dynamics; 2) technological advances; and 3) varying susceptibilities to risk. The authors write, "These factors operate within a complex international system, whereby international cooperation, can be a serious potential attenuator or amplifier of the risk of emerging infection depending on the degree of successful collaboration on such matters as surveillance (that includes animal populations), travel policy, trade restrictions, and enforcement."

An *emerging infectious disease* is an infectious disease that is newly recognized as occurring in humans. A *newly (or "re-") emerging disease* is one that has been recognized before but is newly appearing in a different population or geographic area than previously affected; one that is newly affecting many more individuals; and/or one that has developed new attributes (e.g., resistance or virulence): re-emerging. A *spillover infection* occurs when a reservoir population with a high prevalence of a pathogen comes into contact with an immunologically naïve population (Morens and Fauci, 2013). *Zoonoses* are diseases that are caused by infectious agents of animals that are transmissible to people. Viral agents of this group have been prominent in the media of late (e.g., Ebola virus disease, Zika virus disease, dengue, West Nile virus, etc.). The reasons for increasing incidence and prevalence of viral diseases are becoming clearer as research progresses into the causes and spread of these agents.

Not surprisingly, it is not uncommon for many factors to contribute to a single incident of either emerging or newly (re-)emerging pathogens. Furthermore, incidents can be divided into relatively transient outbreaks that flare up and resolve (e.g., SARS) and sustained pandemics (e.g., AIDS). Sustained epidemics can lead to dynamic, evolving health consequences that require different approaches as affected areas and populations progress from introduction, perhaps through a spillover event, or post-introduction epidemic patterns to more established, mature epidemics. And, of course, epidemics may be shaped, altered, and ultimately mitigated by a growing and expanded array of prevention, mitigation, and response strategies, which often focus on key, affected populations.

The interplay of factors operative in any infectious disease emergence can be diverse and complex, involving aspects as disparate as climate change, industrial and commercial development, ecosystem change, and social inequalities. Considering these factors requires planning and responses that often extend beyond conventional public health activities and policies. Efforts to promote water, sanitation, and hygiene (WASH), and to ameliorate poor access to treatment and prevention services, remain core public health priorities. However, the complexity of emerging infectious disease events requires an understanding of the effects of globalization, politics, human susceptibility, and even disparities in basic human rights (Olson et al., 2015). Furthermore, an effective response to an infectious disease outbreak requires an understanding of the capacity of pathogens, vector populations, and reservoir species to adapt to environmental changes that occur over time (Mills et al., 2010). Recent efforts

to identify and characterize emerging infectious diseases over the last 40 years consistently point to the dominant contribution of zoonotic diseases: a recurring estimate is that over 60% of these emerging infectious diseases have an animal origin (Kilpatrick and Randolph, 2012).This places the "One Health" concept, which recognizes that human health is inextricably connected to the health of animals and their shared environment, at the center of understanding and controlling emerging infectious diseases. The complexities of diseases that may involve multiple hosts and vector species, dynamic evolution, and a complex set of drivers require multidisciplinary approaches. Medical, veterinary, ecological, sociological, economic, microbial ecological, and evolutionary perspectives are essential to meet the challenge of these diseases (Karesh et al., 2012).

Diseases need not infect humans to have severe adverse effects on human health. Epizootics with great impact on animal populations can cause secondary impacts on human populations through the loss of food sources. The introduction of rinderpest virus into the African pastoral peoples in 1890 (Phoofolo, 1993) led to the death through starvation of millions of people. Foot-and-mouth disease (FMD) in the UK in 2001 spread to The Netherlands, France, and Ireland, before being brought under control by widespread culling. The UK alone suffered economic losses of more than US$ 12 billion, and some 6.5 million sheep, cattle, and pigs were slaughtered to stamp out the outbreak (Thompson et al., 2002).Recent epizootics of porcine epidemic diarrhea virus (PEDv) and influenza A viruses among birds caused price increases for pork and egg products, as well as having resulted in the culling of large populations of the affected animals.

The chain of transmission of viral diseases varies with the nature of the virus, the host immune status, and the infective dose received. Knowledge of that chain enables scientists to identify the weak links that lead to interruption of the chain and the termination of epidemics. A classic example of the disruption of transmission is the routine use of rabies vaccine in domesticated animals, and its less frequent use in wildlife, to protect humans from spillover of rabies virus from animals. The reduction, over time, in the number of rabies cases in humans in the USA is directly attributable to vaccination of domestic dogs, cats, wildlife, and other pets (Lembo et al., 2011). More recently, the WHO developed the "Strategic Framework for Elimination of Human Rabies Transmitted by Dogs in the South-East Asia Region," where approximately 45% of human deaths due to rabies virus occur and where 96% of infections are associated with dog bites. The strategy focuses on increasing canine rabies vaccination rates, decreasing the canine population through reproduction control, and improving the use of post-exposure prophylaxis (PEP) for humans bitten by dogs (WHO, 2012)

This chapter will look at four diseases – rabies, influenza A, Ebola virus disease, and Zika virus disease – to give the reader a perspective on re-emerging, emerging, and zoonotic threats. These four were chosen because of their immediacy and their ability to illustrate the interplay of drivers, evolutionary factors, and policy decisions that are central to the understanding and control of these diseases.

7.2 Rabies

Rabies is an ancient disease of mammals with an essentially global distribution. The US Centers for Disease Control and Prevention conducts rabies surveillance in the USA, and data are disseminated annually in the *Journal of the American Veterinary Medical Association* (CDC, 2015a; Birhane et al., 2017). Despite being 100% vaccine preventable, rabies is estimated to kill over 59 000 humans annually, mostly in Africa and Asia. In the USA, human deaths number in single digits each year. In 2015, three human rabies deaths were reported, compared with one in

2014. In 2016, no cases of human rabies in the USA were reported. In the USA, bats are the most common vector for human rabies cases; globally, most human rabies cases are attributable to dog bites each year (WHO, 2012, 2017a).

7.2.1 Natural History

Rabies virus is a single-stranded RNA virus of the genus *Lyssavirus* with a lipid envelope. Its envelope makes the virus susceptible to rapid environmental inactivation and necessitates intimate transmission of the virus, typically by biting. However, the virus can also be transmitted when saliva from an infected animal contacts wounds or mucous membranes (Birhane et al., 2017). Carnivores are the natural hosts of rabies, with striking regional distributions in North America. When raccoon-associated rabies surfaced in the eastern USA, in 1981, early methods of controlling the virus included trapping and culling. However, control of virus transmission in wildlife populations was ultimately successful because of widespread distribution of an oral vaccine using a recombinant vaccinia virus, a self-replicating poxvirus that serves as the vector for the rabies virus gene that is responsible for the production of rabies glycoprotein. The glycoprotein by itself is noninfective and cannot cause rabies but it serves as an "antigen" capable of eliciting an immune response to rabies when the vaccine is swallowed by raccoons, foxes, or coyotes (National Park Service, 2005; Slate et al., 2005).

Rabies virus enters the human population through direct human contact with infected domestic animals and wildlife. Because rabies virus is enzootic in North America and has a variable long incubation period, eradication of rabies on this continent will be challenging. However, because of the enforcement of canine rabies vaccination among dogs, scientists in 2008 determined that molecular, phylogenetic, and epizootiologic evidence showed that domestic dog rabies was no longer enzootic to the USA

(Velasco-Villa et al., 2008). It should be stressed that dogs can and do acquire and transmit rabies viruses. However, the virus specific to dogs has been eliminated from dog-to-dog transmission in the USA, underscoring the need to maintain vaccination of domestic pets.

7.2.2 The Epizoology of Rabies Virus

Before the agent of rabies or the existence of viruses was known, rabies was transmitted experimentally, in 1804, by injecting saliva from a rabid dog into other animals (Jackson and Greenlee, 1993). Thus, the association between the bite and the disease was proven. All species of mammals are susceptible to the rabies virus and capable of transmitting the virus to other animals. However, only a few species are important reservoirs for the disease. Dogs, coyotes, foxes, raccoons, skunks, and some types of insectivorous bats are important sources of exposure to the virus in the USA (CDC, 2011). Once the virus is deposited in peripheral wounds, centripetal passage occurs toward the central nervous system. After viral replication, there is centrifugal spread to major exit portals, most notably the salivary glands. The virus replicates locally in the muscle cells and moves, mediated by viral surface antigens, through the neuromuscular junction to the peripheral nerve. Time in the muscle cells is fairly short, less than 30 hours in many species. The virus migrates to the brain, and the duration of incubation is proportional to the distance from the brain (CDC, 2016a). The two common presentations, furious or dumb, are related to both the species infected and brain structure affected.

Crucial to completion of the cycle of transmission is infection of the salivary glands and alteration of the infected animal's behavior. Animals that are typically shy and nocturnal may approach potential hosts, animal or human, without fear during daylight. Animals showing no signs can spread the virus through licking, thus not providing the victim with any indication of potential exposure. Incubation in humans ranges from 1 to 3 months; however, this may vary greatly, with most clinical signs occurring 4 to 8 weeks after exposure. Once clinical signs appear, death is almost inevitable: experimental rabies-specific treatments have not been repeatable, and care remains only palliative.

Children, because of their inquisitive nature, and individuals who work in professions (veterinary medicine, zoos, animal shelters, research laboratories, etc.) that routinely interact with animals are often at greatest risk for rabies. Public education campaigns are directed at maintaining the rabies vaccination status of dogs, cats, and other many other pets, recognizing risks for exposure, encouraging vaccination of individuals with the greatest potential for exposure, and promoting dog and cat population control (CDC, 2016a). Once exposure to a rabid animal has been confirmed it is crucial to thoroughly wash any bite wound with soap and water and seek health care to determine whether PEP is needed. In 2008, it was approximated that 23 415 courses of PEP were administered in the USA following exposure to the bite of an animal that may have been infected with rabies virus (Christian et al., 2009). For persons previously unvaccinated with rabies vaccine, PEP consists of four 1-mL doses of human diploid cell vaccine or purified chick embryo cell vaccine administered intramuscularly as soon as possible after exposure (day 0). Additional doses then should be administered on days 3, 7, and 14 after the first vaccination. Rabies immune globulin (RIG) is also administered. For previously vaccinated persons, two doses of rabies vaccine are administered on days 0 and 3, and no RIG is given (Rupprecht et al., 2010).

7.2.3 Global Burden

Although human rabies in the USA and other resource-rich countries has been dramatically reduced, it persists as an important and often neglected global health issue. Rabies affects human populations in the Americas, Africa, Australia, Eastern Europe, and Asia (Hampson et al., 2015). It is present in temperate, and even in polar regions, but is mainly endemic in resource-constrained tropical areas. This is particularly unfortunate because this zoonosis is entirely preventable (Rupprecht et al., 2002). Too often, control in developing countries focuses only on pre- and post-exposure prophylaxis, if available, of humans, despite the demonstration that control of rabies in domestic dogs is an effective and less costly approach. It is estimated that, globally, over 95% of human rabies is contracted through bites from domestic dogs. Furthermore, mathematical models suggest that 70% vaccination coverage of domestic dogs is adequate to control rabies in canine populations – a vaccination threshold currently recommended by the WHO (Coleman and Dye, 1996; WHO, 2015). However, in many developing countries, despite the effectiveness of canine rabies vaccination to control human infections, dogs are often ignored by veterinary services and the agricultural public health sectors, which tend to focus on livestock species like cattle due to their recognized economic importance. From a policy perspective, there is a need to expand global rabies networks and organizational partnerships and to replicate and scale up successful, sustainable programs for the prevention and control of rabies, including increasing the availability and affordability of PEP (Lembo et al., 2011; WHO, 2012).

7.3 Avian Influenza

7.3.1 Natural History

Aquatic waterfowl and shorebirds are recognized as the pre-eminent natural host species of influenza A viruses (Webster et al., 1992). From these reservoir species, influenza A viruses have been able to adapt to a variety of animals including domestic and wild avian species and an array of mammalian species including swine, horses, and felids. Influenza A viruses have also adapted to humans, and novel strains have emerged since ancient times to cause global pandemics, although these have only been well characterized over the last 100 years (Taubenberger and Morens, 2009). These pandemics have emerged in dissimilar ways from different geographic point sources and have contained diverse genetic elements derived from a variety of avian and mammalian host species (Taubenberger and Kash, 2010). The number of well-studied influenza A "host switch" events has grown over time, but data seem to reinforce their polygenic nature and the inherent unpredictability of these events and the pandemic emergences that result from them. Considered together, they represent a diversity of solutions to influenza's biological imperative to replicate and transmit to other hosts (Taubenberger and Morens, 2009; Morens and Taubenberger, 2011).

Avian influenza is caused by influenza type A virus (influenza A), which belongs to the family *Orthomyxoviridae*. Avian-origin influenza viruses are broadly categorized based on a combination of two groups of proteins on the surface of the influenza A virus: hemagglutinin, or "H" proteins, of which there are 16 (H1–H16); and neuraminidase, or "N" proteins, of which there are nine (N1–N9). Many different combinations of "H" and "N" proteins are possible. Each combination is considered a different subtype, and related viruses within a subtype may be referred to as a lineage (USDA, 2017).

Viral morphology and immunology reveal one of the clearest examples of form and function in the entire field of virology. The single-stranded RNA genome codes for 10 genes and is arranged in eight segments inside a lipid envelope. RNA has a replication error rate of ~1:10 000, thus essentially assuring that every daughter genome is a mutant. Although several gene products are now targets for vaccine antigens, the surface antigens, hemagglutinin (H) and neuraminidase (N), are essential for infection, for eliciting the immune response, and for evading immunity, as well as serving as vaccine components. In addition to being central targets of the host immune response, the hemagglutinin and neuraminidase proteins are essential functional viral proteins. Hemagglutinin serves as a receptor to cells in the respiratory tract and is responsible for attaching the virus to cells prior to viral penetration. Neuraminidase enzymatically cleaves the sialic acid groups from host glycoproteins allowing assembled virus to be released from the host cell (Shtyrya et al., 2009; Cheng et al., 2012).

A large part of the ability of influenza to infect human populations in annual cycles is determined by host immunity and virus ability to overcome host immunity. The ability of influenza to infect, spread, and cause disease in human and other animal populations hinges on two evolutionary mechanisms: point mutations and genetic reassortment. Influenza is one of the few viral diseases that subject the host to annual infections. Viral evasion of the immune system stems from small mutations in H and N antigens that render pre-existing antibodies less effective. This process, often called antigenic drift, periodically leads to viral strains with greater fitness and transmissibility that achieve dominance over other strains and rapidly spread in human populations causing epidemic transmission. In contradistinction to antigenic drift, the eight-segment structure of the influenza viral genome permits segment exchange (or reassortment) when distinct viruses co-infect the same host cell. The progeny viruses that result from reassortment have a mixture of genetic elements from both parent viruses and may be endowed with transmissibility and virulence characteristics that allow them to evade the human immune system and rapidly spread globally – causing a pandemic. Even if not initially endowed with the capacity to efficiently spread from human to human, this capability could theoretically develop through small point mutations over time (Webster and Govorkova, 2014)

Influenza is an ancient disease of waterfowl, with viral mapping aging the virus back centuries. Waterfowl from over the globe migrate north of the Arctic Circle for breeding and rearing of the young; avian influenza is generally spread throughout the community of birds with no signs of infection. Unlike mammalian infection, the virus in waterfowl is shed in the gut and contaminates the wetlands, persisting in the 39 F/4C water for up to 20 days. Only about 1 bird in 1000 will have a persistent infection and that is enough for the virus to be borne globally with the winter migration. A polar projection of the globe reveals that Europe, Asia, and North America are relatively close, and thus all susceptible to spread of influenza virus. Influenza is naturally spread amongst wildfowl, as seen from records of the H5N1 originating in East Asia starting in the late 1990s (Lee et al., 2015).

Humans are particularly susceptible to develop influenza because we share the influenza virus with several species, most notably pigs and poultry. Indeed, when the "three Ps" (people, poultry, pigs) reside together, the H and N surface proteins on the influenza virus tend to rearrange and subsequently confuse the recognition and memory of an individual's immune system. Traditional cultural practices of herding swine and ducks into the farmer's courtyard and stables exposed the inhabitants to infection. It is assumed that swine became infected from ducks, and then chickens became infected (Emch et al., 2017). At some point the virus was sufficiently adapted to replicate in horses with occasionally disastrous results for cities that relied on horse-drawn public transportation, garbage collection, and fire service. Within modern times, an adaptation of equine influenza has been seen in dogs in the USA, and avian influenza has also adapted to felids (Short et al., 2015)

7.3.2 Recent Outbreaks

Since the late 1990s, avian influenza (A) H5N1 viruses have emerged as major pathogens in domestic poultry in numerous countries and have been transmitted sporadically, or by "spillover" to humans exposed to infected flocks. In humans, from 2003 through mid-2017, the avian influenza A (H5N1) virus caused a limited number of human cases (859), but high mortality (52.7%) (WHO, 2017b). To date there is no evidence of sustained human-to-human community spread. In 2013, low pathogenic avian influenza A (H7N9) viruses emerged in China in domestic poultry, where they caused inapparent infection, that is, low pathogenicity. Despite this low pathogenicity in poultry, the avian influenza A (H7N9) virus has infected more humans than avian influenza A (H5N1), and has a substantial, albeit lower, case-fatality rate (CFR). As of June 2007, there were 1533 human infections with avian influenza A (H7N9) with at least 592 deaths (CFR = 38.6%) reported to the World Health Organization since March 2013 (WHO, 2017c).

Exemplifying the complex genetic events that underlie the emergence of these strains is that both avian influenza A (H5N1) and H7N9 are triple reassortment viruses, with six segments from avian influenza A (H9N2) viruses, which are enzootic in poultry populations in parts of Africa, Asia, and the Middle East. It appears that reassortment with avian influenza A (H9N2) led to a dramatic increase in human infections with H5N1 and H7N9 viruses, suggesting that H9N2 must be considered an important "enabler" of infection (Webster and Govorkova, 2014; WHO, 2017c). In fact, avian influenza A (H9N2) has the ability to infect humans: the first case in a human was detected in 1999 in Hong Kong SAR, and by 2017 there were approximately 30 reported infections with avian influenza A (H9N2), all reported from China, Bangladesh, and Egypt, as well as Hong Kong SAR. In most human cases, signs and symptoms are mild and there has been no evidence of human-to-human transmission (WHO. 2016a).

Among domestic poultry in the USA, primarily chickens and turkeys, avian influenza presents in one of two forms, classified as either "low pathogenic" or "highly pathogenic" based on their genetic features and the severity of the disease they cause. Most poultry influenza viruses are of *low pathogenicity* (LPAI), meaning that they cause no signs or only minor clinical signs of infection in poultry and are spread either through direct contact between healthy and infected birds, or through contact with contaminated equipment and other materials (USDA, 2016). Because of its ability to quickly cause severe financial impact to a commercial poultry operator, for example, decreased egg production and lower feed efficiency, even the presence of LPAI is cause for concern. Depopulation is one method to control LPAI, but local government officials ultimately determine the control methods used for LPAI. *Highly pathogenic avian influenza* (HPAI) viruses cause severe clinical signs and potentially high mortality rates among poultry. A 2015 incursion of HPAI avian influenza A (H5N2) in the Midwest led to the depopulation of over 40 million turkeys and chickens and decreased egg production in the USA, to the point where demand was met by importing eggs from Europe (Greene, 2015). To date, there have been no confirmed human infections with avian influenza A (H5) viruses in the USA, although as noted above, cases have occurred in humans exposed to infected poultry in other parts of the world.

Due in large part to the random nature of point mutations and reassortment events, and its many animal reservoirs, influenza A remains a daunting public health challenge. Pandemic emergence is a particularly unpredictable phenomenon. As Morens and Fauci (2013) have noted, its "appearance in pandemic form, its patterns of pandemic recurrence, the stability of its endemic persistence, its eventual disappearance, and its ability to cause fatalities all appear to be highly complex and poorly understood."

The pandemic that was caused by avian influenza A (H1N1)pdm09 virus provides a prime example of the unpredictability and challenging nature of pandemic influenza. Influenza experts around the world were preparing for the spillover from birds and subsequent spread of avian influenza A (H5N1) in humans. Many predicted that the next pandemic would emerge from a point source in Asia where most poultry-based outbreaks were concentrated, and where high human population density in proximity to poultry farms provided seemingly optimal conditions for an initial spillover event. Instead, the avian influenza A (H1N1)pdm09 influenza virus spread from swine to humans in Mexico. Despite advances in global influenza surveillance, respiratory infection spread and amplified in Mexico without being identified as influenza. Only after its spread to California and Texas was it confirmed to be an outbreak of influenza A. As of August 2010, more than 18 000 human deaths in more than 214 countries or territories had been attributed to this pandemic (WHO, 2010a). In September 2010, WHO monitoring of the pandemic moved into the post-pandemic period, at which time it was to be considered a "seasonal" influenza virus, which continues to this day to circulate globally, with typical seasonal influenza patterns (WHO, 2010b). The swine origin of the virus was another surprising feature of the pandemic and revealed the global inadequacy of surveillance for influenza in swine populations. Because of this pandemic, the importance of swine surveillance was recognized and subsequently addressed through an expansion of the "OFFLU" network, a collaboration between the World Animal Health Organization (OIE) and the Food and Agricultural Organization of the United Nations (FAO), which was originally established to monitor avian influenza, and subsequently swine influenza. The intent of the OFFLU network is for the animal health community to provide early recognition and characterization of emerging influenza viral strains in animal populations, and effective management of known infections, thereby better managing the risk to human health and supporting global food security, animal health and welfare, and other community benefits derived from domestic animals

and wildlife (OFFLU, 2017; Webster and Govorkova, 2014).

Given the preparations for a pandemic attributable to avian influenza A (H5N1), which would be expected to be severe, another unexpected characteristic of the 2009 H1N1 pandemic was its relatively low severity and low CFR. Initial reports suggested that its H protein was antigenically similar to the hemagglutinin protein from the 1918 Spanish influenza H1N1 virus leading to concern that this might be a particularly severe pandemic (Xu et al., 2010). But, the H1N1pdm09 strain proved to relatively mild. In fact, the WHO found that the overwhelming majority of humans infected with avian influenza A (H1N1)pdm09 experienced uncomplicated influenza-like illness, with full recovery within a week, even without medical treatment (WHO, 2009). H1N1 influenza presentations were commonly severe in younger persons who were immunologically naive to H1N1 strains that had circulated during and after the Spanish flu pandemic. This also explains the relatively mild impact this pandemic had on the elderly. Infection with this strain was also associated with severe disease in pregnant women and the obese. Overall it is estimated to have killed over 100 000 persons worldwide (Simonsen et al., 2013). The 2009 pandemic also confirmed that despite improvement in preparation of influenza vaccines, the process still took more than 6 months for vaccine rollout and was inadequate to address the first wave of the pandemic (Jack, 2009; McKenna, 2010). Another example of a virus that needs to be closely monitored is highly pathogenic avian influenza A (H5N8), detected in 2016 and currently circulating among a widening range of poultry flocks, presumably being transmitted by wild birds. In 2017, avian influenza A (H5N8) was detected in Africa, Asia, Europe, and the Middle East resulting in the depopulation of hundreds of millions of poultry, but no human infections with the H5N8 virus have been reported. However, increasing surveillance efforts for this virus must continue to be implemented globally in an effort to detect early human infections. The capacity for avian influenza A (H5N8) to cause a pandemic is unclear but the threat of a pandemic always exists if one human is able to sustainably transmit any influenza virus to another.

Influenza research focuses on the discovery of a long-lasting vaccine that does not rely on the mutable H or N antigens. Efforts are underway to develop a universal flu vaccine that is based on the highly conserved stalk of the H protein and the ectodomain of the M2 protein that is embedded in the lipid envelope with its ectodomain exposed on the surface (Pinto and Lamb, 2006; Cheng et al., 2012). A major controversy in influenza research is "enhancement of function" research, which seeks to discover what changes could make influenza more dangerous for people. Opponents of this research fear that the virus could escape the laboratory and cause a global pandemic. At present, no laboratory assays can reliably predict the virulence, transmissibility, or clinical severity of potential pandemic strains, making the development of such assays an important research goal. In addition, new classes of antiviral agents that attack different parts of the life cycle are needed so that combination therapies could be developed to augment influenza control efforts and to prevent the emergence of drug-resistant strains.

From a policy standpoint, the recent explosive spread of avian influenza A (H5N8) and its unknown impact on humans, and the emergence of the pandemic attributable to influenza A (H1N1)pdm09 virus originating from swine, suggest that animal and human surveillance must be strengthened and that biosecurity must be regularly practiced. Resources must be directed toward resource-challenged countries in which epizootics among poultry continue to occur and biosecurity is not financially feasible. To summarize, global epidemiologic and laboratory capacity to detect and characterize influenza viruses that emerge in local contexts must be strengthened.

7.4 Zika Virus

The ready availability of antibiotics after World War II greatly facilitated virus isolation in cell culture and subsequently the identification of geographically limited viruses from disparate environments that caused morbidity ranging from vague flu-like symptoms to much more serious clinical presentations. This also led to the definition of the arthropod-borne ("arbo-") viruses, and the many viral families they constituted. These viruses, now numbered in the hundreds and typically named after site of isolation, share similar natural histories, as is seen with the causative agents of West Nile disease, dengue, chikungunya, and now Zika virus.

Yellow fever demonstrated the global distribution of arboviruses and provided the general pattern for globalization of dengue, chikungunya, and West Nile virus. The mosquito vector, the wide-ranging *Aedes* spp., and the virus were brought to the New World from Africa aboard slave ships and merchant vessels (Smith, 2013). The disease advanced at the speed of human travel – the speed of a sailing ship. Disease still advances at the speed of human travel, albeit via intercontinental air flights at over 500 miles per hour.

Zika virus was isolated from a sentinel rhesus monkey in the Zika forest of Entebbe, Uganda, in 1947 and the first human cases were identified in 1952 in Uganda and Tanzania (Simpson, 1964). The virus slowly migrated east across South Asia without causing much disease and appeared on Yap Island, Micronesia, in 2007, where it caused clinical disease characterized by rash, conjunctivitis, and arthralgia, and infected approximately 73% of Yap residents aged 3 years or older. This outbreak represented the first detection of transmission of Zika virus outside of Africa and Asia (Duffy et al., 2009). Starting in 2013, the virus was responsible for thousands of infections throughout the Pacific islands and was implicated in an increase of Guillain–Barré syndrome in those same populations (Oehler et al., 2014). Zika virus was undetected in the Americas until March 2015, when Brazil notified WHO of an unknown viral-like illness. In April of that same year, a Brazilian state laboratory tested samples that were positive for Zika virus, and in May, the national laboratory confirmed the presence of the virus in a patient's blood sample, confirming virus circulation among humans (WHO, 2017d). There was little doubt that the virus would arrive in North America due to the routine and frequent intercontinental travel between Brazil and the USA.

The sudden and cumulative changes in the virulence of Zika virus may be explained by a mutation that occurred sometime during the infection on the island of Yap. There is phylogenetic evidence that the virus that initially entered Brazil in 2013 is descended from the French Polynesian ZIKV strain (Faria et al., 2016). The impact of the virus was hard to discern until the infection reached the much larger population centers of Brazil where approximately 5000 cases of microcephaly provided a sufficient epidemiologic link of infection and microcephaly (Johansson et al., 2016).

However, it is by no means certain that the magnitude and severe outcomes associated with the current global pandemic of Zika virus are because of viral mutational changes. de Melo Freire et al. (2015) demonstrated that the recent Asian lineage, when compared with the African lineage, was associated with significant NS1 codon usage to human housekeeping genes, an adaptation that could facilitate viral fitness resulting in enhanced replication and increased viral titers. However, further studies are necessary to determine whether these or other viral genetic modifications mediated a true shift in viral pathogenesis (Lessler et al., 2016).

One alternative hypothesis to explain the recent explosive spread of Zika virus in the Americas is that it is driven by chance – the accidental introduction of the virus into a large immunologically naive Brazilian population. However, given the frequency of international travel, it is unclear why such introductions did not occur earlier. Some

have postulated that in 2015–2016, temperature and rainfall increases stemming from El Niño could have contributed to Zika virus spread through an extension of the geographic range and population size of its chief vector, the *Aedes* mosquitoes. Others have posited that immunological interactions with other flaviviruses, such as dengue virus, may be facilitating the spread and severity of the clinical response to Zika virus infection during this recent pandemic. More severe presentations of dengue fever are known to occur through antibody-dependent enhancement mechanisms when a host previously exposed to one serotype of dengue virus is infected with a different serotype (Lessler et al., 2016). Yet another potential cause of the recent dramatic spread of Zika virus in the Americas is a possible genetic change in the mosquito vector. Although there is no evidence for this, it is known that some genetic variants of *A. aegypti* are more competent than others at transmitting flaviviruses (Black et al., 2002).

Anxiety about the rapid spread of a virus through an immunologically naive population is exacerbated by evidence of virally induced fetal malformations. The ability of viruses to cross the placental barrier is well recognized in humans and animals. However, Zika virus is the first arbovirus recognized to cross the placenta in humans. As is well documented in cattle, the stage of gestation when infection occurs is related to site and degree of damage. Because this is a "new" virus, the correlation of trimester of gestation at infection and damage induced are not well established for Zika virus infection. The causal relationship of Zika virus and microcephaly has been established (Johansson et al., 2016).

Although impressive gains have been made in our understanding of the current Zika virus health crisis, there is still much to learn. John Maurice identified several knowledge gaps, discussed at recent WHO emergency committee meetings (Maurice, 2016). These included the effect of strain variation on clinical disease severity, an incomplete understanding of the neuropathology of Zika virus, including consequences of *in utero* exposures in infants born without overt microcephaly, the persistence of virus infection, the risk of infection during different phases of gestation, and the identification of strains of *Aedes* mosquitoes responsible for transmission and their sensitivity to insecticides. Another key question is whether Zika virus will establish an endemic presence following its introduction in affected areas and whether vaccines can be developed and tested quickly enough to have a meaningful impact on the course of this evolving pandemic. Since the majority of infections are inapparent, surveillance for this infection is challenging and dependent on the promotion of rapid-cycle research to enable the development of biological assays to identify infection with Zika virus. Of particular concern is the ongoing presence of the *Aedes* mosquitoes, for which there is no sustainable control mechanism. *A. aegypti* and *A. albopictus*, the two most competent *Flavivirus* vectors, are both present in the USA and both capable of transmitting virus (CDC, 2016b). Increasing surveillance, laboratory capacity, and funding for vector control mechanism research requires political will and robust, sustainable funding.

7.5 Ebola Virus Disease (EVD)

Ebola virus seems to be a highly niche-adapted virus requiring a complex web of interactions to lead to human disease. The virus is a member of the small family of *Filoviridae*, which are filamentous viruses with five known genera. *Filoviridae* members have nucleic acid arranged in an elongate nucleocapsid with the genome, of about 19 000 nucleotides, coding for seven genes that resemble the organization of the *Paramyxoviridae* (Feldman and Klenk, 1996). Although the Marburg agent had been known since 1967 due to laboratory acquired infections of 31 people working with African grivet monkeys, Ebola virus hemorrhagic fever was not recognized until 1976 when a Marburg-like virus was isolated from an outbreak of hemorrhagic fever in Zaire near the Ebola River. The pattern of infection has not changed since those early cases. The natural history of Ebola virus was, however, much harder to describe. Today the natural reservoir of Ebola is believed to be fruit bats (Leirs et al., 1999). Ebola virus causes illness in humans and nonhuman primates and is caused by infection with a virus of the family *Filoviridae*. There are five detected Ebola virus species to date: Ebola virus (*Zaire ebolavirus*), Sudan virus (*Sudan ebolavirus*), Taï Forest virus (*Taï Forest ebolavirus*, formerly *Côte d'Ivoire ebolavirus*), Bundibugyo virus (*Bundibugyo ebolavirus*), and Reston virus (*Reston ebolavirus*), which does not cause disease in humans, but does in nonhuman primates.

The natural cycle of the virus seems to be a silent reservoir in fruit bats and possibly in insectivorous bats, with ground species such as primates or duiker antelope being infected only infrequently. Infection in wildlife may come from consumption of dead or sick bats, their incompleted meals, or their excreta. Scavenging mammals may be quite susceptible to infection, and health agencies sometimes get alarms of duiker or primate die-offs as a prelude to human infection. People in poorer parts of Africa may scavenge or salvage protein from dead animals or may hunt "bushmeat," a generic term for whatever the hunter gets. Human infection probably occurs as the harvester dresses the animal and then becomes the index case for the village. Human-to-human transmission follows and can lead to large numbers of affected people. In some past Ebola outbreaks, primates were also affected by Ebola and multiple spillover events occurred when people touched or ate infected primates (CDC, 2016b).

Initial signs and symptoms of infection with Ebola virus are so indistinct that many diseases are included in a clinician's differential diagnosis list, potentially resulting in insufficient personal protective measures and potentially infection of health-care workers (HCWs). In fact, delay in diagnosis and nosocomial transmission were early features of the 2014 West African EVD epidemic. The first case, which occurred on December 26, 2013, in a 2-year-old boy in Milandou, Guinea, is believed to have originated as a spillover from an epizootic in wildlife. That case and subsequent cases in other parts of Guinea, Sierra Leone, and Liberia went undiagnosed until March 23, 2014, when an astute health official at the WHO requested that a specimen be sent from the Ministry of Health in Guinea to the Institut Pasteur, and Ebola virus etiology was confirmed. By that point, Ebola virus had been spreading for 3 months, a time period equivalent to the longest previous African epidemic. The virus spreads by contact with infected fluids and enters the next host by wounds or mucosal exposure. By the end of the outbreak, in March 2016, it had been the largest outbreak of EVD ever reported, with a total of 28 646 laboratory-confirmed, probable, and suspected cases, from Guinea, Liberia, Sierra Leone, Nigeria, Mali, and Senegal. The remainder of any cases reported resulted from travel (WHO, 2016b). In the 2014 West Africa Ebola epidemic, epidemiologists remarked that Ebola virus seemed designed to target health-care workers. In fact, in Liberia by August 2014 there had been 10 clusters of EVD reported among HCWs (Matanock et al., 2014). The basic reproduction number, R_0, which indicates how contagious an infectious disease is, was high for two groups of people: HCWs and family members of those infected. HCWs needed to suspect EVD as the likely cause of clinical presentations with even nondescript symptoms (Hageman et al., 2016). Family members had to be informed about the dangers of burial rituals, which often involved washing and kissing the corpse.

The 2014 West African EVD outbreak remains a stark reminder that poor healthcare infrastructure, particularly in resource-poor countries, can have devastating global consequences when challenged with a virulent pathogen such as the *Zaire ebolavirus*. This reminder was visited, yet again, when in May 2017 the Democratic Republic of the Congo's Ministry of Health confirmed an outbreak of EVD, the eighth outbreak of EVD since 1976. Despite the outbreak's location being extremely remote, a coordinated response from multiple partners resulted in only five confirmed cases (four fatal) of EVD of 105 suspected cases (WHO, 2017d).

The WHO was singled out for its slow response in the early stages of the West African outbreak, and there has been a call for essential WHO reforms (Moon et al., 2015; Frieden et al., 2014; Coltart et al., 2017). Perhaps the most difficult lesson of the West African Ebola virus outbreak is that to succeed against this and other emerging threats, we must find the political will to support the building of local public health capacity in all nations of the world. The notion of neglected tropical diseases is a deeply ingrained and helpful construct but until we find a way to support the neglected countries that harbor and give rise to these emerging diseases, we will be severely hindered in our efforts to control them.

7.6 Summary

It is imperative that humanitarian-focused efforts of developed countries, agencies, and other international stakeholders invest in implementing policies that can be driven at the local level to actively prevent, detect, and respond to disease and emerging disease threats – which is the aim of the US Global Health Security Agenda (CDC, 2016c). The USA works with partner institutions on Prevent, Detect, Respond "action packages" to provide focus and structure to effectively respond to infectious disease threats around the world, including actions mentioned earlier in this chapter, for example, promoting biosecurity systems, developing laboratory capacity, and improving access to medical and nonmedical countermeasures, among other objectives (https://www.ghsagenda.org/packages). Without specific objectives to guide the reduction of disease burden among animal and human populations, the threat of emerging infectious diseases will persist.

Acknowledgments

The authors gratefully acknowledge the extensive contributions of Kira A. Christian, DVM, MPH, DACVPM, and John A. Herrmann, DVM, MPH, DACT, in the preparation of this chapter.

References

Abraham, T. (2009). Risk and outbreak communication: lessons from alternative paradigms. *Bull WHO* 87, 604–607.

Birhane, M.G., Cleaton, J.M., Monroe, B.P., et al. (2017). Rabies surveillance in the United States during 2015. *J Am Vet Med Assoc* 250(10), 1117–1130.

Black, W.C. 4th, Bennett, K.E., Gorrochótegui-Escalante, N., et al. (2002). Flavivirus susceptibility in Aedes aegypti. *Arch Med Res* 33(4), 379–388.

CDC (Centers for Disease Control and Prevention) (1996). Pneumocystis pneumonia––Los Angeles. *Morb Mortal Wkly Rep.* 45(34), 729–733.

CDC (Centers for Disease Control and Prevention) (2011). How is rabies transmitted? Atlanta, GA: CDC. Available at: https://www.cdc.gov/rabies/transmission/exposure.html (accessed 20 April, 2017).

CDC (Centers for Disease Control and Prevention) (2015a). Human Rabies. Atlanta, GA: CDC. Available at: https://www.cdc.gov/rabies/location/usa/surveillance/human_rabies.html (accessed 10 May, 2017).

CDC (Centers for Disease Control and Prevention) (2015b). Ebola Virus Disease Transmission. Atlanta, GA: CDC. Available at: https://www.cdc.gov/vhf/ebola/transmission/index.html (accessed 15 July, 2017).

CDC (Centers for Disease Control and Prevention) (2016a). World Rabies Day. Atlanta, GA: CDC. Available at: https://www.cdc.gov/worldrabiesday/(accessed 20 April, 2017).

CDC (Centers for Disease Control and Prevention) (2016b). Estimated range of *Aedes albopictus and Aedes aegypti* in the United States, *2016.* Atlanta, GA: CDC. Available at: https://www.cdc.gov/zika/pdfs/zika-mosquito-maps.pdf (accessed 6 July, 2017).

CDC (Centers for Disease Control and Prevention) (2016c). The Global Health Security Agenda. Atlanta, GA: CDC. Available at: https://www.cdc.gov/globalhealth/security/ghsagenda.html (accessed 6 July, 2017).

CDC (Centers for Disease Control and Prevention) (2017). *Legionella* (Legionnaire's Disease and Pontiac Fever). Atlanta, GA: CDC. Available at: https://www.cdc.gov/legionella/about/history.html (accessed 15 May, 2017).

Cheng, V.C., To, K.K., Tse, H., Hung, I.F., and Yuen, K.Y. (2012). Two years after pandemic influenza A/2009/H1N1: what have we learned? *Clin Microbiol Rev* 25(2), 223–263.

Christian, K.A., Blanton, J.D., Auslander, M., and Rupprecht, C.E. (2009). Epidemiology of rabies post-exposure prophylaxis––United States of America, 2006–2008. *Vaccine* 27(51), 7156–7161.

Coleman, P.G. and Dye, C. (1996). Immunization coverage required to prevent outbreaks of dog rabies. *Vaccine* 14(3), 185–186.

Coltart, C.E., Lindsey, B., Ghinai, I., et al. (2017). The Ebola outbreak, 2013–2016: old lessons for new epidemics, *Philos Trans R Soc Lond B Biol Sci* 372(1721).

de Melo Freire, C.C., Iamarino, A., de Lima Neto, D.F., Sall, A.A., and de Andrade Zanotto, P.M. (2015). Spread of the pandemic Zika virus lineage is associated with NS1 codon usage adaptation in humans, *bioRxiv*, pp. 1–8; doi: 10.1101/032839.

Duffy, M.R., Chen T.-H., Hancock, W.T., et al. (2009). Zika virus outbreak on Yap Island, Federated States of Micronesia. *N Engl J Med* 360(24), 2536–2543.

Emch, M., Dowling-Root, E., and Carrel, M. (2017). *Health and Medical Geography*, 4th edn, London: Guilford Press.

Faria, N.R., Azevedo, R.D.S.V.S., Kraemer. M.U.G., et al. (2016). Zika virus in the Americas: Early epidemiological and genetic findings. *Science* 352(6283), 345–349.

Feldman, H. and Klenk, H.-D. (1996). *Medical Microbiology*, 4th edn. Galveston: University of Texas.

Fineberg, H.V.W. and Wilson, M.E. (2010). Emerging Infectious Diseases. International Risk Governance Council, Lausanne. Available at: http://irgc.org/wp-content/uploads/2012/04/Emerging_Infectious_Diseases_Fineberg_and_Wilson-2.pdf (accessed April 20, 2017).

Frieden, T.R., Damon, I., Bell, B.P., Kenyon, T., and Nichol, S. (2014). Ebola 2014––new challenges, new global response and responsibility. *N Engl J Med* 371(13), 1177–1180.

Gradmann, C. (2014). A spirit of scientific rigour: Koch's postulates in twentieth-century medicine. *Microbes Infect* 16(11), 885–892.

Greene, J.L. (2015). Update on the highly-pathogenic avian influenza outbreak of 2014–2015. *Congressional Research Service* 7-5700, R4414.

Hageman, J.C., Hazim, C., Wilson, K., et al. (2016). Infection prevention and control for Ebola in health care settings – West Africa and United States. *MMWR Suppl* 65(3), 50–56.

Hampson, K., Coudeville, L., Lembo, T., et al. (2015). Estimating the global burden of endemic canine rabies. *PLoS Negl Trop Dis* 9(4), e0003709.

Henderson, D.A. (2011). The eradication of smallpox––an overview of the past, present, and future. *Vaccine* 29(Suppl. 4), D7–9.

Institutes of Medicine (2009). *Sustaining Global Surveillance and Response to Emerging Zoonotic Diseases.* Washington, DC: National Academies Press.

Jack, A. (2009). The problem with flu vaccines. *BMJ* 338, 1298–1299.

Jackson, A.C. and Greenlee, J.E. (1993). Rabies. Neurology Medlink. Available at: http://www.medlink.com/article/rabies#Zinke_1804 (accessed April 15, 2017).

Johansson, M.A., Mier-y-Teran-Romero, L., Reefhuis, J., Gilboa, S.M., and Hills, S.L. (2016). Zika and the risk of microcephaly. *N Engl J Med* 375, 1–4.

Karesh, W.B., Dobson, A., Lloyd-Smith, J.O., et al. (2012). Ecology of zoonoses; natural and unnatural histories. *Lancet* 380, 1936–1945.

Keogh-Brown, M.R. and Smith, R.D. (2008). The economic impact of SARS: how does the reality match the predictions? *Health Policy* 88(1), 110–120.

Kilpatrick, A.M. and Randolph, S.E. (2012). Drivers, dynamics, and control of emerging vector-borne zoonotic diseases. *Lancet* 380, 1946–1955.

Lee, D.H., Torchetti, M.K., Winker, K., Ip, H.S., Song, C.-S., and Swayne, D.E. (2015). Intercontinental spread of Asian-origin H5N8 to North America through Beringia by migratory birds, *J Virol* 89(12), 6521–6524.

Leirs, H., Mills, J.N., Krebs, J.W., et al. (1999). Search for the Ebola virus reservoir in Kikwit, DR: Reflections on a vertebrate collection. *J Infect Dis* 179(s. 1), S155–S163.

Lembo, T., Attlan, M., Bourhy, H., et al. 2011, Renewed global partnerships and redesigned roadmaps for rabies prevention and control, *Vet Med Int* 2011, Art. No. 923149.

Lessler, J., Chaisson, L.H., Kucirka, L.M., et al. (2016). Assessing the global threat from Zika virus. *Science* 353(6300), aaf8160.

Matanock, A., Arwady, M.A., Ayscue, P., et al. (2014). Ebola virus disease cases among health care workers not working in Ebola treatment units––Liberia, June–August, 2014. *Morb Mortal Wkly Rep* 63(46), 1077–1081.

Maurice, J. (2016). The Zika virus public health emergency: 6 months on. *Lancet* 388(10043) 449–450.

McKenna, M. (2010). H1N1 lessons learned vaccine production foiled, confirmed experts' predictions. Centre for Infectious Disease Research and Policy. Available at: http://www.cidrap.umn.edu/news-perspective/2010/04/h1n1-lessons-learned-pandemic-underscored-influenzas-unpredictability (accessed December 1, 2017).

Mills, J., Gage, K.L., and Khan, A.S. (2010). Potential Influence of climate change on vector-borne and zoonotic diseases: a review and proposed research plan. *Environ Health Perspect* 118(1), 1507–1514.

Moon, S., Sridhar, D., Pate, M.A., et al. (2015). Will Ebola change the game? Ten essential reforms before the next pandemic. The report of the Harvard-LSHTM Independent Panel on the Global Response to Ebola. *Lancet* 386(10009), 2204–2221.

Morens, D.M. and Fauci, A.S. (2013). Emerging infectious diseases: threats to human health and global stability. *PLoS Pathog* 9(7), e1003467.

Morens, D.M. and Taubenberger, J.K (2011). Pandemic influenza: certain uncertainties. *Rev Med Virol* 21(5), 262–284.

National Park Service (2005). *Rabies and Rabies Control in Wildlife*. Washington, DC: NPS.

Oehler, E., Watrin, L., Larre, P., et al. (2014). Zika virus infection complicated by Guillain–Barré syndrome––case report, French Polynesia, December 2013. *Euro Surveill* 19(9), 1–3.

OFFLU (2017). *Mission and objectives, 2017*. Geneva: OFFLU.

Olson, S.H., Benedum, C.M., Mekaru, S.R., et al. (2015). Drivers of emerging infectious disease events as a framework for digital detection. *Emerg Infect Dis* 21(8), 1285–1292.

Ortblad, K.F., Lozano, R., and Murray, C.J. (2013). The burden of HIV: Insights from the GBD 2010, *AIDS, vol.* 27, pp 2003–2017.

Phoofolo, P. (1993). Epidemics and revolutions: the rinderpest epidemic in late nineteenth-century southern Africa. *Past and Present* 138(1), 112–143.

Pinto, L.H. and Lamb, R.A. (2006). The M2 proton channels of influenza A and B viruses. *J Biol Chem* 281(14), 8997–9000.

Rupprecht, C.E., Briggs, D., Brown, C.M., et al. (2010). Use of a reduced (4-dose) vaccine schedule for postexposure prophylaxis to prevent human rabies: recommendations of the Advisory Committee on Immunization Practices. *MMWR* 59(Rr-2), 1–9.

Rupprecht, C.E., Hanlon, C.A., and Hemachuha, T. (2002). Rabies re-examined. *Lancet Infect Dis* 2(6), 327–343.

Short, K.R., Richard, M., Verhagen, J.H., et al. (2015). One health, multiple challenges: The inter-species transmission of influenza A virus. *One Health* 1, 1–13.

Shtyrya, Y.A., Mochlova, L.V., and Bovin, N.V. (2009). Influenza virus neuraminidase: structure and function. *Acta Naturae* 1(2), 26–32.

Simonsen, L., Spreeuwenberg, P., Lustig, R., et al. (2013). Global mortality estimates for the 2009 influenza pandemic from the GLaMOR project: a modeling study. *PLoS Med* 10(11), e1001558.

Simpson, D.I. (1964). Zika virus infection in man. *Trans R Soc Trop Med Hyg* 58, 335–338.

Slate, D., Rupprecht, C.E., Rooney, J.A., Donovan, D., Lein, D.H., and Chipman, R.B. (2005). Status of oral rabies vaccination in wild carnivores in the United States. *Virus Res* 111, 68–76.

Smith, B.G. (2013) *Ship of Death: a Voyage That Changed the Atlantic World*. New Haven: Yale University Press.

Smith, R.D. (2006). Responding to global infectious disease outbreaks: lessons from SARS on the role of risk perception, communication and management. *Soc Sci Med* 63(12), 3113–3123.

Taubenberger, J.K. and Kash, J.C. (2010). Influenza virus evolution, host adaptation and pandemic formation. *Cell Host Microbe* 7(6), 440–451.

Taubenberger, J.K. and Morens, D.M. (2009). Pandemic influenza – including a risk assessment of H1N1. *Rev Sci Tech* 28, 187–202.

Thompson, D., Muriel, P., Russell, D., et al. (2001). Economic costs of the foot-and-mouth disease outbreak in the United Kingdom in 2001. *Rev Sci Tech* 44, 675–687.

USDA (United States Department of Agriculture) (2016). Low pathogenicity avian influenza (LPAI). Available at: https://www.aphis.usda.gov/aphis/ourfocus/animalhealth/animal-disease-information/avian-influenza-disease/defend-the-flock/defend-the-flock-lpai-info (accessed December 1, 2017).

USDA (United States Department of Agriculture) (2017). Highly pathogenic avian influenza. Washington, DC: USDA. Available at: https://www.aphis.usda.gov/aphis/ourfocus/animalhealth/animal-disease-information/avian-influenza-disease/defend-the-flock/2017-hpai (accessed December 1, 2017).

Velasco-Villa, A., Reeder, S.A., Orciari, L.A., et al. (2008). Enzootic rabies elimination from dogs and reemergence in wild terrestrial carnivores, United States. *Emerg Infect Dis* 14(12), 1849–1854.

Webster, R.G. and Govorkova, E.A. (2014). Continuing challenges in influenza. *Ann N Y Acad Sci* 1323, 115–139.

Webster, R.G., Bean, W.J., Gorman, O.T., Chambers, T.M., and Kawaoka, Y. (1992). Evolution and ecology of influenza A viruses. *Microbiol Rev* 56, 152–179.

WHO (World Health Organization) (1978). Ebola haemorrhagic fever in Zaire, 1976. *Bull World Health Organ* 56(2), 271–293.

WHO (World Health Organization) (2003). *Summary of probable SARS cases with onset of illness from 1 November 2002 to 31 July 2003*. Geneva: WHO.

WHO (World Health Organization) (2009). *Clinical features of severe cases of pandemic influenza*. Geneva: WHO.

WHO (World Health Organization) (2010a). *Pandemic (H1N1) 2009 – update 112*. Geneva: WHO.

WHO (World Health Organization) (2010b). *Influenza updates*. Geneva: WHO.

WHO (World Health Organization) (2012). *Strategic Framework for Elimination of Human Rabies Transmitted by Dogs in the South-East Asia Region*. New Delhi: WHO.

WHO (World Health Organization) (2015). *Human and dog rabies vaccines and immunoglobulins: Report of a meeting*. Geneva: WHO.

WHO (World Health Organization) (2016a). *Influenza at the human–animal interface: Summary and assessment*. Geneva: WHO.

WHO (World Health Organization) (2016b). *Ebola Situation Report*. Geneva: WHO.

WHO (World Health Organization) (2017a). *Rabies*. Geneva: WHO.

WHO (World Health Organization) (2017b). *Cumulative number of confirmed human cases for avian influenza A(H5N1) reported to WHO, 2003–2017*. Geneva: WHO.

WHO (World Health Organization) (2017c). *Human infection with avian influenza A(H7N9) virus – China*. Geneva: WHO.

WHO (World Health Organization) (2017d). *Ebola outbreak Democratic Republic of the Congo 2017*. Geneva: WHO.

Xu, R., Ekiert, D.C., Krause, J.C., Hai, R., Crowe, J.E. Jr, and Wilson, I.A. (2010). Structural basis of preexisting immunity to the 2009 H1N1 pandemic influenza virus. *Science* 328(5976), 357–360.

8

Reigning Cats and Dogs: Perks and Perils of Our Courtship with Companion Animals

Sandra L. Lefebvre[1] and Robert V. Ellis[2]

[1] *American Veterinary Medical Association, Schaumburg, IL, USA*
[2] *University of Cincinnati College of Medicine, Cincinnati, OH, USA*

8.1 Introduction

The strength of the bond between people and their companion animals is reflected in trends in human behavior and the pet products and services industries. Eighty percent of the online population in Argentina and Mexico and 73% of the online population in Russia in 2015 (GfK, 2016), 65% of US households in 2014 (American Pet Products Manufacturers' Association, 2017), 63% of Australian households in 2013 (Australian Veterinary Association, 2016), 57% of Canadian households in 2014 (Alberta Agriculture and Forestry, 2014), and 52% of UK households in 2015 (People's Dispensary for Sick Animals, 2016) had at least one pet. Pets have become increasingly popular in other countries as well (ZENOAQ, 2013) (The Korea Bizwire, 2014; Anon., 2012; Bruha, 2015; GfK, 2016) and in some situations seem to be preferred to children (Evans and Buerk, 2012). Cats and dogs are the most common companion animals in most countries, with others, such as rabbits and caged birds, found in 3% or fewer households (Pet Food Manufacturers' Association, 2015; American Veterinary Medical Association, 2012). Our affection toward these pets is growing, with many owners now considering their pets as members of the family. Thirty

percent of dog owners and 61% of cat owners in the USA and Australia reported sleeping with their pets in a 2004 telephone survey (Laflamme et al., 2008). In the same survey, 26% of cat owners and 22% of dog owners reported eating with their pets.

Human-type services and products for pets, including birthday parties, weddings, blessings, funerals, costumes, bakery products, holiday gifts, and greeting cards, are transitioning from novelty to the norm. Indeed, the US pet care industry, one of the largest in the world, was expected to top $69.36 billion in 2017 (American Pet Products Manufacturers' Association, 2017). Services are also being developed to provide care for pets and, therefore, peace of mind for elderly owners or those with terminal illness (Veterinary Practice News Editors, 2015). In addition, policies are being developed for pets in the workplace, healthcare facilities, and other environments where humans interact, such as restaurants, retail stores, swimming pools, hotels, and public transportation.

However, this close coexistence also opens the door to hazards and harms for both parties. The World Health Organization considers health as having physical, mental, and social dimensions (World Health Organization, 2006). If considered with respect to the household, the health effects we

Beyond One Health: From Recognition to Results, First Edition.
Edited by John A. Herrmann and Yvette J. Johnson-Walker.
© 2018 John Wiley & Sons, Inc. Published 2018 by John Wiley & Sons, Inc.

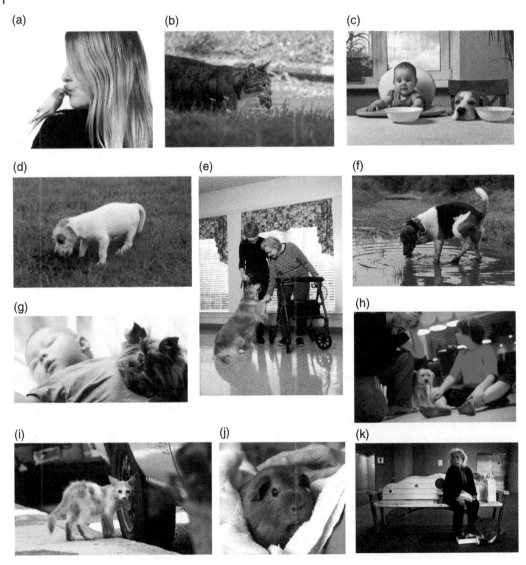

Figure 8.1 Examples of the relationships among humans, companion animals, and the environment. Humans can share close contact with pets in much the same way they do with their fellows, supporting each other (e,j,k), eating together (c), sleeping together (g), and sharing kisses (a). When appropriate pet care is provided and hygiene is practiced, human and pet health can thrive. However, this close contact provides opportunities for contamination of indoor and outdoor environments and pathogen sharing (b,d,f). In the presence of negligence (i) or animal or interpersonal violence (h), humans and pets can also share suffering. *Sources:* (a) ©Multiart/iStock; (b) ©joegolby/iStock; (c) ©igorr1/iStock; (d) ©nattawat thathun/iStock; (e) ©iofoto/iStock; (f) ©Baz251286/iStock; (g) ©kirza/iStock; (h) ©funstock/iStock; (i) ©Gerivori/iStock; (j) ©suemack/iStock; (k) ©epicurean/iStock.

have on each other, both beneficial and harmful, can be conceptualized as being intertwined with the effects of the environment (Figure 8.1). The environment in this context is not just limited to inside the home or outdoors but also to settings in which companion animals might participate in activities designed to leverage the healing properties of human-animal action, such as hospitals, long-term care facilities, schools, or prisons.

"One Health," as it relates to pets and their families, is beginning to evolve from concept to action, as initiatives in the USA set specific targets for the veterinary public health community to achieve (Ehnert, 2015; 2020 Healthy Pets, Healthy Families Coalition of Los Angeles County, 2014). Such targets include but are not limited to dog bite prevention, disaster preparedness, decreased prevalence of obesity in pet owners and pets, decreased prevalence of in-home cigarette smoking, increased prevalence of pet sterilization, increased vaccination of pets, and increased parasite prevention by pet owners.

The purpose of this chapter is to review the benefits and hazards of pet ownership and related interactions among people, pets, and the environment. The focus will primarily be on owned (rather than feral or stray) dogs and cats, with acknowledgment that other species such as rabbits or birds also enhance our lives and bring unique hazards of their own. For the sake of brevity, the geographic scope of discussions regarding infectious diseases will be primarily limited to North America, with acknowledgment that disease risks vary among and within continents, countries, states or provinces, and even local communities, as well as among cultures. Relationships with companion animals used outside the home for work, sport, or other purposes of benefit to humans will be briefly discussed, as these jobs introduce new hazards but also share many qualities with household pets.

8.2 Benefits and Hazards of Human-Pet Relationships

8.2.1 Physical and Mental Health

8.2.1.1 Impacts on Humans

Pets have played a key role in human life for thousands of years. Humans first domesticated dogs from wolves up to 27 000 years ago to in order to improve success in hunting and for protection within hunter gatherer communities (Skoglund et al., 2015; Perri,

2016). Cats were domesticated around 10 000 years ago at the time humans began to cultivate crops and were likely used to control rodent populations (Vigne, 2004). Over the years, pets have been used for hunting, guarding/protection, herding, companionship, idolized, and even as an emergency food source. In Western societies, the current most common use of pets by far is as companions, whether it is to keep us company, for ornament or status symbol, or as a helping animal.

As a companion, the benefits of pets to our physical and emotional well-being are well documented. Dog ownership is associated with higher levels of physical activity compared to non-pet owners (Yabroff et al., 2008; Cutt, 2007; Cutt et al., 2008). See Section 8.2.2 for a more complete discussion of this topic. Whether it is due to the "hygiene hypothesis" or due to changes in our intestinal microbiome, there are now numerous studies that show a benefit of early childhood exposure to pets and a decrease in the incidence of allergies and asthma (Domingeez-Bello and Blaser, 2015). A Swedish study showed that children exposed to dogs and farm animals in the first year of life had a decreased risk of asthma in their preschool and school years (Fall et al., 2015). A Finnish study showed that children less than 1 year of age who had dog contact in the home had fewer upper respiratory tract infections (URIs) and a lower incidence of antimicrobial use than similar-aged children with no dog contact (Bergroth et al., 2012). Cat contact within the home was also associated with fewer URIs, although the magnitude of that decrease was smaller than for dog contact. A study from the UK showed that pet ownership during pregnancy and childhood was associated with a 52% decreased risk of atopic asthma at 7 years of age, but a slightly increased risk of non-atopic asthma (Collin et al., 2015). This risk was mostly seen with rabbit and rodent ownership. While there is good evidence for the role of pet exposure early in life and a decreased incidence of developing asthma and severe allergies, the evidence for removal of pets from the home that contains an asthmatic or severe allergy sufferer is lacking and is mostly based on expert opinion such as the National, Heart, Lung, and Blood Institute's Guideline for the Diagnosis and Management of Asthma (Custovic and van Wijk, 2005; Anon., 2012). In developing this guideline, the recommendation to remove pets from the home was assigned category D, meaning the panel's consensus judgment was that it was deemed valuable but there was insufficient clinical literature to give it a stronger recommendation.

Multiple studies have shown that pet owners are healthier than non-pet owners. Data from Germany and Australia indicate that pet owners have 15% fewer annual doctor visits (Headey and Grabka, 2007). Some studies have shown that pet ownership is associated with lower blood pressure, lower cholesterol and triglycerides, improved cardiovascular reactivity to stress, and, in some studies, an improved 1-year survival rate following cardiovascular disease (Levine & al, 2013). The American Heart Association, in their statement on Pet Ownership and Cardiovascular Risk, recommends that "pet ownership, particularly dog ownership, may be reasonable for the reduction in cardiovascular disease risk" and gives it a "B" level of evidence (Levine & al, 2013).

Mental health benefits of pet ownership are also well documented as far back as Florence Nightingale, the founder of modern nursing, who wrote that small animals reduced anxiety in children and adults living in psychiatric institutions (Connor and Miller, 2000). We share a strong bond with companion animals, particularly with dogs. Dogs can discriminate the emotional expressions of human faces and people can reliably interpret the meaning of a dog bark (Muller, 2015; Pongrácz et al., 2005). It is common to hear stories of how a pet helped a person get through a rough time such as a loss of a loved one or getting the diagnosis of a severe medical condition. Most studies involving mental health lie in the realm of animals involved in animal-assisted activities or interventions; however, there are

some involving pet ownership. Pet owners had improved cardiovascular response to mental stress (Allen et al., 2001). Pet owners diagnosed with AIDS reported less depression than non-pet owners (Siegel et al., 1999). In adults over 60 years of age, pet owners were 35% less likely to report loneliness (Stanley et al., 2014). In one survey, 50% of psychiatrists and psychologists surveyed reported that they have prescribed a pet for their patients (Ernst, 2014). Animal-assisted activities involving dogs in nursing homes have been shown to reduce loneliness and decrease agitation, aggression, and depression in dementia patients (Ernst, 2014). In the hospital, heart failure patients who receive canine-assisted ambulation walked sooner, walked farther, and were more motivated than those not randomly assigned to work with the animals (Abate et al., 2011).

The potential benefits of pet ownership far outweigh the small but real risks. Even in high-risk populations, such as those who are immunocompromised, experts do not recommend rehoming or relinquishment of pets (https://aidsinfo.nih.gov/contentfiles/lvguidelines/adult_oi.pdf) (Tomblyn et al., 2009). However, health hazards do exist and should be considered in order to minimize risks to humans. Common health hazards of pet ownership include bites and scratches, injuries/trauma, zoonoses or infections that can be transmitted to and from animals, and emotional distress from the loss of a pet.

Animal bites are a common hazard of pet ownership, with an annual incidence of about 4.7 million in the USA, accounting for 1% of emergency department visits and 9500 hospitalizations (Holmquist and Elixhauser, 2010; Anon., 2003). There are 10–20 deaths from animal bites each year in the USA, and the hospitalizations alone cost $54 million annually (Holmquist and Elixhauser, 2010; Anon., 2003). Dogs account for 85–90% of the bites, cats 5–10%, and rodents 2–3%. Greater than 70% of biting dogs are known to the victim (Holmquist and Elixhauser, 2010; Anon., 2003). About half the dog bites and 89% of the cat bites were provoked, as reported by the victim (Gandhi et al., 1999; Patrick and O'Rourke, 1998; Anon., 2003). Postal workers in the USA suffer over 6500 dog bites a year (Anon., 2016a). Any dog can bite and no one breed of dog is overrepresented in the number of bites; however, larger breeds can cause more damage and thus account for more emergency room visits and hospitalizations (Bradley, 2014; Anon., 2014). In the USA pit bulls are more frequently impacted in severe and fatal attacks but this is likely due to their popularity in certain communities, reporting biases, and their frequent use as a fighting dog. Other geographic areas will have different breeds that are more involved in severe attacks, for example, sledding dogs in many areas of Canada and the mastiff in Rome, Italy. One problem with studies looking at dog breed and bites is accuracy of breed identification. Most studies rely on media reporting or victim identification, which are often inaccurate. This difficulty in identifying a breed type is highlighted in a study looking at adoption agency breed identification compared to DNA breed identification (Voith et al., 2009). This study showed that only 25% of dogs contained genetic evidence of the agencies' identified breed. Dog breed is a poor predictive factor of aggression, and breed bans have not been shown to be effective in reducing the rate or severity of bite injuries (Anon., 2014).

The American Veterinary Medical Association (AVMA) and the National Animal Care and Control Association have well-established guidelines to help health officials, national, state, and local communities set up programs, laws, and ordinances to decrease the health hazards of animal bites (Anon., 2001). Recommendations by the AVMA task force and the Animal and Society Institute to prevent animal bites include the following (Bradley, 2014; Anon., 2001):

- Choose a pet carefully based on the living situation.
- Socialize and train pets at a young age. A trained pet is more confident, less fearful, and less likely to bite.
- Neuter pets, particularly at a young age, to decrease aggression and bites.
- Maintain regular veterinary check-ups and keep pets healthy. When a pet is feeling ill or painful they are more likely to bite.
- Teach children proper behavior around pets. Children are often too aggressive with pets, have quick, jerky, and unpredictable movements, often put their face in the face of a pet, and often climb on a pet. These behaviors can lead to a bite.
- Be alert for the warning signs an animal is giving off. In a dog this includes ears back, brow lifted, lip curved, eyes wide, growl, licking of the lips, and the tail tucked between the legs. Not all dogs will exhibit all of these signs.
- Babies and small children should never be left alone with a pet.

Outside of bite-related injuries, few data exist regarding the burden of pet-related injuries. The Centers for Disease Control and Prevention (CDC) has analyzed fall injuries due to dogs and cats and estimated that over 86 000 fall injuries related to dogs and cats happen each year, representing a rate of 29.7 per 100 000 population (Stevens et al., 2009). This accounts for over 26 000 fractures a year in the USA. Eighty-eight percent of these falls were related to dogs, with 31% due to falling or tripping over the animal, 21% due to being pushed or pulled over by the pet, and 9% due to falling over a pet item such as a bowl or toy. Recommended preventive strategies include raising public awareness of such risks, recognizing that pets and pet items can cause falls, and obedience training for dogs.

Poor sleep is another human health hazard of pet ownership. Co-sleeping with a pet is very common in the USA, with 62% of cat owners, 62% of small-dog owners, 41% of medium-dog owners, and 32% of large-dog owners reporting that they regularly sleep with their pet (American Pet Products Manufacturers' Association, 2017). Nightly sleep disturbance was reported in 20–53% of pet owners who sleep with their pet; they were more likely to take longer to fall asleep and wake up tired, but there were no significant differences in the self-reported sleep length or feeling tired during the day (Smith et al., 2014; Krahn et al., 2015).

8.2.1.2 Impacts on Pets

The physical and mental health benefits that companion animals derive from their relationships with people have received comparatively less scientific study, although some might appear obvious. The needs of companion animals can be considered in the context of the five freedoms of animal welfare over which humans have control (Box 8.1) (Farm Animal Welfare Council, 2009). As applied to pets, these freedoms speak to the need for nutritious food; fresh, clean water; a sense of comfort and safety (freedom from intentional or accidental harm); adequate healthcare, including disease prevention, diagnosis, and treatment; shelter; exercise; social opportunities with humans or conspecifics (e.g., through training activities, socialization classes, or playing together); and other species-specific needs. Specific needs can vary among and even within species, for companion animals can be as individual as their owners (Ellis et al., 2013; Stafford, 2007; Rolls, 2013; Peron and Grosset, 2014).

When pet owners provide for these needs, the pets enjoy an optimal quality of life and the owners enjoy their companionship for a potentially longer period. The average lifespan of pet dogs in the USA has increased 4% in the past 10 years, and the average lifespan of pet cats has increased 10% (Banfield Pet Hospital, 2013). The increase in lifespans of dogs and cats in other countries such as Japan is even more dramatic (Kozuka, 2014) – from 7.6 years in 1985 to 13.3 years in 2012 for dogs, and from 11 years to 13.5 years for cats in Japan. The precise mechanisms underlying this improved longevity are unknown and are likely multifactorial, possibly involving increases in the prevalence of pet sterilization; improvements in diet formulation, disease prevention, and general care or healthcare provided; and owner sensitivity to end-of-life decisions, among other things.

Human acts of affection toward pets also appear to benefit animals. For example, just as petting dogs has physiological and emotional benefits for humans, so can petting behavior have beneficial effects for dogs. For example, several experimental trials have shown that even in presumably stressful settings such as animal shelters, human interaction or petting sessions can decrease circulating cortisol (a purported surrogate marker of perceived stress in animals; Dhabhar et al., 2012) in dogs and cardiac indicators of emotional arousal, and improve behavioral test results, suggesting a reduction in perceived stress, although the immunological consequences of this decrease remain unclear (Coppola et al., 2006; Dudley et al., 2015; Bergamasco et al., 2010; Menor-Campos et al., 2011).

Unfortunately, although the five freedoms may seem intuitive and most new pet owners likely start out with an earnest intent to ensure some or all of the freedoms are met, these freedoms can also prove challenging to achieve in the household environment, even for the best-intended owners. And failure to meet a pet's needs can elicit a stress response in the animal, which, as in people, can cause untoward physiological, behavioral, and psychological changes (Mills et al., 2014) that can threaten the pet's general well-being and manifest as health and behavioral problems. Such problems can challenge the owner-pet bond and lead to relinquishment or euthanasia (Patronek et al., 1996; Kwan and Bain, 2013). Interestingly, although it may seem intuitive that owners who are more attached

---

Box 8.1 Five freedoms of animal welfare, as proposed by the British Farm Animal Welfare Council

- Freedom from hunger and thirst
- Freedom from discomfort
- Freedom from pain, injury, or disease
- Freedom to express normal behavior
- Freedom from fear and distress

to their pets would be less likely to relinquish them to an animal shelter, several studies have failed to support this presumption (Shore et al., 2003; DiGiacomo et al., 1998; Douglas, 2005).

Animal hoarding represents an example of the human-animal bond gone awry, involving derangements to mental health, animal welfare, and public health. This poorly understood phenomenon is distinguished from owning or caring for a larger than typical number of pets in that the intentions are not to help the animals but to satisfying a human need to accumulate animals and control them, with this need superseding the needs of the animals involved (http://vet.tufts.edu/hoarding/about). A typical hoarder acquires more than the typical number of companion animals; is unable to provide even their basic needs, with this neglect often resulting in starvation, illness, and death (Williams and Viscusi, 2016; Reinisch, 2009); and is "in denial of the inability to provide this minimum care and the impact of that failure on the animals, the household and human occupants of the dwelling" (http://www.aspca.org/animal-cruelty/animal-hoarding). The prevalence of this condition is unknown, but hoarding is believed to be widespread. Hazards to hoarders, their co-residents, and public health in general can include fire hazards (e.g., due to rundown or crowded living conditions), lack of basic utilities such as running water or electricity, infestation with rodents or insects, and exposure to and spread of zoonotic diseases through urine, feces, and other contaminants. Buildup of pet excrement can also cause other problems such as irreparable damage to buildings, release of noxious aerosols and gases, and offensive odors (http://vet.tufts.edu/hoarding/about). Furthermore, the response to animal hoarding cases places a heavy demand on community resources, requiring a sustained, cross-jurisdictional, multi-agency effort (Castrodale et al., 2010).

As for the typical pet owner, keeping cats and dogs indoors may reduce their risk of infectious disease and vehicular and other trauma; however, evidence is increasing that, particularly for cats, strictly or primarily indoor housing can increase the risk of other adverse health conditions such as lower urinary tract disease, obesity, or hyperthyroidism (Buffington, 2002) and of unwanted behaviors. In the situation of lower urinary tract disease, case-control studies have shown that the risk increases in a dose-dependent manner with increasing degree of indoor confinement (Walker et al., 1977; Reif et al., 1977). The adverse health conditions may be attributable to characteristics inherent to indoor housing, such as an inability to express natural behaviors or preferences (e.g., climbing, scratching, hunting, resting, or hiding) and the presence of perceived threats or challenges. Urinary problems pose a particular challenge to the human-companion animal bond because they can lead to elimination in places owners deem inappropriate, which is the most common reason why cats are surrendered to animal shelters (Patronek et al., 1996). The presence of multiple pets in the home can also be an important source of stress for some but not all cats and other companion animals. For these reasons and others, various methods of environmental enrichment have been proposed to help cats behave as naturally as possible within the home. A thorough summary of those methods can be found elsewhere (Herron and Buffington, 2010).

Being an obligate social species, dogs do not cope well with isolation (Heath and Wilson, 2014), and leaving dogs at home alone can trigger separation anxiety, from which 14–17% of pet dogs are believed to suffer (Horowitz, 2008). Besides being linked to an increased severity and frequency of dermatological problems for affected dogs (Dreschel, 2010), separation anxiety can also strain the dog-owner relationship through the resulting property destruction, indoor elimination, and unwanted vocalization (barking and whining). In addition, a low frequency of owner play sessions with dogs (never or once a day) has been associated with a lower likelihood of dogs behaving in a friendly manner toward strangers or being obedient, and a greater likelihood of dogs showing aggression toward visitors (Tami et al., 2008). Dogs also have a strong need for exercise; however, as few as 40% (both genders) or 53% (males) of dog owners have reported walking their dog in the past week (Cutt et al., 2007). In addition to the adverse effects of lack of exercise on dog health, a short daily walk length (<0.5 hours/day) has been associated with a greater likelihood of dogs fearing strangers and a lower likelihood of them being obedient (Tami et al., 2008), thereby threatening relationships between dogs and people.

Birds are also susceptible to health problems related to neglect and confinement. Undesirable behaviors such as aggression toward humans, screaming, or feather picking are common according to bird owners (Gaskins and Bergman, 2011), but are apparently not such a problem that they would consider relinquishment or euthanasia. Interestingly, chronic egg laying, second only to feather picking as the most common behavior problem reported by veterinarians (but not by owners), can result from owners cuddling and petting birds, further reinforcing the fact that even well-intended owners can contribute to behavior problems in their pets.

Evidence from The Netherlands and the UK suggests the manner in which pet rabbits are housed and cared for may adversely affect their welfare to the point that it may shorten their lifespan (Rooney et al., 2014; Schepers et al., 2009). Specific bad practices include provision of small hutches, solitary housing (preventing socialization), and inappropriate diets. A large proportion (61%) of owned rabbits in a UK study were reported to display specific signs of fear when handled by their owners, such as struggling, freezing, biting, scratching, or kicking (Rooney et al., 2014).Twenty-five percent of limb fractures in rabbits in a Japanese study were attributed to accidental falls due to human error, and 2% were caused by trampling by humans (Sasai et al., 2015). This and other findings

suggest that some rabbit owners lack proper handling skills. It follows that people with less common pets such as birds, ferrets, small rodents, amphibians, reptiles, or recently domesticated wildlife (e.g., hedgehogs or sugar gliders) also lack the necessary knowledge for proper husbandry, nutrition, and handling, posing a threat to the health and welfare of the pets (McLaughlin and Strunk, 2016) and also potentially that of those in contact with the pet. This situation regarding nutrition is further complicated by the general lack of data on nutrient requirements of many species kept as pets.

As previously alluded to, owner-perceived behavioral problems or the need to seek behavioral advice increase the likelihood that dogs and cats will be relinquished to animal shelters (Patronek et al., 1996; Fatjó et al., 2015). Whether a pet is surrendered for euthanasia because of behavior problems can vary by country (Lambert et al., 2015). Many of these behaviors are a result of a failure to allow the pet to behave naturally (e.g., barking, chewing, or scratching) or to provide for their needs (e.g., hyperactivity). A simple remedy for many problems could be obedience training and behavioral counseling, which has been shown to strengthen the relationship between people and their dogs (Clark and Boyer, 1993).

Although feeding is a benefit that pets derive from their relationship with humans, opportunities exist for well-intended owners to inadvertently contribute to nutritional deficiencies, injury, or infectious disease for their pets. And infection of pets can consequently lead to infection of those who share their households. Food choices by owners are not just a reflection of their awareness and personal beliefs regarding nutritional needs but also of social and cultural factors (Michel, 2006). Feeding practices can also reflect parenting styles of owners (German, 2015).

8.2.2 Overweight and Obesity

Infectious diseases aside, perhaps the most obvious manner in which human and companion animal health is inextricably linked is through the chronic disease of obesity. Human overweight and obesity is a global phenomenon. According to the World Health Organization, the prevalence of obesity in humans has more than doubled since 1980 (World Health Organization, 2015). Prevalence estimates for overweight and obesity in cats and dogs range 34% to 59% and 27% to 39%, respectively (German, 2015), and that prevalence appears to be increasing (Banfield Pet Hospital, 2012). This increase is important because of hypothesized or established associations between obesity and other diseases such as diabetes mellitus, heart disease, arthritis, respiratory disorders, metabolic syndrome, and other chronic diseases in humans and companion animals alike. Existing ambiguities concerning relationships between obesity and adverse health outcomes in people and pets may be attributable to a failure to distinguish between overweight and obesity in most studies.

Lack of physical activity or a sedentary lifestyle along with a calorie-dense diet are risk factors for overweight or obesity in both parties (Nijland et al., 2010), although humans can choose to change lifestyles and diets to prevent obesity in themselves and their dogs. Dry diet (which owners may choose over canned diets for convenience) and restricted or no access to the outdoors were identified as independent risk factors for overweight or obesity at 1 year of age in cats in a UK longitudinal study (Rowe et al., 2015). In a UK cross-sectional study, overweight cats were significantly more likely to have overweight owners than were non-overweight cats (Heuberger and Wakshlag, 2011); however, a study in The Netherlands found that owner body mass index had no relationship with overweight in their cats after other factors were controlled for (Nijland et al., 2010). For dogs in the UK study, that relationship was identified only for owners who were at least 60 years of age, but for dogs in The Netherlands study, the correlation was significant regardless of owner age. Similarly, overweight parents are more likely to have obese or overweight children than non-overweight parents (Danielzik et al., 2004). Factors other than indulgent feeding practices that have been associated with overweight or obesity in cats include apartment dwelling, inactivity, middle age, male sex, and neutering (Scarlett et al., 1994). Factors for dogs include food type, feeding of treats or snacks, restricted activity, neutering, living in single-dog households, and feeding frequency (Mao et al., 2013; Robertson, 2003; Lefebvre et al., 2013).

It follows that shared exercise between humans and their pets, particularly dogs, could reduce the risk of overweight or obesity or increase the physical fitness of both parties (Yabroff et al., 2008). That notion has spurred the development of numerous programs designed to increase fitness or reduce the risk of overweight and obesity through encouragement of dog walking (US Dept of Health and Human Services, 2015). There are numerous anecdotal accounts of where an obese person with multiple chronic medical conditions credits their dog adoption as saving their life (Box 8.2). Is there evidence that dog ownership reduces obesity? Dog ownership itself does not appear to influence the likelihood of human obesity, at least for children (Westgarth et al., 2012). However, a recent meta-analysis revealed that dog owners are more physically active than non-dog owners (Christian et al., 2013). That meta-analysis did not include a cross-sectional study in which no difference in amount of moderate or vigorous physical activity was identified between dog owners and non-dog owners (Richards, 2016). An additional benefit of dog walking for people and dogs is the opportunity for social interaction with conspecifics.

8.2.3 Feeding Practices and Illness

8.2.3.1 Human Illness Related to Pet Feeding Practices

With respect to diet, debate has been heated regarding the health benefits and concerns to

There are numerous stories of a person saving the life of a pet from a pound or adoption center only to find that their new pet also saves their life as well. One of these stories, the Eric and Peety Mutual Adoption, was featured on National Public Radio (Shute, 2016). Eric was a middle-aged obese sedentary man with several chronic medical conditions including obesity and diabetes. His doctor told him that he was going to die unless he made some major lifestyle changes. After talking to a nutritionist he decided to adopt a dog. He went to the local shelter and asked for a middle-aged over-weight dog so they would have something in common. Eric described the first time they saw each other and they gave each other a look that said "Really? I'm going to be stuck with you?" Nonetheless, Eric and Peety went home together and began to take walks together. Over the next year Eric lost 140 pounds and Peety lost 25. Eric's chronic medical conditions improved. Eric even began to run and has now completed a marathon. The full story can be found at http://www.npr.org/sections/health-shots/2016/03/10/469785736/he-rescued-a-dog-then-the-dog-rescued-him.

humans and pets alike related to the feeding of raw foods of animal origin and other raw foodstuffs to dogs and cats, with both sides of the debate citing evidence to support or malign this practice. Proponents of raw diets, whether commercial or homemade, cite their personal observations of the nutritional superiority of this feeding approach and various published but largely unscientifically substantiated integumentary, digestive, orthopedic, and immune benefits (Billinghurst, 1993; Lonsdale, 2001; Schultze, 1998). In a prospective cohort study, dogs that consumed raw diets were at considerably less risk of extraintestinal infections involving the skin, eyes, ears, or urinary tract, as reported by their owners (Lefebvre et al., 2009a). Personal mistrust of the pet food industry, exacerbated by highly publicized recalls of adulterated, imbalanced, or contaminated processed pet foods, also contributes to the argument in support of homemade diets in general (Michel et al., 2008; Rumbeiha and Morrison, 2011).

Given the uncommonness of reports of pets becoming ill from consumption of raw diets, the deep concern related to this practice is likely not so much that they cause health concerns for the pets that consume them (potential nutritional deficiencies aside) but rather that this practice could adversely affect human health, particularly that of the very young, very old, or immuno-compromised. And certainly, the same debate could pertain to humans choosing to eat or accidentally ingesting raw or undercooked foods of animal origin, as parasites known to infect food animals such as *Taenia* spp. (found in beef and pork and the cause of cysticercosis), *Trichinella* spp. (found in pork, bear meat, and meat of other potential food animal species), and *Toxoplasma gondii* (found in pork, lamb, and venison, which are believed to be the primary source for human infection, and not cats directly).

Several reports exist of microbial contamination of raw foods of animal origin and of animals shedding pathogens after consuming such foods. An example of potential unwanted effects on humans of feeding raw diets to pets and potential environmental contamination as a result is found in a longitudinal study that revealed that the incidence of *Salmonella* shedding in a specific population of dogs fed raw meat was 0.61 cases/dog-year, which was almost eight times as high as the incidence for dogs not fed raw meat (0.08 cases/dog-year) (Lefebvre et al., 2009a).

Just as processed foods intended for human consumption can become contaminated and serve as a source of illness for humans and companion animals, so can processed pet foods and treats. For example, *Salmonella-*

contaminated pig ear and dried beef treats for dogs was implicated in outbreaks of human salmonellosis in Alberta, Canada (Pitout et al., 2003; Clark et al., 2001). Whether humans became ill from handling the treats or the dogs that ate the treats remains unclear. Dogs that consume pig ear treats were reported to have a higher risk of shedding salmonellae than dogs that did not consume the treats, controlling for other factors, in another study (Lefebvre et al., 2009a). It is also unclear whether any dogs became ill in the Alberta outbreaks.

Pets and their owners are both susceptible to foodborne illness, and efforts are underway to leverage existing data for foodborne-disease surveillance programs (US Food and Drug Administration, 2016). An oft-cited example is detection of neurobehavioral changes in cats (referred to as "dancing cats") in Minamata, Japan, that preceded an outbreak of severe neurological disease in the local townsfolk, which was later linked to ingestion of seafood contaminated with methylmercury (Tsuchiya, 1992). Melamine-adulterated wheat gluten and rice protein concentrates from China that were used in the manufacturing of pet food in the USA caused the deaths of several pet dogs and cats and prompted the recall of more than 150 brands of pet food in the USA in 2007 (US Food and Drug Administration, 2014; World Health Organization, 2016a). This was followed by melamine adulteration of milk and infant formula products and other foodstuffs in China, leading to illness for hundreds of thousands of infants (Branigan, 2008).

An outbreak of salmonellosis in dog owners and dogs in the USA and Canada was attributed to contaminated commercially produced dry dog food (Imanishi et al., 2014), with young children at greatest risk, while another outbreak in humans in the USA was linked to locally manufactured chicken jerky pet treats (Cavallo et al., 2015). The US Food and Drug Administration, in conjunction with the Veterinary Laboratory Investigation and Response Network (Vet-LIRN), has also investigated chicken, duck, or sweet potato

jerky treats, many imported from China, as a source of Fanconi-like illness (a disease in which the kidneys are unable to reabsorb essential electrolytes causing bone disease and other metabolic derangements) in more than 5800 dogs, 25 cats, and three people (US Food and Drug Administration, 2015).

8.2.3.2 Pet Illness Related to Feeding Practices

Owners can contribute to nutritional deficiencies of dogs, cats, rabbits, birds, and other companion animals when they choose to prepare or devise their own diets, leading to clinical disease. Classic examples include the pet cat who is fed canned tuna and consequently develops taurine deficiency-associated cardiomyopathy (Pion et al., 1992), the puppy fed a raw ground beef-based diet that develops rickets (Taylor et al., 2009), or the pet parakeet fed an all-seed diet that develops hyperparathyroidism and bone disease (Arnold et al., 1974). Such dietary deficiencies in the past were attributable in large part to a lack of data regarding the nutritional needs of companion animals; however, with the development of nutritional guidelines for companion animals (National Research Council Ad Hoc Committee on Dog and Cat Nutrition, 2006; FEDIAF, 2011, 2013; Harrison, 1998), a lack of owner awareness, education, or resources is likely the primary reason. These matters are complicated by the enthusiastic reactions that owners can get when they feed their pets (and children), which can provide pleasure for both parties, strengthening the bond between them but potentially adversely affecting their overall health when feeding is done on the basis of pet response rather than nutrition.

Some evidence also suggests that commercially prepared pet foods can increase the risk of certain chronic diseases in pets. For example, several epidemiologic studies have revealed a potential role of canned cat foods in the development of hyperthyroidism in cats, the strongest of which have involved controlling for other factors such as age and sex (Edinboro et al., 2004; Wakeling et al.,

2009; Olczak et al., 2005). However, the mechanisms underlying this association, whether involving nutrient composition, iodine content, or potential contaminants or toxicants found in food sources, additives, or the cans themselves, remain unclear.

Injuries can result from the physical properties of foods fed. Bones, bone fragments, and raw hides can get lodged in the esophagus or gastrointestinal tract of dogs and cats, causing mild to severe problems (Thompson et al., 2012; Gianella et al., 2009; Augusto et al., 2005). Pets can also become infected or intestinally colonized by consuming microbially contaminated raw foods of animal origin and other foodstuffs (Schlesinger and Joffe, 2011), but reports of dogs and cats becoming ill from consuming raw foods of animal origin are rare. A pathogenic strain of *Yersinia enterocolitica* was recovered from the diarrheic feces of two dogs that frequently were fed raw pork in Finland (Fredriksson-Ahomaa et al., 2001). Outbreaks of salmonellosis in groups or colonies of working and high-performance dogs that consumed raw foods of animal origin have also been reported (Caraway et al., 1959; Morley et al., 2006). On the other hand, several reports exist of pets becoming ill from commercial pet foods (ConsumerAffairs, 2016).

8.2.4 Infectious Disease Transmission

8.2.4.1 Companion Animal-to-Human Transmission

Zoonotic diseases have a high burden on health, with the CDC reporting that they account for three out of every five new cases of human sickness and listing no less than 70 diseases that can be spread from pets to people, with about 75% of newly reported human infections emerging from animal reservoirs (Day et al., 2012). Table 8.1 lists information on the major zoonotic diseases. A few of the most common and those with high public health concern are discussed further here. Depending on the disease, zoonoses can be spread by direct contact such as petting, ani-

mal licking, and contact with urine or feces, or indirect through vectors such as fleas or ticks.

Rabies is one of the most feared zoonotic infections, with a nearly 100% mortality rate once symptoms are present. It is a major cause of global mortality, claiming approximately 26 400 to 61 000 lives per year, with 95% of cases occurring in Africa and Asia (World Health Organization, 2013). The USA typically has 1–3 human cases each year and as such, lay media often report that rabies is a minimal threat to people. However, even in the USA, it continues to be a threat that requires significant public health efforts to maintain this control, with annual cost of $245–510 million (Anon., 2015a). Each year in the USA, there are over 6000 animal cases of rabies including 200 cats and almost 100 dogs (Monroe et al., 2016). Despite laws and ordinances in most areas requiring all dogs and cats to be vaccinated against rabies, 65% of dogs and 92% of cats associated with bites were not vaccinated (Patrick and O'Rourke, 1998). Post-exposure prophylaxis (PEP) is indicated for all individuals possibly exposed to rabies (Tables 8.2 and 8.3), and includes human rabies immunoglobulin and four rabies vaccines on days 0, 3, 7, and 14. The cost of PEP is over $3000 in the USA (Manning et al., 2008; Rupprecht et al., 2010). Improved pre-exposure control is many times more efficient than waiting to give PEP. The CDC estimates the cost per human life saved is $10 000 to $100 million depending on the circumstances.

Rabies preventive efforts should be an interdisciplinary approach including awareness and education of animal owners, education of health providers such as physicians and veterinarians, animal vaccination programs, enforcement of vaccination laws, and strict control over the stray animal population (Brown et al., 2016). It is essential to educate the public on what is considered a potential exposure to rabies. Any mammal can carry rabies, but certain species such as raccoons, bats, skunks, and foxes are much more likely to be infected. Saliva and neural tissue are considered infective material. One

Table 8.1 Epidemiologic characteristics of various infectious organisms with established potential for transmission from dogs, cats, birds, and rabbits to humans.

| Organism | Prevalence of infection or seropositivity in North America (%) | | Geographic distribution | Route of transmission to humans | Ongoing surveillance or reporting of human cases in North America or the World | Susceptible human groups | Signs of infection | | Key preventive strategies for pet owners |
	Companion animals	Humans					Humans	Companion animals	
Ancylostoma spp. and *Uncinaria stenocephala* (hookworms)	Dogs: 1.2% Cats: 0.3%	Rare	Tropical climates, particularly resource-poor communities	Penetration of unprotected skin by larvae found in fecally contaminated soil (i.e., CLM)	None	Children (because of behaviors)	Self-limiting raised erythemic lesions and severe pruritus; rarely, abdominal discomfort and diarrhea	No signs; in severely infected, vomiting, anorexia, cachexia, distended abdomen, severe anemia	● Anthelmintic treatment (deworming) for pets ● Avoid skin contact with potentially fecally contaminated surfaces
Bartonella henselae	Cats: 30–50% are seropositive; kittens, stray, and shelter cats at highest risk	0.2–90% seropositive; 22 000 new cases of infection/year in USA	Unknown; cat-scratch disease found worldwide	Cat scratches/bites; rubbing eyes after handling cats; possibly flea bites (not established)	None	Children <15 years; immunocompromised	Bacillary angiomatosis or peliosis (cat-scratch disease); swollen lymph nodes; Parinaud's ocular glandular syndrome	No signs in most; sometimes uveitis or chondritis	● Flea preventives for cats ● Keep cats indoors ● Refrain from activities promoting cat scratches/bites
Bordetella bronchiseptica	Dogs: 2% (3% of puppies) Rabbits: 52%	Rare, in immuno compromised	Worldwide	Aerosol or direct contact with respiratory secretions of infected dog	None	Immuno compromised	Pneumonia, sinusitis, or bronchitis	Respiratory disease, pneumonia	● Vaccination of dogs ● Avoid close contact with dogs or rabbits with respiratory signs

(*Continued*)

Table 8.1 (Continued)

Organism	Prevalence of infection or seropositivity in North America (%)		Geographic distribution	Route of transmission to humans	Ongoing surveillance or reporting of human cases in North America or the World	Susceptible human groups	Signs of infection		Key preventive strategies for pet owners
	Companion animals	Humans					Humans	Companion animals	
Brucella canis	Dogs: sporadic; 1–8% in USA; more common in strays. Cats: resistant	Infection rare	Worldwide	Mucosal contact with body fluid/secretions, particularly of aborted pups and their dams	WAHID, NNDSS, CNDSS	Veterinary staff or dog breeders	Fever, dyspnea, sore throat, septicemia; infection can last from weeks to years	Abortion; rarely prostatitis, uveitis, or discospondylitis	• Avoid contact with body fluids of whelping dogs
Campylobacter jejuni or *C. coli*	Dogs: 1% Cats: 2%	6% of human cases attributed to pets	Worldwide	Fecal-oral; raw or undercooked foods of animal origin	WAHID, FoodNet, NESP	Children and young adults	Bloody, self-limiting diarrhea; Guillain–Barré syndrome; bacteremia in people with AIDS	Diarrhea or no signs	• Hand hygiene • Prompt, proper disposal of pet feces • Avoid raw or undercooked foods of animal origin
Capnocytophaga canimorsus	Normal oral flora in dogs and cats	Rare	Worldwide	Bites or scratches; contact with saliva	None	Alcoholics; immunocompromised	Meningitis, septic arthritis, disseminated intravascular coagulopathy, thrombocytopenia, purpura	None	• Refrain from activities promoting cat scratches/bites
Cheyletiella spp.	Prevalence unknown in rabbits, dogs, and cats	Unknown	Worldwide	Close contact	None	Pet groomers, veterinary staff, kennel workers, or people in high-density pet settings	Self-limiting papular, pruriginous dermatitis	Exfoliative dermatitis	• Ectoparasite preventives for pets

Organism	Prevalence in pets	Human cases	Geographic distribution	Transmission	Surveillance	At-risk populations	Clinical signs (humans)	Clinical signs (pets)	Prevention
Cryptosporidium canis or *C. felis*	Dogs: 2–6% Cats: 1–8%	450 cases of cryptosporidiosis/year in Canada Approx. 10 000 cases of cryptosporidiosis/year in USA Cases only rarely attributable to pets	Worldwide	Fecal-oral; ingestion of fecally contaminated substances, including water; low infective dose	NNDSS, CNDSS, FoodNet, CryptoNet, NESP	Children <4 years old; elderly; immuno compromised	Watery diarrhea, death in immunocompromised (chronic intestinal disease >1 month is AIDS-defining); dog strain not pathogenic to humans	Diarrhea or no signs; adults rarely affected because of immunity	• Prompt, proper disposal of pet feces
Dipylidium caninum	Dogs: 2% Cats: 5%	Unknown; occasional cases reported	Wherever dogs and fleas coexist	Ingestion of infected fleas	None	Infants and young children	Asymptomatic or digestive ailments (e.g., diarrhea and colic), abdominal distension	Anal irritation/pruritus	• Flea preventives and anthelmintic treatment (deworming) for pets
Echinococcus granulosus	Dogs: unknown; 6–11% in some high-prevalence regions	Cystic disease uncommon (<48 cases/10 years in Canada)	Southern South America, the Mediterranean; southwestern Asia	Fecal-oral	WAHID	People working or living around sheep (intermediate host for parasite)	Often asymptomatic; slowly enlarging cysts in the liver, lungs, and other organs cause site-specific symptoms	Typically no clinical signs	• Prompt, proper disposal of pet feces • Avoid raw or undercooked foods of animal origin
Echinococcus multilocularis	Dogs: 0.5% (up to 12% in Native American communities)	Alveolar disease rare (16 cases/10 years in Canada)	Northern Hemisphere	Fecal-oral (eggs on dog's muzzle); raw foods of animal origin	WAHID	Children around multiple dogs; people in northern territories/Alaska	Respiratory disease; cysts in liver and lungs; case fatality rate >50%		• Prompt, proper disposal of pet feces • Avoid raw or undercooked foods of animal origin
Fleas (*Ctenocephalides felis*)	6% of dogs, 11% of cats	Unknown	Worldwide	Contact with infested pets or their environment	None	Dog and cat owners	Flea bites that cause pruritus and irritation, particularly around ankles/legs	Severe pruritus, self-excoriation, alopecia, allergic dermatitis, anemia in extreme infestations	• Flea preventives for pets

(Continued)

Table 8.1 (Continued)

Organism	Prevalence of infection or seropositivity in North America (%)		Geographic distribution	Route of transmission to humans	Ongoing surveillance or reporting of human cases in North America or the World	Susceptible human groups	Signs of infection		Key preventive strategies for pet owners
	Companion animals	Humans					Humans	Companion animals	
Francisella tularensis	Dogs: <0.1% seropositive; higher in endemic areas (e.g., south central USA) Cats: largely unknown; up to 6% seropositive (strays in endemic regions)	0.06 cases/100 000 people in the USA; small proportion of human cases attributed to cats (large proportion to tick bites)	Northern Hemisphere	Dog ticks; cat bites/scratches; contact with respiratory/ ocular secretions; low infective dose	NNDSS, CNDSS	Rabbit or muskrat hunters/trappers (lagomorphs/rodents are principal source); people in areas with high tick concentrations and who spent a lot of time outdoors; people who work closely with animals	Respiratory disease; ulceroglandular disease if bitten	Respiratory disease, septicemia in cats; no signs in dogs	• Ectoparasite control for pets • Insect repellent/ protective clothing for people • Keep cats indoors • Vaccination of high-risk people
Leptospira interrogans	Dogs: 8% seropositive Cats: rare	0.02 to 0.05 cases/100 000 people in the USA	Most widespread disease worldwide (absent in polar regions)	Exposure to urine or feces of infected animals or contaminated water through skin abrasions or via mucosae; low infective dose	WAHID, NNDSS	People exposed to multiple dogs through their jobs (e.g., kennel worker or veterinarian)	Respiratory disease, fever, myalgia, liver and renal failure; self-limiting in most	Pyrexia, vomiting, conjunctivitis, pneumonia	• Vaccination of dogs • Avoid contact with dog (and other animal) urine or potentially urine-contaminated water
Pasteurella multocida	Dogs: 15–50% Cats: 50–75% Rabbits: 55%	Unknown; a few case reports of severe disease from pets	Worldwide	Scratches or bites, direct or indirect contact with respiratory secretion, possibly aerosol	None	People who have close contact with pets	Abscess (common), septic arthritis, osteomyelitis, meningitis, endocarditis, pneumonia	"Snuffles" (chronic upper respiratory tract disease), septicemia, death in rabbits; normal flora in dogs and cats	• Refrain from activities promoting cat scratches/bites • Refrain from allowing pets to lick humans' wounds

Rabies	Dogs: 80 to 100 cases/year Cats: >300 cases/year	1 to 3 cases/year, occasionally by dog bite/contact outside the USA	Approx 60 000 human cases/year worldwide, >99% transmitted by dogs	Scratches or bites	WAHID, NNDSS, CNDSS	People who work with feral or free-roaming dogs and cats of unknown or no vaccination history	Typically fatal progressive disease of the central nervous system	Altered behavior, encephalitis, paralysis, death	• Vaccination of pets
Trichophyton mentagrophytes and *Microsporum* spp. (dermatophytes/ringworm)	Dogs: 0% to <1% Cats: 0.6–13% (most common in kittens)	Generally unknown; 8% of veterinarians/5 years	Worldwide	Direct contact or fomites	None	Children, people with HIV, people who work with multiple cats	Tinea corporis, tinea capitis, onychomycosis; cutaneous and disseminated mycosis in people with AIDS	90% of infected cats have no signs; focal alopecia, scaling, and crusting	• Keep cats indoors • Hand hygiene • Refrain from direct contact with known infected cats (and have them treated)
Salmonella spp.	Dogs: 1–3% Cats: 1% High prevalence in puppies and kittens Pet reptiles: 4–50%	1% of human salmonellosis cases in the USA attributed to companion animals	Wordwide	Fecal-oral; raw or undercooked foods of animal origin	WAHID, NNDSS, FoodNet, NESP	Children, elderly	Diarrhea; septicemia, meningitis, endocarditis, neurological signs in immunocompromised (recurrent septicemia is AIDS-defining)	Diarrhea or no signs	• Proper disposal of pet feces • Hand hygiene • Avoid raw or undercooked foods of animal origin
Sarcoptes scabiei	Dogs, cats, and rabbits: unknown One of most common causes of skin disease in dogs	Unknown; 30% of dogs with sarcoptic mange infect their owners	Worldwide	Direct contact, fomites	None	No particular group	Self-limiting itchiness or rash	Severe pruritus, self-excoriation, scabs; alopecia	• Ectoparasite preventives for pets • Hand hygiene

(Continued)

Table 8.1 (Continued)

Organism	Prevalence of infection or seropositivity in North America (%)		Geographic distribution	Route of transmission to humans	Ongoing surveillance or reporting of human cases in North America or the World	Susceptible human groups	Signs of infection		Key preventive strategies for pet owners
	Companion animals	Humans					Humans	Companion animals	
Toxocara canis or *T. cati* (roundworms)	Dogs: 1–2% Cats: 1.3% High prevalence in puppies and kittens	750 cases of OLM/year; seroprevalence of 2–7% in adults	Highest prevalence in developing countries	Fecal-oral; possibly contact with eggs on fur	None	Toddlers, particularly those exposed to multiple dogs	Respiratory disease, VLM, OLM	Abdominal distension, gastrointestinal disturbance	• Anthelmintic treatment (deworming) for pets • Prompt, proper disposal of pet feces • Hand hygiene
Toxoplasma gondii	Cats: 30–80% seropositive	30–40% seropositive	Worldwide (one of the most widespread of all zoonoses)	Fecal-oral transmission of sporulated oocysts; raw or undercooked foods of animal origin	WAHID	Pregnant women and their fetuses; immunocompromised	Encephalitis, hydrocephalus (fetus), organomegaly, posterior uveitis in immunocompromised (infection of the brain is AIDS-defining); no signs in healthy adults	Adult cats, no signs or uveitis; kittens, diarrhea	• Avoid raw or undercooked foods of animal origin • Prompt, proper disposal of pet feces • Hand hygiene
Yersinia enterocolitica	Rare	Rare	Worldwide (less common in tropical areas)	Fecal-oral likely; contaminated or unpasteurized milk, fecally contaminated water, raw or undercooked foods (pork)	FoodNet, NESP	Children <2 years old; immunocompromised	Fever, abdominal pain, vomiting, diarrhea; more severe disease such as septicemia possible	Diarrhea, vomiting	• Hand hygiene • Proper disposal of feces

| Yersinia pestis | Dogs: 0.1% Cats: 0.05% Pet rabbits: unreported | Cats are common source for human infection in endemic regions (e.g., southwestern USA) | Endemic in certain regions of nearly all continents; absent in Australia, New Zealand, and New Guinea | Fleas; cat scratches/bites; respiratory droplets; contact with exudates; cats consuming infected rodents | IHR (pneumonic only), CNDSS | Veterinarians or those caring for sick cats | Bubonic (swelling of peripheral lymph nodes), septicemic, or pneumonic plague | Respiratory disease; high case fatality rate | • Keep pets indoors or prevent them from roaming or hunting when outdoors • Rodent control • Flea preventives for pets |

CLM, cutaneous larva migrans; CNDSS, Canadian Notifiable Diseases Surveillance System; IHR, International Health Regulations (require report to WHO); NESP, National Enteric Surveillance Program; NNDSS, (US) Nationally Notifiable Diseases Surveillance System; OLM, ocular larva migrans; VLM, visceral larva migrans; WAHID, World Animal Health Information Database; WHO, World Health Organization.

Sources: Acha and Szyfres, 2003; Banfield Pet Hospital, 2016; CDC, 2016; World Health Organization, 2016b; Public Health Agency of Canada, 2016; Day et al., 2012.

Table 8.2 Centers for Disease Control and Prevention (CDC) rabies post-exposure prophylaxis (PEP) guidelines for various animal bites.

Type of animal bite	Evaluation and disposition of animal	Recommendations
Dog, cat, ferret	Healthy; observe animal for 10 days	Vaccination should not be initiated unless the animal develops clinical signs of rabies
	Rabid (or suspected)	Vaccination should begin immediately
	Unknown (e.g., escaped)	Public health officials should be consulted; immediate vaccination should be considered
Raccoon, skunk, fox, other carnivore, bats	Regarded as rabid unless the animal tests negative	Consider immediate vaccination; if the animal is being tested, delay vaccination until results are available
Livestock, horses	Consider individually	Public health officials should be consulted; most livestock in the USA are vaccinated for rabies
Rodent, rabbit, hare, other mammal	Consider individually	Public health officials should be consulted; bites of rabbits, hares, and small rodents (e.g., squirrels, hamsters, guinea pigs, gerbils, chipmunks, rats, mice) almost never require post-exposure rabies prophylaxis

Adapted from Manning et al., 2008. The Canadian guidelines are very similar (Anon., 2015b).

Table 8.3 World Health Organization (WHO) rabies post-exposure prophylaxis (PEP) guidelines.

Category	Type of exposure	Treatment recommendation
I	Touching or feeding animals, licks on intact skin	No treatment
II	Nibbling of uncovered skin, minor scratches or abrasions without bleeding, licks on broken skin	Vaccine only
III	Single or multiple transdermal bites or scratches, contamination of mucous membrane with saliva from licks, exposure to bat bite or scratch	Vaccine and immunoglobulin

Adapted from the World Health Organization (http://www.who.int/rabies/human/postexp/en).

often overlooked situation by patients is waking up with a bat in the room or finding a bat in the room of a young child who has been unattended. Patients and families often do not realize that this is considered a possible rabies exposure and PEP is recommended. There are several CDC case reports on people developing rabies after handling a bat or having bats in the home and not seeking medical care to receive PEP. Improved education for health professionals is needed. Many healthcare providers are often unsure what to do in evaluating whether to give PEP

or not. This often leads to over- or under-use of PEP. National guidelines on rabies prevention recommend that healthcare providers contact local or state health departments to help determine whether to give PEP, but the quality of help by these health departments is highly variable.

Toxoplasmosis is caused by a parasite prevalent worldwide that is carried by cats and shed in the feces. Oocysts shed in the feces take 1–5 days to sporulate and become infective and can survive in the environment for years (Lopez et al., 2000). Most human cases occur from eating undercooked meat, and toxoplasmosis is the second leading cause of foodborne deaths in the USA, accounting for approximately 750 deaths per year. Most human cases are asymptomatic, but severe infections can cause damage to the brain, eyes, and other organs. It can be passed from mother to baby congenitally causing learning disabilities, chorioretinitis, or even death. In the USA the seroprevalence is approximately 20%, while in some European countries it is as high as 60–85% (Jones et al., 2003). The young, fetuses, and immunocompromised individuals are at highest risk. Infections can be acute or latent, especially in individuals who become immunocompromised. Prevention should be focused on educating individuals about toxoplasmosis, particularly pregnant women and those who are immunocompromised (Lopez et al., 2000). The CDC does not recommend that pregnant women or immunocompromised patients need to give up a pet cat or avoid cats. Other recommendations include: cook meats thoroughly; wash fruit and vegetables; wear gloves when gardening; change the litter box daily and have a non-pregnant person change the litter box if possible; wear gloves when changing the litter box; keep cats indoors; avoids stray cats; don't feed a cat a raw food diet; and keep outdoor sand boxes covered.

Bartonellosis is a heterogeneous group of infections that include cat-scratch disease, trench fever, carrion disease, and Oroya fever. *Bartonella henselae*, the cause of cat-scratch disease, is associated with pet cats. A cat can spread it by biting or scratching an individual. There are approximately 25 000 cases annually in the USA, with a seroprevalence rate of 4–6% (Skerget et al., 2003). Approximately 40% of cats carry *B. henselae*, and as high as 90% of kittens less than 1 year of age. Cats are usually asymptomatic carriers. Fleas are the actual source of the infection, and the cat inoculates a person with a bite or scratch that is contaminated with flea dirt (feces). Infections can also be transmitted directly to a person through a flea or tick

bite. Most human infections are mild and self-limited; however, severe infections can cause splenomegaly, bacillary angiomatosis, and Parinaud's oculoglandular syndrome. The best way to prevent this is to educate people on flea control in cats, including the proper routine flea medicine, avoiding rough play, and avoiding stray cats (M. Pennisi et al., 2013).

Worms such as *Toxocara canis* (dog roundworm), *T. cati* (cat roundworm), *Ancylostoma caninum* (hookworm), and *Baylisascaris procyonis* (raccoon roundworm) are common preventable zoonotic infections. Most have a fecal-oral transmission although hookworms can penetrate through the skin causing cutaneous larva migrans. There are approximately 10 000 human cases annually in the USA, and 20% of dogs and 80% of puppies carry *T canis* in the USA (Lee et al., 2010). Human infections are often asymptomatic, but the worms can migrate out of the gastrointestinal tract to organs and muscles causing visceral or ocular larva migrans. Preventive measures consist of regular veterinary care for pets including: fecal sample testing; regular use of heartworm medication for dogs and cats; washing hands after playing outside; keeping children from playing in areas that may be soiled with animal stool; cleaning a pet's living area at least once a week, particularly of dog feces; covering outdoor sand boxes and avoiding uncovered sand boxes; and teaching children to keep their hands out of their mouth when playing outside and not to put dirt or soil in their mouth (Lee et al., 2010).

Ringworm is caused by several types of fungus that are common worldwide. While ringworm can be zoonotic, most human cases are caused by species that are anthropophilic, meaning that they are adapted to humans and are usually transmitted from person to person (Anon., 2013). *Microsporum canis* is the major source of zoonotic dermatophytosis. Most animals that are infected, including humans, dogs, and cats, are symptomatic. The classic tinea corporis lesion is annular with a raised scaly border, central clearing, and mild erythema. Cats and dogs as well as human scalp lesions have an annular area of alopecia. Notable exceptions to this rule are Yorkshire Terriers and Persian cats, which can be asymptomatic carriers. Since the majority of human infections are not zoonotic, asymptomatic pets of infected owners usually do not need to be treated.

8.2.4.2 Human-to-Companion Animal Transmission

A final yet important example of how relationships with humans may adversely affect pet health and welfare involves infectious disease. Although the transmission of infectious disease from companion animals to people has received much attention in the past, the reverse situation is only now garnering interest – that is, infection of pets by contact with people who are infected, colonized, or transient carriers of infectious organisms. Reports of many such instances were recently summarized in a literature review (Messenger et al., 2014). The range of infectious organisms to which companion animals may be exposed expands if the owner works in the healthcare industry. The most common "reverse zoonosis" affecting companion animals in the review was methicillin-resistant *Staphylococcus aureus* (MRSA), and mathematical modeling predicts that humans are the most important source of this organism for dogs in particular (Heller et al., 2010) (Box 8.3). However, the fact that most reports of reverse zoonoses pertain to MRSA could simply reflect publication bias associated with prevailing concerns about antimicrobial resistance and hospital-associated infections.

Transmission of infections from humans to companion animals has been suspected or presumed to have occurred for other organisms. The nature of this type of transmission can be further classified to assume three forms (Mayr, 1989):

- Reciprocal transmission between humans and companion animals, e.g., *Campylobacter jejuni* (Damborg et al., 2005), various strains of *Escherichia coli* (Beutin, 1999), *Trichophyton rubrum* (Kushida and Watanabe, 1975; Van Rooij et al., 2012), or *Microsporum* spp.
- Transmission primarily from humans, e.g., the 2009 pandemic H1N1 influenza virus (to dogs, cats, and ferrets) (Lin et al., 2012; Sponseller et al., 2010; Swenson et al., 2010) (Box 8.4); *Mycobacterium tuberculosis* (to birds, cats, and dogs) (Morakova et al., 2011; Pavlik et al., 2005) (Table 8.4).
- Infections in which humans are the primary host but for which pets have served as dead-end hosts, e.g., herpes simplex virus type 1 (to rabbits) (Grest et al., 2012; Müller et al., 2009); mumps virus (to dogs) (Noice et al., 1959); and *Entamoeba histolytica* (cats) (American Association of Veterinary Pathologists, 2014).

In situations involving organisms for which humans are believed to be the primary host, microbiological or molecular confirmation that companion animals are infected with the same strain or clone as the person or people with whom they had contact strongly suggests that reverse zoonosis occurred. However, unequivocal or strongly suspected cases of reverse zoonoses involving multi-host organisms such as *Salmonella* or *Campylobacter* resulting in disease (vs colonization or temporary carriage) in this regard are challenging to identify, as that would require ruling out other potential sources such as food, other animals, or the environment, and also molecular comparison of microbial isolates recovered from affected parties.

8.2.5 Pets, People, and Antimicrobial Resistance

In addition to the aforementioned concerns of disease associated with foodstuffs, concern has been expressed that pets could serve as reservoirs for human infection or colonization with antimicrobial-resistant microorganisms and vice versa (Guardabassi et al., 2004; Lloyd, 2007). The same types of antimicrobials used

Box 8.3 Human-to-dog transmission of methicillin-resistant *Staphylococcus aureus* (MRSA)

Bronwyn E. Rutland, BSc (VB,) BVMS (Hons), DACVIM. See Rutland et al. (2009).

Bella, an 8-year-old spayed female Labrador Retriever, was brought to the veterinarian because of cellulitis of the ventral neck that had failed to respond to oral cephalexin treatment. Three months prior, Bella had undergone a tibial plateau-leveling osteotomy procedure; the implant from that surgery had been removed a few weeks before the cellulitis developed (Figure 8.2).

Bella lived with an elderly man who had multiple comorbid diseases and a history of prolonged corticosteroid treatment. Prior to her surgery, Bella's owner had been diagnosed with invasive pulmonary aspergillosis and had been treated with voriconazole for a month, after which he had developed cellulitis caused by MRSA, for which he had been hospitalized twice.

Bella's own cellulitis rapidly progressed, and her condition deteriorated dramatically. The swelling on her neck became necrotic and the skin sloughed. Histological evaluation of a biopsy sample revealed severe vasculitis and deep dermatitis. Systemic inflammatory response syndrome developed, and Bella failed to respond to treatment. Humane euthanasia was elected.

MRSA was cultured from Bella's neck, blood, and stifle joint. Subsequent pulsed-field gel electrophoresis confirmed the bacterium was the same strain that had infected her owner. The owner was a carrier (nasal swabs) during the time Bella had developed her illness, and he had developed his MRSA

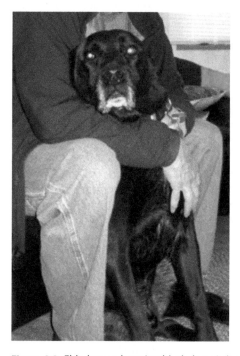

Figure 8.2 Elderly man hugging black dog.: A dog was suspected to have acquired a fatal MRSA infection through licking the hand of her elderly owner, who had been previously hospitalized for MRSA cellulitis. *Source:* ©JessieEldora/iStock.

infection prior to Bella becoming ill. Bella and her owner spent a lot of time together, and Bella had been known to lick her owner's hand. This was the presumed course of spread (although unable to be proven). The tragic outcome represents a rare case of a fatal infection in a pet that was acquired from its owner.

to treat humans are used to treat companion animals, and both parties can become infected with the same opportunistic pathogens such as *Staphylococcus aureus*, *E. coli*, or *Enterococcus* spp., and many of the same bacterial pathogens such as *Salmonella* spp. in which antimicrobial resistance can occur. Resistance of these pathogens to previously effective antimicrobials complicates and delays resolution of infections and restricts the range of antimicro-

bials to which the responsible bacteria are susceptible. Moreover, the genes through which resistance is conferred may be transferred among bacteria of pet and human origin, whether on or in the people and pets or within the environment (Guardabassi et al., 2004). Although several studies have been reported that show companion animals and humans share similarly resistant microorganisms, few have shown that this is true within

Box 8.4 Reverse zoonosis of pandemic H1N1 influenza A in a multi-cat household

Dr Christiane V. Löhr, Dr Med. Vet., PhD, Diplomate ACVP. See Löhr et al. (2010).

Abbey, a 2.5-year-old, female spayed domestic longhair cat from a household of three indoor-only cats, was brought to the veterinarian repeatedly over a 3-day period, initially for signs of lethargy, anorexia, and occasional wheezing that progressed over the 3 days to dyspnea. Results of physical examinations, bloodwork, and radiography suggested the most likely diagnosis was bacterial pneumonia secondary to aspiration. Abbey was treated with antimicrobials and a bronchodilator and returned home. Three days later, Abbey was brought back to the veterinarian, by which point, dyspnea was obvious. Thoracic radiography revealed a worsening of lung disease, with alveolar change extending into ventral portions of caudal lung lobes, worsening in right middle lobe, and persistence of changes in cranial lung lobes. A nasal swab was obtained for virus isolation, and Abbey was hospitalized and treated with supplemental oxygen. However, respiratory function deteriorated rapidly, and the cat was subsequently humanely euthanized and submitted to the local veterinary diagnostic laboratory for postmortem examination (Figure 8.3).

Postmortem and histopathological examination revealed diffuse, severe, acute bronchointerstitial, fibrinonecrotizing pneumonia. Virus isolation from a piece of fresh lung identified influenza A virus, and molecular screening and typing confirmed the pandemic (H1N1) 2009 influenza A virus. No virus was isolated from the nasal swab.

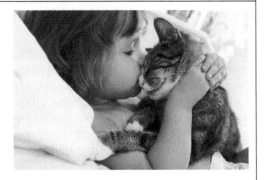

Figure 8.3 Child kissing cat. A cat was suspected of having acquired a fatal H1N1 influenza A infection following close contact with an infected child. *Source:* ©ehaurylik/iStock.

After discussing the results with the referring veterinarian, the investigating veterinary pathologist subsequently contacted Abbey's owner for additional information about the clinical circumstances. It turned out that a child in the family had been very ill with flu-like symptoms a week prior to the cat developing lethargy and anorexia. Abbey had very affectionately snuggled up with the sick child. Only after the demise of the cat did results confirm pH1N1 2009 influenza A in the child. No other person in the household showed any signs of respiratory disease.

After Abbey's death, the remaining two cats in the household developed signs of mild respiratory distress. Serological testing confirmed seroconversion for pandemic H1N1 2009 influenza A virus, consistent with infection of these two cats also. It was unclear whether the two surviving cats contracted their infection from the child or the deceased cat.

the same household. An example of the latter is a study in which owners of dogs that received antimicrobial treatment for deep pyoderma caused by multidrug-resistant *Staph. intermedius* were found to be colonized with identical organisms (Guardabassi,

et al., 2005). Given the lack of reported cases of human or pet infection with the same resistant organisms within the same household, the role of the human-companion animal relationship in the spread of antimicrobial resistance remains unclear.

Table 8.4 Reported cases of infectious diseases in companion animals with molecular or other strong evidence to support humans as the source.

Report	Case location	Organism recovered	Human source	Animal affected	Nature of animal's infection	Suspected or confirmed transmission route	Nature of supporting evidence
Rutland et al., 2009	Canada	MRSA	76-year-old male owner treated with vancomycin for cellulitis caused by MRSA	8-year-old Labrador Retriever	Cellulitis and generalized abscessation of the neck, progressing to septic shock and death	Through the dog's open orthopedic surgical wound after close contact with owner	Isolate from dog was molecularly indistinguishable from isolate from owner's; owner's infection preceded the dog's
Erwin et al., 2004; Hackendahl et al., 2004	USA	*Mycobacterium tuberculosis*	71-year-old female owner with tuberculosis	3.5-year-old Yorkshire Terrier	Chronic cough, weight loss, and vomiting	Owner allowing dog to lick her face	Isolate from dog was molecularly indistinguishable from owner's; owner's infection preceded the dog's; humans are reservoir hosts
Schmidt et al., 2008	Germany	*Mycobacterium tuberculosis*	Male owner with pulmonary tuberculosis who had completed anti-tuberculosis treatment 2.5 years earlier	Adult African Grey parrot	Emaciation, sublingual edema and nodules causing dysphagia, and osteolytic changes in the right wing; eventual euthanasia	Owner feeding the bird prechewed food	Histopathologic findings with tuberculosis and molecular confirmation that the strains recovered from the bird and owner had identical patterns; owner's infection preceded the bird's
Löhr et al., 2010	USA	2009 pandemic H1N1 influenza virus	Female with 10-day history of severe respiratory disease, confirmed via eventual hospitalization to be caused by H1N1	8-year old female Domestic Shorthair cat	Moderate-to-severe bronchointerstitial pneumonia resulting in euthanasia	Direct contact with owner while she was sick	Molecular confirmation of virus in lung homogenate from cat; hospital confirmed H1N1 infection in owner (technique not stated)

(Continued)

Table 8.4 (Continued)

Report	Case location	Organism recovered	Human source	Animal affected	Nature of animal's infection	Suspected or confirmed transmission route	Nature of supporting evidence
Martin and Anderson, 1997	USA	Stealth virus	Two owners (a couple) with flu-like illness	Dog (no further details given)	Neurological signs	Degree of contact or possible transmission route not stated	Cytopathic effect of viral isolate identical between owners and dog; the owners' illnesses appear to have preceded the dog's
Noice et al., 1959	USA	Mumps virus	Several juvenile family members with the mumps	Dog 1: 6-month-old Dachshund; Dog 2: 3-month-old Boston Terrier	Dog 1: inappetence and swollen parotid glands; Dog 2: extremely enlarged parotid glands, dysphagia and pain while swallowing	Exposure to droplets while on beds and in rooms of sick children	Virus isolation from dogs' (and not children's) saliva
Müller et al., 2009	Germany	Herpes simplex virus type 1	Owner with concurrent severe labial and facial herpesvirus infection	8-month-old male rabbit	Anorexia, runny eye, bruxism, hypersalivation, and ataxia leading eventually to euthanasia	Nose-to-nose and nose-to-mouth contact with owner	Histologic characterization and molecular confirmation of virus identity for rabbit; exclusive contact of rabbit with owner (for whom viral genetic sequencing was not performed); owner's infection preceded rabbit's
Castrejón and Sánchez, 2010	Mexico	Leptospira spp.	35-year-old male with leptospirosis	Puppy (age and breed unreported)	Pneumonia, vomiting, diarrhea, abdominal pain, hematuria, rapidly deteriorating to death	Puppy licked up blood that accidentally spilled from his owner's IV catheter	Serological tests revealed antibody against Leptospira interrogans icterohaemorrhagiae and L. canicola in blood samples from the owner and dog

MRSA, methicillin-resistant Staphylococcus aureus.

Within the home, people and pets can be expected to share microbial flora to a certain degree (Song et al., 2013). A few small-scale cross-sectional studies have been conducted into the prevalence of various potential pathogens within the home environment and their relationship with pet ownership. For example, *Clostridium difficile* ribotype 027, which can cause severe diarrhea in pets and people alike, was identified in environmental samples from 31% of sampled households in Ontario, Canada, and strains isolated from dogs differed from those in the environment, suggesting dogs were not the primary source (Weese et al., 2010). Furthermore, contaminated households could provide a source of MRSA infection for all members (Davis et al., 2012).

Ample evidence exists to suggest that indiscriminate or noncompliant use of antimicrobials prescribed for humans or companion animals may increase the likelihood of antimicrobial resistance in normal bacterial flora. Few owners fully comply with veterinary instructions for antimicrobial administration to their pets, and this is particularly true for drugs requiring frequent administration (i.e., more than twice a day) (Adams et al., 2005). For humans, compliance also decreases with increasing dose administration (Claxton et al., 2001). For cats perhaps more so than dogs, the opportunity exists for straining the human-animal bond when veterinary medication is required, as pets learn to resist or even fight medications and avoid their owners. Therefore, attempts to do something beneficial for pets may result in strained relationships. A similar situation exists for cats, which are taken for veterinary checkups far less often than dogs. Interestingly, although cats outnumber dogs in US households, they are approximately a fifth as likely to visit the veterinarian (Banfield Pet Hospital, 2014). Owners cite their cats' resistance to carriers and transport as important factors preventing them from visiting the veterinarian (Volk et al., 2014).

8.2.6 Social and Community Health

People, dogs, cats, birds, and rabbits have a mutual need for some extent of social interaction or companionship and mental stimulation. People can provide opportunities for play and mental stimulation for their pets, and pets can do the same in return. When these opportunities are provided at the community level, such as through off-leash dog parks, pet training classes, pet picnic parties, or fundraising runs or walks involving pets, whole groups of people and pets benefit. Other programs that are specifically tailored to improve the well-being of pets and people include programs involving inmate training of dogs and other animals. Whether these correctional programs involve juvenile offenders training abused and abandoned dogs, female offenders training puppies, or hardened male offenders training difficult-to-home shelter dogs, reported benefits to society include lower recidivism rates and, therefore, lower societal costs of institutionalization (Strimple, 2003). Animals (mostly dogs) who complete these programs go on to find permanent homes as pets, assistance animals, or residents in long-term care facilities, when they otherwise may have been euthanized. Inmate participants develop marketable skills leading to employment after release (Box 8.5).

Another aspect of the human-companion animal relationship outside the home concerns situations in which pets are brought to places typically reserved for human activity and interaction. A prime example is taking pets to work, which is becoming increasingly popular but is not without adverse consequences for workers, pets, and the work environment. From the perspective of hazards to humans, pet dander is among the most common types of human allergies, and air contamination with dander could create an uncomfortable or hazardous environment for affected co-workers (Asthma and Allergy Foundation of America, 2015). Pets do not typically undergo the stringent screening

---

Box 8.5 PAWS for Life

*Sources: Fitzgerald,2014; Karma Rescue (*http://krpawsforlife.tumblr.com*)*

Paws For Life, a program offered by the non-profit Karma Rescue, matches dogs at risk of euthanasia at high-kill shelters with inmates serving life-term sentences at the high-security California State Prison in Los Angeles County (http://krpawsforlife.tumblr.com). Karma volunteers instruct inmates on how to train the dogs to pass the Canine Good Citizen test, thereby increasing the likelihood that the dogs will be successfully adopted. As a result, the inmates receive unconditional love and develop compassion and a sense of purpose as well as skills. The dogs develop behaviors that facilitate bonding with their new owners, with the expectation that the dogs will enrich the lives of those owners and their community (Figure 8.4).

But the benefits don't stop there. In an interview with Dr Patricia Fitzgerald of the Huffington Post, one inmate said, "It gave me another chance at unconditional love. It's changed the entire yard, there is a lot of peace with the C.O.s [Correctional Officers] and other inmates. It brought everybody closer."

Positions in the program are limited. Interested inmates, who must have committed to their own rehabilitation by upholding an environment free of violence, disruption, and illegal drug use, were required to undergo a competitive process involving interviews and essay writing.

In 2014, 14 inmates trained five shelter dogs, who stayed at the prison throughout the 12-week program. The program concluded with a graduation ceremony, where inmates receive a certificate of completion and dogs receive Canine Good Citizen status. Afterward, inmates met with adoptive families to provide tips on care. Success of the first class of Paws for Life has led to plans to continue the program with even more dogs.

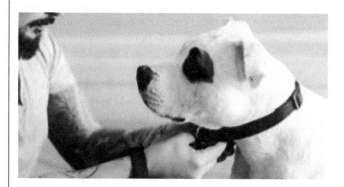

Figure 8.4 Younger man with collared dog. Prison dog-training programs offer inmates unconditional love, skills, and a sense of compassion and purpose. In return, hard-to-adopt shelter dogs get a new shot at finding a forever home and enriching the lives of others. *Source:* ©vgajic/iStock.

---

required for visitation of healthcare facilities, so opportunities also exist for workplace contamination through urinary or fecal soiling and associated infectious agents or through physical harm to people in the form of bites and scratches by anxious or fearful pets. In addition, pets cannot be presumed to enjoy workplace visits, as strange environments and people can pose significant sources of stress to pets. Furthermore, co-workers simply may not enjoy or may even fear interaction with pets, and the presence of pets may cause distractions for owners and co-workers alike.

8.2.7 Domestic Health and Violence

A discussion of the One Health concept as it concerns relationships among companion animals, their owners, and the environment that they share would be incomplete without mention of the increasing efforts of law enforcement, social services, animal protection agencies, and eventually veterinarians, to recognize and establish procedures for ensuring that instances of domestic violence, child abuse, or animal abuse are investigated fully to ensure safety of all parties in acknowledgment of the link among the three (Unti, 2008). The US Federal Bureau of Investigation announced in 2016 that it has begun collecting "detailed data from participating law enforcement agencies on acts of animal cruelty, including gross neglect, torture, organized abuse, and sexual abuse," acknowledging that these incidents are often precursors to larger crimes (Federal Bureau of Investigation, 2016). An entire discipline (veterinary forensic pathology) is emerging as the need grows for forensic evaluation of suspicious animal deaths caused by humans (similar to investigation of suspicious human deaths) (McDonough et al., 2015).

An environment of domestic violence can have a profound impact on the human victims, their families, and their pets. In such environments, the family pet often serves as emotional support for abuse victims, helping them cope (Flynn, 2000). Indeed, such victims can delay leaving their abusive situation out of fear that their pets will be harmed or even killed in their absence (Gallagher et al., 2008; Faver and Strand, 2003). Their fears appear well founded, as 71% of abused women, identified as current or past pet owners in a US study, reported that the abuser had threatened, hurt, or killed a pet (Ascione, 1998). And the abusive cycle appears to be self-perpetuating: in the same study, 32% of abused women with children had a child that had either hurt or killed a pet.

The link between animal cruelty and interpersonal violence expands beyond the home. For example, an association has been established between sexual (vs nonsexual) murderers and a childhood history of cruelty to animals and potentially to children as well (Kressler et al., 1986). Animal abusers have also been shown to be more likely than non-animal abusers to commit interpersonal violence and other antisocial acts (Arluke et al., 1993). Although commitment of animal cruelty does not necessarily presage commitment of acts against humans it is a behavior for which sufficient evidence exists to raise alarm bells in this regard.

8.3 Interactions Among Humans, Pets, and the Environment

8.3.1 Working Dogs

Working dogs, canine athletes, pets used for emotional support, and pets that participate in animal-assisted activities and interventions – all share the possibility of becoming exposed to hazards outside the home as a result of their activities that regular house pets would not encounter. These animals can also:

- become bridges to bring pathogens into the home, or
- help to disperse pathogens among the community, or
- act as sentinels for human hazard detection.

In addition, such animals are subjected to unique stressors with the potential to adversely affect their welfare.

The hazards are perhaps most obvious for certain groups of working dogs; those used for bomb or cadaver detection, search and rescue, or military or police activities share potentially hazardous environments with their handlers. For example, military dogs that worked for US forces during the Vietnam

War reportedly had a high risk for development of testicular seminoma or dysfunction. Vietnam War veterans also had a significant decrease in sperm quality (Hayes et al., 1990).

Although the effects of animal-assisted interventions on people have been well researched, the effects on the participating animals have received little attention. The opportunity for distress and harm to these animals is not negligible; indeed, screening tests for participating animals involve evaluating their responses to novel, invasive, and startling stimuli and ability to suppress natural behaviors such as exploring their environment (Therapy Dogs International, 2008). Several studies have been conducted into the effects of animal-assisted interventions on salivary cortisol concentration or behavioral signs of stress in participating dogs, with some findings supporting the hypothesis that participation is stressful for dogs under certain specific circumstances or for particular dogs but not for other circumstances or dogs (Ensminger, 2014). Small sample sizes (≤21 dogs) and highly specific scenarios limit the generalizability of any findings, and existing studies have included only dogs when cats, birds, and rabbits are also used for this purpose. Anecdotal reports of physical harms and fatigue to residential animals also exist (Iannuzzi and Rowan, 1991). Additional research is required to better understand these impacts.

Pets used in therapeutic ways can also become contaminated or colonized with human healthcare-associated pathogens such as *Clostridium difficile* and multidrug-resistant bacterial species that are otherwise normal flora such as *Staph. aureus* or *E. coli* (Lefebvre et al., 2009b). Such organisms are serious causes of morbidity and death in humans in North American healthcare facilities and are common environmental contaminants in such settings. Animal-assisted activities and interventions therefore may provide a conduit through which pathogens could spread from healthcare facilities into the community. It should be noted that there have been no reports of human infection through contact with such animals; however, a resident cat in a human geriatric ward was implicated in spreading MRSA among patients (Scott et al., 1988), so the possibility exists.

8.3.2 Environmental Toxicants

Another hazard within the home, tobacco smoke, can threaten the health of all inhabitants, regardless of species. For example, an association has been identified between environmental tobacco smoke (ETS) and atopic dermatitis in children (Yi et al., 2012) and in dogs (Ka et al., 2014). An experimental study also revealed cytological evidence of airway changes in dogs with ETS exposure (Roza and Viegas, 2007), although the clinical implications of such changes are unclear. ETS exposure is suspected of contributing to asthma or other respiratory diseases in cats (Cornell Feline Health Center, 2014), although such a relationship has not been scientifically established. Although more data are available for dogs in this respect, findings are conflicting or inconclusive (Hawkins et al., 2010; Yamaya et al., 2014). Pet birds with ETS exposure have greater plasma concentrations of cotinine, a nicotine metabolite, than do birds without this exposure (Cray et al., 2005); however, the health consequences of this finding are unknown.

For cats, which are fastidious groomers, the concern of ingestion of smoke-associated residues also exists; however, if this were true, then one would expect the risk of ETS-related diseases to be higher in long-haired cats than in short-haired cats, which does not appear to be the case on the basis of evidence to date (Bertone et al., 2002; 2003). Just as in human medicine, causal relationships between ETS and various forms of cancer in cats have been suspected but not definitively established (Snyder et al., 2004; Jelinek and Vozkova, 2012), and the evidence for dogs is weakly suggestive (e.g., nonsignificant odds ratios that include 1) (Reif et al., 1998, 1992) or nonsupportive (Coggins, 2001; Bukowski et al., 1998), with considerably less research on the subject for companion animals compared with the amount performed for humans.

Pets and young children can have a greater degree of exposure to potentially hazardous chemicals that accumulate in household dust or on flooring or that already exist in items; either group may ingest these chemicals simply by virtue of how they interact with the environment. Other home environment factors explored for associations with disease in companion animals include use of indoor coal or kerosene heaters, which is a risk factor for sinonasal cancer in dogs (Bukowski et al., 1998).

Some people have suggested that pets be used as sentinels of exposure to cancer-causing agents within or outside the home. A benefit of this approach is that the lifespan of pet cats and dogs is considerably shorter than that of humans, allowing for detection of hazards to the health of both parties. Epidemiologic findings that link pollutants, chemicals, or other physical environmental hazards to human disease are generally strengthened by similar findings in pets. The evidence in this regard is uncommon and sometimes weak. For example, a small study found no association between serologic evidence of exposure to polybrominated diphenyl ethers (PBDEs – found in flame-retardant materials and hypothesized to cause endocrine dysfunction) and hyperthyroidism in cats, but the investigators suggested that because serum concentrations in the cats were as much as 100 times as great as median concentrations in US adults, cats could serve as sentinels for human exposure (Dye et al., 2007). This would be important because PDBE exposure has been found to have adverse effects on neurobehavioral development in children (Eskenazi et al., 2013). Findings of a more recent Australian study also failed to support a role of PBDEs in feline hyperthyroidism (Chow et al., 2015).

8.3.3 Pets and the External Environment

The relationship between pets and their people can be extended to include the environment outside the home, highlighting some additional hazards to the environment and other creatures within it. Allowing cats and dogs outdoors to express their natural behaviors can have an adverse impact on the environment and wildlife. Free-roaming cats, both owned and unowned, contribute to a considerable number of deaths to birds, small wild mammals, and possibly wild amphibians and reptiles, both in the USA (Loss et al., 2013) and likely elsewhere as well. Allowing dogs on recreational trails in wildlife protection areas results in a significant decrease in habitat use by wild mammals such as squirrels, prairie dogs, and bobcats (Lenth and Knight, 2008). Even walking dogs on a leash in natural areas has been found to cause a significant reduction in bird abundance and diversity, with ground-dwelling birds the most affected (Banks and Bryant, 2007).

Fecal contamination of the environment by pet dogs and cats with outdoor access has long been established as increasing the risk of human exposure worldwide to various zoonotic parasites with a life stage involving the environment such as *Toxocara canis* or *T. cati* or *Toxoplasma gondii*, creating a health hazard for humans and companion animals alike. Used clay-based cat litter and plastic bags containing dog feces can burden landfill or sewer systems. Flushing of cat litter down the toilet has also been hypothesized to put marine life at risk for *T. gondii* infection as the resilient parasite finds its way into waterways and oceans (McGrath, 2014).

Allowing pets outdoors increases their risk of exposure to infectious organisms and environmental hazards such as pollutants or toxicants that have health implications for humans as well. This is particularly true for dogs and cats kept outdoors, and even greater for those allowed to freely roam.

Saprozoonoses are a special type of zoonoses involving infectious agents that depend on inanimate reservoirs or development sites in addition to vertebrate hosts to maintain their natural cycle (Schwabe, 1984). The zoonoses included in this category vary from textbook to textbook, but for the purposes of this chapter, examples involving companion animals and humans alike include blastomycosis, coccidiomycosis, and histoplasmosis, which are fungal infections for which soil or decaying organic matter is believed to be a primary source of the infectious spores. Geographic distribution of saprozoonotic organisms ranges from limited (e.g., regions with sandy, acidic soil close to freshwater sources in the Americas for blastomycosis or arid regions in the Americas for coccidiomycosis) to worldwide (histoplasmosis) (Acha and Szyfres, 2003). Transmission of associated diseases between companion animals and humans is rare and has typically involved injection via dog bites or occupational exposure (Gnann et al., 1983; Ramsey, 1994). Where these diseases are of particular interest from a One Health perspective is that when the risk of exposure is increased for companion animals, so it is increased for their owners or handlers (Herrmann et al., 2011; Baumgardner and Burdick, 1991; Morgan and Salit, 1996). And this increase in risk typically results from environmental conditions conducive to pathogen growth (e.g., temperature and humidity) and degree of outdoor activity. Consequently, pets can serve as sentinels for human exposure, particularly when those pets are allowed to freely explore the outdoors.

Other zoonoses in which a contaminated environment largely plays a role include leptospirosis, cryptosporidiosis, giardiasis, and hantavirus pulmonary syndrome. As an example of this, leptospirosis is caused by spirochetes, with 100–200 cases annually in the USA, about half of which are from Hawaii. It is likely underreported as most infections are mild and self-limited. Transmission can be direct between animals or indirect from contaminated water. Infections can be sporadic or associated with outbreaks usually involving a contaminated water source. Severe infections can cause kidney damage, liver failure, meningitis, and death. Preventive measures include vaccinating dogs, avoiding stagnant water, preventing pets from drinking stagnant water, increased community rodent control measures, avoiding contact with animal urine, and disinfecting urine-contaminated surfaces (Sykes et al.,

2011). Knowledge of endemic areas and how these zoonoses relate to contaminated environments and how they are spread can help public health officials improve control of these zoonoses and educate people on ways to protect themselves.

Another consideration is that when pets themselves become contaminated with hazardous chemicals through exposure outside the home, they can bring residues into the home and expose people to them through petting and other interactions (Morgan et al., 2008).

Curiosity is rising into the potential for pets to serve as sentinels for chronic environmental hazards such as carcinogens. The underlying premise is that pets intimately share our environments and, given their shorter lifespan, may develop clinical signs of intoxication or cancer more rapidly than humans might. However, for diseases such as cancer with a multifactorial etiology, establishment of definitive associations has proven challenging, as it also has for human diseases, and the existing evidence is somewhat weak. An excellent albeit dated critical review of studies that have examined associations between potential environmental hazards and cancer development in dogs is available elsewhere (Bukowski and Wartenberg, 1997). Examples provided in that review include an association between topical application of insecticide and bladder cancer in dogs, home exposure to electromagnetic fields and lymphoma in dogs, and owner exposure to asbestos and mesothelioma in their dogs. Recent evidence from a case-control study involving 263 dogs with biopsy-confirmed malignant lymphoma suggests that use of professionally applied lawn pesticides increased the odds of malignant lymphoma by 40%, controlling for other factors (Takashima-Uebelhoer et al., 2012). Another recent study found that dogs in a household less than 1 km away from a natural gas well in Pennsylvania were three times more likely to have a health condition (dermal, respiratory, ocular, neurological, gastrointestinal, reproductive, geriatric, neoplasms, musculoskeletal, or other ailments as classified by a veterinarian) as were dogs living further away, prompting the investigators to suggest continued monitoring of disease in dogs and other animals to infer the effects of natural gas exploration on surrounding communities (Slizovskiy et al., 2015). Although the value of comparison between cancers in pets and their owners has been considered (Schneider, 1970), no such studies have been reported.

Allowing pets to roam free increases the risk of the pet coming into contact with and spreading serious infections to people. One such infection is plague (caused by *Yersinia pestis*), which has recently had a resurgence in the number of human cases in the USA (Kwit et al., 2015). Dogs and cats can pick this up from contact with wild rodents or infected fleas and can subsequently spread it to humans they contact. Tularemia is another zoonosis that can be brought into the home in this manner. Cats and outdoor rabbits are particularly sensitive. Humans typically become infected by contact with infected animals, tick bites, or environmental aerosolizing activities (Pedati et al., 2015).

8.3.4 Disaster Preparedness

Natural disasters resulting in short-term or permanent displacement of owners and their pets present multiple challenges, which emergency response programs have only recently begun to acknowledge and address (HR 3858 (109th Congress), 2006; Heath and Linnabary, 2015). In 2006, the US Pets Evacuation and Transportation Standards (PETS) Act was signed into law, authorizing the Federal Emergency Management Agency "to provide rescue, care, shelter, and essential needs for individuals with household pets and service animals, and to the household pets and animals themselves following a major disaster or emergency" (AVMA, 2016).

Pet owners can struggle with the decision to either evacuate and leave their pets behind or remain in unsafe conditions, resulting in failure to evacuate or evacuation with subsequent attempts to re-enter an unsafe home to rescue the pets (Heath and Champion, 1996; Heath et al., 2001a). Evacuation without a pet can also cause extreme anxiety for an owner until the safety of their pet can be assured. Studies have shown that people who are attached to their pets are more likely to take them with them when they evacuate their homes during or following natural disasters (Heath et al., 2001b).

Major disasters such as large-scale hurricanes (e.g., Hurricane Katrina along the Gulf Coast of the USA in 2005) can also result in translocation of unclaimed pets alone and pet owners with their pets, sometimes to homes thousands of miles away (Levy et al., 2007), providing opportunities for spread of vector-borne zoonotic pathogens (e.g., *Dirofilaria immitis* and West Nile virus) from endemic regions to new locations (Levy, et al., 2011). People familiar to dogs and cats (and snakes) are more likely to be bitten by these animals during disruptions caused by hurricanes than are strangers or rescue workers (Warner, 2010).

In addition to large-scale translocation of animals in the wake of natural disasters, such translocation can also occur through people who rescue or import dogs and cats for various reasons from other countries, bringing with them pathogens and their arthropod vectors. South Korea, for example, imports a large percentage of pet cats and dogs from other countries, including China, the USA, and Russia (The Korea Bizwire, 2014). Illegal importation of animals intended as pets, ranging from puppies (Galpérine et al., 2004) to turtles (Brianti et al., 2010), also increases opportunities for disease and vector spread to nonendemic areas. For example, a UK outbreak of babesiosis in dogs that had never traveled outside of England has been hypothesized to be attributable to inadvertent importation of infected vectors (*Dermacentor* ticks) with dogs rescued from abroad (Swainsbury et al., 2016).

Both travel and rehoming of dogs have been attributed with spreading leishmaniasis, a vector-borne zoonosis for which sand flies are the established vector, across Europe

(Pennisi, 2015). Although dogs are the primary host, cats can also become infected through sand fly bites. Chagas disease, endemic to Latin America and caused by *Trypanosoma cruzi*, has been spreading into the dog population of the southern USA, presaging the possibility of human infection through contact with excrement of the vector – infected blood-sucking triatomine ("kissing") bugs (Raghavan et al., 2015). In addition, dogs infected with the zoonotic nematode *Onchocerca lupi* have been imported into Canada from the southwestern USA, where infection is endemic, raising concern that the parasite could establish a new geographic range, particularly given that the vectors – black flies – are also found in Canada (Verocaie et al., 2016).

8.3.5 Climate Change

Climate and environmental changes are other factors changing the landscape of several zoonotic diseases because of their impact on the agents, vectors, and hosts. Factors such as deforestation, human movement and encroachment on previously unpopulated areas, temperature and rainfall, road construction, and contamination of natural bodies of water all have the potential to change the risk of human and pet exposure to infectious agents (Patz et al., 2000). An example that has been associated with climate change is Lyme disease, caused by infection with *Borrelia burgdorferi*, the prevalence and geographic distribution of which is expanding in North America, concurrent with the geographic spread of associated tick vectors (*Ixodes scapularis* and *I. pacificus*) and primary hosts (white-tailed deer) (Eisen et al., 2016). The seroprevalence of *Borrelia burgdorferi* exposure in dogs in the USA increased by 21% between 2009 and 2013, and the geographic range of areas at high risk for human infections appears to be expanding (Kugeler et al., 2015). Results of statistical modeling have also suggested that the geographic distribution of plague (*Yersinia pestis*) and tularemia (*Francisella*

tularensis) is changing in the USA as a result of climate change (Nakazawa et al., 2007).

8.3.6 Zoonotic Disease Surveillance for Both People and Pets

As suggested in the discussion of saprozoonoses (see Section 8.3.3), pets can and do serve as sentinels of zoonotic disease in humans, particularly when pets are at a greater risk of exposure to zoonotic pathogens than people because of their behaviors. They are important in this respect because not only can companion animals be sources of zoonotic infections, but also they can serve as intermediate hosts between wildlife reservoirs and humans, or as harbingers of emerging diseases. It is through surveillance of Lyme disease in dogs and people that we have begun to appreciate its spread into new geographic areas within North America, presumably owing to the changing geographic distribution of the primary host (white-tailed deer) and the disease vector (black-legged ticks) (Banfield Pet Hospital, 2014; CDC, 2015).

Multiple national and international surveillance programs already exist for specific infectious diseases of people, many of which are zoonotic and some of which might be transmitted by pets. These include but are not limited to the Canadian Notifiable Diseases Surveillance System, US National Enteric Surveillance Program, US Nationally Notifiable Diseases Surveillance System, and World Animal Health Information Database (Day et al., 2012) (see Table 8.1). However, these programs are not uniform in scope; some involve active surveillance, and others passive surveillance. No international health agency is mandated to coordinate surveillance of diseases in companion animals (exceptions include rabies and leishmaniasis), making it more difficult to establish a One Health surveillance system that incorporates companion animal species as well. Although national or regional surveillance programs (including those of corporate medicine and diagnostic laboratories, and organizations such as the Companion Animal Parasite Council) might be used to establish a companion animal-related program, no standardization exists among them regarding nomenclature, disease definition, or diagnostic approach. To further complicate matters, private laboratories consider their data proprietary, even in aggregate, as do some veterinary medical corporations and will not share it with researchers or public health agencies (Uchtmann et al., 2015).

Despite the challenges inherent to establishing a One Health surveillance program, such as identification of funding sources and responsible agencies and addressing legal concerns (Stärk et al., 2015), efforts are underway to share infectious disease data between veterinary and human hospitals or diagnostic laboratories to identify increases in the incidence or prevalence of certain companion animal-associated zoonoses or the emergence of new diseases. However, given that the prevalence of many companion animal-associated zoonoses is currently unknown, and therefore a baseline has not been established, considerable work is necessary before any such program yields data that are actionable rather than simply academic in nature. The One Health Surveillance Working Group of the International Society for Disease Surveillance is but one such example, and their scope is global. This group aims to engage in the "collaborative, on-going, systematic collection and analysis of data from multiple domains to detect health related events and produce information which leads to actions aimed at attaining optimal health for people, animals, and the environment" (ISID, 2016).

8.4 Conclusion

Our world is enriched by companion animals, and in most circumstances, any hazards arising from the interaction among them, us, and the environment are a small price to pay for the privilege of their company. Most hazards are preventable or can be mitigated through commonsense practices, particularly if both owner and pet are healthy.

From a One Health perspective, communication between veterinarians, human healthcare providers, and health officials is key to optimizing the health of the human and pet population. Our current system, especially in the USA, lacks the requisite communication, with each field acting in their own silo. When physicians are surveyed they feel that veterinarians should take the lead in educating people when it comes to pet-related health hazards, but this is problematic in that non-pet owners are exposed to animals and pets as well (Grant and Olsen, 1999). Furthermore, many people with chronic medical conditions that directly affect their animal-related risk do not feel comfortable disclosing this to the veterinarian thus preventing adequate discussion of risk and prevention (St Pierre et al., 1996). A survey from Tucson, Arizona, showed that 86% of physicians felt that it was important to educate patients about pet-related health hazards but only 17% reported regularly counseling families (Villar et al., 1998). Physicians also reported that they were "very uncomfortable" with educating patients on pet-related health hazards (Grant and Olsen, 1999). A survey of veterinarians and physicians in Tennessee showed that 93% of physicians indicated that they never or rarely discussed zoonoses with HIV-infected patients, 100% of veterinarians indicated that they never or rarely contacted physicians for advice on zoonoses risk, and only 26% and 33% of veterinarians and physicians respectively were able to identify the zoonoses posing the greatest risk for HIV patients. This shows a need for better training for the physician work force in medical school, residency, and in continuing medical education. The Association of American Veterinary Medical Colleges and the Association for Prevention Teaching and Research recently partnered to create a new interprofessional curriculum on One Health topics to help fill this gap (Anon., 2016b). Despite the fact that many One Health publications call for enhanced communication between human and veterinary medicine, on a day-to-day frontline basis, this is an unusual occurrence. In order for this to happen, a greater emphasis needs to be placed on One Health issues with targeted interventions that are shown to change physician and veterinary behavior. These strategies could be evidenced based systematic guidelines, clinical paths, or financial incentives. Traditional continuing medical education has not been shown to be a good driver of change at least in human physicians.

Pet-owner practices to promote health of the human-pet-environment relationship:

- Collect and properly dispose of pet waste on a timely basis.
- Practice hand hygiene regularly, particularly after potential contact with pet excrement.
- Prevent pets from licking or contacting surface wounds.
- Prevent pets from drinking from potentially contaminated water sources such as puddles or lakes and from consuming the excrement of other animals.
- Refrain from kissing pets or letting them lick you when you're ill.
- Supervise young children when in the presence of any animals.
- Provide pets with their basic needs.
- Provide pets with adequate healthcare, including annual or more frequent veterinary checkups and preventive services such as vaccines and antiparasitic medications.
- Seek professional advice for pet training or behavioral concerns.
- When trying to determine the source of an infection, tell your physician or veterinarian about the:
  - travel history of you and your pet;
  - the presence of pets in the home.

Institutional practices to promote health of the human-pet-environment relationship:

- Mandate and earmark funding to support the establishment of reporting and surveillance systems for diseases shared between humans and companion animals.
- Provide tangible incentives for private laboratories, human and veterinary healthcare facilities, public health agencies, and others to share data to advance human, companion animal, and environmental health.
- Train veterinarians and physicians to inquire about the health of all household members when trying to identify the source of an infection.
- Train veterinarians and physicians to inquire about pets or children in the home when domestic violence, elder abuse, child abuse or neglect, or animal abuse or neglect is suspected and to report such suspicions to appropriate authorities.
- Require public health courses in veterinary schools and zoonotic disease courses in medical school.
- Require primary care physicians to inquire about pet ownership and animal contact as a routine, standard-of-care question.
- Provide access to healthcare for all people, and promote routine, preventive veterinary care for all pets.

Disclaimer

The names of all patients in vignettes have been changed to ensure patient confidentiality.

References

2020 Healthy Pets, Healthy Families Coalition of Los Angeles County (2014). *Healthy Pets, Healthy Families Initiative*. Los Angeles: 2020 Healthy Pets, Healthy Families Coalition.

Abate, S., Zucconi, M., and Boxer, B. (2011). Impact of canine-assisted ambulation on hospitalized chronic heart failure patients' ambulation outcomes and satisfaction: a pilot study. *J Cardio Nurs* 26(3), 224–230.

Acha, P. and Szyfres, B. (2003). *Zoonoses and Communicable Diseases Common to Man and Animals*, 3rd edn. Washington, DC: Pan American Health Organization.

Adams, V. et al. (2005). Evaluation of client compliance with short-term administration of antimicrobials to dogs. *J Am Vet Med Assoc* 225(4), 567–574.

Alberta Agriculture and Forestry (2014). Consumer corner: Canadian pet market outlook, 2014. Available at: http://www1. agric.gov.ab.ca/$department/deptdocs.nsf/ all/sis14914 (accessed March 5, 2016).

Allen, K., Shykoff, B., and Izzo, J. (2001). Pet ownership, but not ACE inhibitor therapy, blunts home blood pressure responses to mental stress. *Hypertension* 38, 815–820.

American Association of Veterinary Pathologists (2014). Entamoeba histolytica. Available at: http://www.aavp.org/wiki/ catprotozoa/coccidia-apicomplexan/ sarcodina/entamoeba-histolytica/(accessed March 10, 2016).

American Pet Products Manufacturers' Association (2017). Pet industry market size & ownership statistics. Available at: http://www. americanpetproducts.org/press_industrytrends. asp (accessed December 5, 2017).

American Veterinary Medical Association (2012). US pet ownership and demographics sourcebook (2012). Available at: https:// www.avma.org/kb/resources/statistics/ pages/market-research-statistics-us-pet-ownership-demographics-sourcebook.aspx (accessed March 5, 2016).

Anon. (2001). A community approach to dog bite prevention: American Veterinary Medical Association task force on canine aggression and human-canine interactions. *JAVMA* 218(11), 1732–1749.

Anon. (2003). Nonfatal dog bite--related injuries treated in hospital emergency departments - United States, 2001. *MMWR* 52(26), 605–610.

Anon. (2012). Rising dog ownership in India driving demand for petfood, accessories. Available at: http://www.petfoodindustry. com/articles/2874-rising-dog-ownership-in-india-driving-demand-for-petfood-accessories (accessed March 5, 2016).

Anon. (2013). Dermatophytosis. Available at: http://www.cfsph.iastate.edu/Factsheets/pdfs/ dermatophytosis.pdf (accessed April 8, 2016).

Anon. (2014). Dog bite risk and prevention: the role of breed. Available at: https://www.avma. org/KB/Resources/LiteratureReviews/Pages/ The-Role-of-Breed-in-Dog-Bite-Risk-and-Prevention.aspx (accessed April 8, 2016).

Anon. (2015a). CDC: Cost of Rabies Prevention. Available at: http://www.cdc. gov/rabies/location/usa/cost.html (accessed April 8, 2016).

Anon. (2015b). Canadian Immunization Guide: Part 4 - Active Vaccines: Rabies Vaccine. Available at: http:// healthycanadians.gc.ca/publications/ healthy-living-vie-saine/4-canadian-immunization-guide-canadien-immunisation/index-eng.php?page=18 (accessed October 24, 2016).

Anon. (2016a). Postal service releases annual dog attack city rankings. Available at: https://about.usps.com/news/national-releases/2016/pr16_039.htm (accessed April 8, 2016).

Anon. (2016b). AAVMC/APTR One Health Case Studies. Available at: http://www. aavmc.org/One-Health/Case-Studies.aspx (accessed April 8, 2016).

Arluke, A., Levin, J., Luke, C., et al. (1993). The relationship of animal abuse to violence and other forms of antisocial behavior. *J Interpers Violence* 14(9), 963–975.

Arnold, S. et al. (1974). Nutritional secondary hyperparathyroidism in the parrakeet. *Cornell Vet* 64(1), 37–46.

Ascione, F. (1998). Battered women's reports of their partners' and their children's cruelty to animals. *J Emot Abuse* 1(1), 119–133.

Asthma and Allergy Foundation of America (2015). Allergy facts and figures. Available at: http://www.aafa.org/page/allergy-facts. aspx (accessed May 10, 2016).

Augusto, M., Kraijer, M., and Pratschke, K. (2005). Chronic oesophageal foreign body in a cat. *J Feline Med Surg* 7(4), 237–240.

Australian Veterinary Association (2016). Pet ownership statistics. Available at: http://www.ava.com.au/news/media-centre/hot-topics-4 (accessed March 4, 2016).

AVMA (American Veterinary Medical Association) (2016). PETS Act (FAQ). Available at: https://www.avma.org/KB/Resources/Reference/disaster/Pages/PETS-Act-FAQ.aspx (accessed August 30, 2016).

Banfield Pet Hospital (2012). *State of Pet Health 2012 Report*. Portland, OR: Banfield Pet Hospital.

Banfield Pet Hospital (2013). *State of Pet Health 2013 Report*. Portland, OR: Banfield Pet Hospital.

Banfield Pet Hospital (2014). *State of Pet Health 2014 Report*. Portland, OR: Banfield Pet Hospital.

Banfield Pet Hospital (2016). *State of Pet Health 2016 Report*. Portland, OR: Banfield Pet Hospital.

Banks, P. and Bryant, J. (2007). Four-legged friend or foe? Dog walking displaces native birds from natural areas. *Biol Lett* 3(6), 611–613.

Baumgardner, D. and Burdick, J. (1991). An outbreak of human and canine blastomycosis. *Rev Infect Dis* 13(5), 898–905.

Bergamasco, L. et al. (2010). Heart rate variability and saliva cortisol assessment in shelter dog: human-animal interaction effects. *Appl Anim Beh Sci* 125(1–2), 56–68.

Bergroth, E. et al. (2012). Respiratory tract illnesses during the first year of life: effect of dog and cat contacts. *Pediatrics* 130(2), 211–220.

Bertone, E., Snyder, L., and Moore, A. (2002). Environmental tobacco smoke and risk of malignant lymphoma in pet cats. *Am J Epidemiol* 156(3), 268–273.

Bertone, E., Snyder, L., and Moore, A. (2003). Environmental and lifestyle risk factors for oral squamous cell carcinoma in domestic cats. *J Vet Intern Med* 17(4), 567–562.

Beutin, L. (1999). Escherichia coli as a pathogen in dogs and cats. *Vet Res* 30(2–3), 285–298.

Billinghurst, I. (1993). *Give Your Dog a Bone: The Practical Commonsense Way to Feed Dogs for a Long, Healthy Life*. Alexandria, NSW: SOS Print + Media Group.

Bradley, J. (2014). Dog bites: problems and solutions. Policy Paper. Animals and Society Institute.

Branigan, T. (2008). Chinese figures show fivefold rise in babies sick from contaminated milk. *The Guardian*, 2 December. Available at: https://www.theguardian.com/world/2008/dec/02/china (accessed December 5, 2017).

Brianti, E. et al. (2010). Risk for the introduction of exotic ticks and pathogens into Italy through the illegal importation of tortoises, *Testudo graeca*. *Med Vet Entomol* 24(3), 336–339.

Brown, C. et al. (2016). Compendium of animal rabies prevention and control, 2016. *JAVMA* 248(5), 505–517.

Bruha, P. (2015). The Brazilian pet market. Available at: http://thebrazilbusiness.com/article/the-brazilian-pet-market (accessed March 4, 2016).

Buckland, E. et al. (2013). A survey of stakeholders' opinions on the priority issues affecting the welfare of companion dogs n Great Britain. *Anim Welf* 22, 239–253.

Buffington, C. (2002). External and internal influences on disease risk in cats. *J Am Vet Med Assoc* 220(7), 994–1002.

Bukowski, J. and Wartenberg, D. (1997). An alternative approach for investigating the carcinogenicity of indoor air pollution: pets as sentinels of environmental cancer risk. *Environ Health Perspect* 105(12), 1312–1319.

Bukowski, J., Wartenberg, D., and Goldschmidt, M. (1998). Environmental causes for sinonasal cancers in pet dogs, and their usefulness as sentinels of indoor cancer risk. *J Toxicol Environ Health A* 54(7), 579–591.

Caraway, C., Scott, A., Roberts, N., and Hauser, G. (1959). Salmonellosis in sentry dogs. *J Am Vet Med Assoc* 135, 599–602.

Castrejón, O. and Sánchez, B. (2010). [Man to dog leptospirosis transmission]. *Enf Inf Microbiol* 30(3), 106–109.

Castrodale, L. et al. (2010). General public health considerations for responding to animal hoarding cases. *J Environ Health* 72(7), 14–18.

Cavallo, S. et al. (2015). Human outbreak of Salmonella typhimurium associated with exposure to locally made chicken jerky pet treats, New Hampshire, 2013. *Foodborne Pathog Dis* 12(5), 441–446.

CDC (Centers for Disease Control and Prevention) (2015). Lyme disease maps. Available at: http://www.cdc.gov/lyme/stats/maps.html (accessed August 30, 2016).

CDC (Centers for Disease Control and Prevention) (2016). Healthy pets healthy people. Available at: https://www.cdc.gov/healthypets (accessed August 28, 2016).

Chow, K. et al. (2015). Evaluation of polybrominated diphenyl ethers (PBDEs) in matched cat sera and house dust samples: investigation of a potential link between PBDEs and spontaneous feline hyperthyroidism. *Environ Res* 136, 173–179.

Christian, H. et al. (2013). Dog ownership and physical activity: a review of the evidence. *J Phys Act Health* 10(5), 750–759.

Clark, C. et al. (2001). Characterization of Salmonella associated with pig ear dog treats in Canada. *J Clin Microbiol* 39(11), 3962–3968.

Clark, G. and Boyer, W. (1993). The effects of dog obedience training and behavoural counseling upon human-canine relationship. *Appl Anim Behav Sci* 37(2), 147–159.

Claxton, A., Cramer, J., and Pierce, C. (2001). A systematic review of the associations between dose regimens and medication compliance. *Clin Ther* 23(8), 1296–1310.

Coggins, C. (2001). A review of chronic inhalation studies with mainstream cigarette smoke, in hamsters, dogs, and nonhuman primates. *Toxicol Pathol* 29(5), 550–557.

Collin, S. et al. (2015). Pet ownership is associated with increased risk of non-atopic asthma and a reduced risk of atopy in childhood: finding from a UK birth cohort. *Clin Exp Allergy* 45(1), 200–210.

Connor, K. and Miller, J. (2000). Animal-assisted therapy: an in-depth look. *Dimens Crit Care Nurs* 19(3), 20–26.

ConsumerAffairs (2016). Pet food recalls and warning. Available at: https://www.consumeraffairs.com/pet-food-recalls-and-warnings (accessed April 10, 2016).

Coppola, C., Grandin, T., and Enns, R. (2006). Human interaction and cortisol: can human contact reduce stress for shelter dogs? *Physiol Behav* 87(3), 537–541.

Cornell Feline Health Center (2014). Feline asthma: a risky business for many cats. Available at: http://www.vet.cornell.edu/fhc/Health_Information/Asthma.cfm (accessed May 11, 2016).

Cray, C., Roskos, J., and Zielezienski-Roberts, K. (2005). Detection of cotinine, a nicotine metabolite, in the plasma of birds exposed to secondhand smoke. *J Avian Med Surg* 19(4), 277–279.

Custovic, A. and van Wijk, R. (2005). The effectiveness of measures to change the indoor environment in the treatment of allergic rhinitis and asthma: ARIA update. *Allergy* 60(9), 1112–1115.

Cutt, H. (2007). Dog ownership, health and physical activity: a critical review of the literature. *Health Place* 13(1), 261–272.

Cutt, H., et al. (2008). Understanding dog owners' increased levels of physical activity: results from RESIDE. *Am J Public Health* 98(1), 66–69.

Damborg, P., Olsen, K., Møller Nielsen, E., and Guardabassi, L. (2005). Occurrence of Campylobacter jejuni in pets living with human patients infected with C. jejuni. *J Clin Microbiol* 42(3), 1363–1365.

Danielzik, S. et al. (2004). Parental overweight, socioeconomic status and high birth weight are the major determinants of overweight and obesity in 5–7 year-old children: baseline data of the Kiel Obesity Prevention Study (KOPS). *Int J Obes Relat Metab Disord* 28(11), 1494–1502.

Davis, M. et al. (2012). Household transmission of meticillin-resistant Staphylococcus aureus and other staphylococci. *Lancet Infect Dis* 12(9), 703–716.

Day, M. et al. (2012). Surveillance of zoonotic infectious disease transmitted by small companion animals. *Emerg Infect Dis* 18(12) (online).

Dhabhar, F., Malarkey, W., Neri, E., and McEwen, B. (2012). Stress-induced redistribution of immune cells––from barracks to boulevards to battlefields: a tale of three hormones––Curt Richter Award winner. *Psychoneuroendocrinology* 37(9), 1345–1368.

DiGiacomo, N., Arluke, A., and Patronek, G. (1998). Surrendering pets to shelters: the relinquishers' perspective. *Anthrozoos* 11(1), 41–51.

Domingeez-Bello, M. and Blaser, M. (2015). Asthma: Undoing millions of years of coevolution in early life? *Sci Transl Med* 7(307), 307fs39.

Douglas, D. (2005). *Benefits to Pets From the Human-Animal Bond: A Study of Pet Owner Behaviors and Their Relation to Attachment.* Wichita, Kansas: Wichita State University.

Dreschel, N. (2010). The effects of fear and anxiety on health and lifespan in pet dogs. *Appl Anim Behav Sci* 125(3–4), 157–162.

Dudley, E., Schiml, P., and Hennessy, M. (2015). Effects of repeated petting sessions on leukocyte counts, intestinal parasite prevalence, and plasma cortisol concentration of dogs housed in a county animal shelter. *J Am Vet Med Assoc* 247(11), 1289–1298.

Dye, J. et al. (2007). Elevated PBDE levels in pet cats: sentinels for humans? *Environ Sci Technol* 41(18), 6350–5356.

Edinboro, C. et al. (2004). Epidemiologic study of relationships between consumption of commercial canned food and risk of hyperthyroidism in cats. *J Am Vet Med Assoc* 224(6), 879–886.

Ehnert, K. et al. (2015). The Healthy Pets Healthy Families initiative as an example of one health in action. *J Am Vet Med Assoc* 247(2), 143–147.

Eisen, R., Eisen, L., Ogden, N., and Beard, C. (2016). Linkages of weather and climate with Ixodes scapularis and Ixodes pacificus (Acari: Ixodidae), enzootic transmission of Borrelia burgdorferi, and Lyme disease in North America. *J Med Entomol* 53(2), 250–261.

Ellis, S. et al. (2013). AAFP and ISFM feline environmental needs guidelines. *J Feline Med Surg* 15(3), 219–230.

Ensminger, J. (2014). Does therapy work stress dogs? Should therapy dogs be allowed off leash? Available at: http://doglawreporter. blogspot.com/2014/10/does-therapy-work-stress-dogs-should.html (accessed March 8, 2016).

Ernst, L. (2014). Animal-assisted therapy: an exploration of its history, healing benefits, and how skilled nursing facilities can set up programs. *Annals of Longer Term Care: Clinical Care and Aging* 22(10), 27–32.

Erwin, P. et al. (2004). Mycobacterium tuberculosis transmission from human to canine. *Emerg Infect Dis* 10(12), 2258–2260.

Eskenazi, B. et al. (2013). In utero and childhood polybrominated diphenyl ether (PBDE) exposures and neurodevelopment in the CHAMACOS study. *Environ Health Perspect* 121(2), 257–262.

Evans, R. and Buerk, R. (2012). Why Japan prefers pets to parenthood. *The Guardian*, 8 June.

Fall, T., Lundholm, C., Örtqvist, A.K., et al. (2015). Early exposure to dogs and farm animals and the risk of childhood asthma. *JAMA Pediatr*, 169(11), e153219.

Farm Animal Welfare Council (2009). Five freedoms. Available at: http://webarchive. nationalarchives.gov.uk/20121007104210/ http:/www.fawc.org.uk/freedoms.htm (accessed March 14, 2016).

Fatjó, J. et al. (2015). Epidemiology of dog and cat abandonment in Spain (2008–2013). *Animals (Basel)* 5(2), 426–441.

Faver, C. and Strand, E. (2003). To leave or stay? Battered women's concern for vulnerable pets. *J Interpers Violence* 18(12), 1367–1377.

Federal Bureau of Investigation (2016). Tracking animal cruelty: FBI collecting data on crimes against animals. Available at: https://www.fbi.gov/news/stories/-tracking-animal-cruelty (accessed December 5, 2017).

FEDIAF (European Pet Food Industry Federation) (2011). *Nutritional Recommendations for Complete and Complementary Pet Food for Dogs and Cats*. Brussels, Belgium: FEDIAF.

FEDIAF (European Pet Food Industry Federation) (2013). *Nutritional Recommendations for Feeding Pet Rabbits*. Brussels, Belgium: FEDIAF.

Fitzgerald, P. (2014). Who rescued whom? Shelter dogs and prison inmates give each other a new "leash" on life. Available at: http://www.huffingtonpost.com/dr-patricia-fitzgerald/who-rescued-who-shelter-dogs-and-prison-inmates-give-each-other-a-new-leash-on-life_b_5760042.html (accessed October 25, 2016).

Flynn, C. (2000). Woman's best friend: pet abuse and the role of companion animals in the lives of battered women. *Violence Against Women* 6(2), 162–177.

Fredriksson-Ahomaa, M., Korte, T., and Korkeala, H. (2001). Transmission of Yersinia enterocolitica 4/O:3 to pets via contaminated pork. *Lett Appl Microbiol* 32(6), 375–378.

Gallagher, B., Allen, M., and Jones, B. (2008). Animal abuse and intimate partner violence: researching the link and its significance in Ireland – a veterinary perspective. *Ir Vet J* 61(10), 658–667.

Galpérine, T. et al. (2004). [The risk of rabies in France and the illegal importation of animals from rabid endemic countries.] *Presse Med* 33(12 Pt 1), 791–792.

Gandhi, R., Liebman, M., Stafford, B., and Stafford, P. (1999). Dog bite injuries in children: a preliminary survey. *Am Surg* 65(9), 863–864.

Gaskins, L. and Bergman, L. (2011). Surveys of avian practitioners and pet owners regarding common behavior problems in psittacine birds. *J Avian Med Surg* 25(2), 111–118.

German, A. (2015). Style over substance: What can parenting styles tell us about ownership styles and obesity in companion animals?. *Br J Nut*. 113(Suppl.), S72–S77.

Gianella, P., Pfammatter, N., and Burgener, I. (2009). Oesophageal and gastric endoscopic foreign body removal: complications and follow-up of 102 dogs. *J Small Anim Pract* 50(12), 649–654.

Gnann, J.J., Bressler, G., Bodet, C., and Avent, C. (1983). Human blastomycosis after a dog bite. *Ann Intern Med* 98(1), 48–49.

Grant, S. and Olsen, C. (1999). Preventing zoonotic diseases in immunocompromised persons: the role of physicians and veterinarians. *Emerg Infect Dis* 5(1), 159–163.

Grest, P. et al. (2012). Herpes simplex encephalitis in a domestic rabbit (Oryctolagus cuniculus). *J Comp Path* 126, 308–311.

Guardabassi, L., Schwarz, S., and Lloyd, D. (2004). Pet animals as reservoirs of antimicrobial-resistant bacteria. *J Antimicrob Chemother* 54(2), 321–332.

Guardabassi, L., Loeber, M., and Jacobson, A. (2005). Transmission of multiple antimicrobial-resistant Staphylococcus intermedius between dogs affected by deep pyoderma and their owners. *Vet Microbiol* 98(1), 23–27.

Hackendahl, N., Mawby, D., Bemis, D., and Beazley, S. (2004). Putative transmission of Mycobacterium tuberculosis infection from a human to a dog. *J Am Vet Med Assoc* 225(10), 1573–1577.

Harrison, G. (1998). Twenty years of progress in pet bird nutrition. *J Am Vet Med Assoc* 212(8), 1226–1230.

Hawkins, E., Clay, L., Bradley, J., and Davidian, M. (2010). Demographic and historical findings, including exposure to environmental tobacco smoke, in dogs with chronic cough. *J Vet Intern Med* 24(4), 825–831.

Hayes, H., Tarone, R., Casey, H., and Huxsoll, D. (1990). Excess of seminomas observed in Vietnam service U.S. military working dogs. *J Natl Cancer Inst* 82(12), 1042–1046.

Headey, B. and Grabka, M. (2007). Pets and human health in Germany and Australia: national longitudinal results. *Soc Indic Res* 80(2), 297–311.

Heath, S. and Champion, M. (1996). Human health concerns from pet ownership after a tornado. *Prehosp Disaster Med* 11(1), 67–70.

Heath, S. and Linnabary, R. (2015). Challenges of managing animals in disasters in the US. *Animals (Basel)* 5(2), 173–192.

Heath, S. and Wilson, C. (2014). Canine and feline enrichment in the home and kennel: a guide for practitioners. *Vet Clin North Am Small Anim Pract* 44(3), 427–449.

Heath, S., Kass, P., Beck, A., and Glickman, L. (2001a). Human and pet-related risk factors for household evacuation failure during a natural disaster. *Am J Epidemiol* 153(7), 659–665.

Heath, S., Voeks, S., and Glickman, L. (2001b). Epidemiologic features of pet evacuation failure in a rapid-onset disaster. *J Am Vet Med Assoc* 218(12), 1898–1904.

Heller, J., Kelly, L., Reid, S., and Mellor, D. (2010). Qualitative risk assessment of the acquisition of Meticillin-resistant staphylococcus aureus in pet dogs. *Risk Anal* 30(3), 458–472.

Herrmann, J., Kostiuk, S., Dworkin, M., and Johnson, Y. (2011). Temporal and spatial distribution of blastomycosis cases among humans and dogs in Illinois (2001-2007). *J Am Vet Med Assoc* 239(3), 335–343.

Herron, M. and Buffington, C. (2010). Environmental enrichment for indoor cats. *Compend Contin Educ Vet* 32(12), p. E4.

Heuberger, R. and Wakshlag, J. (2011). Characteristics of ageing pets and their owners: dogs v. cats. *Br J Nutr* 106(Suppl.), S150–153.

Holmquist, L. and Elixhauser, A. (2010). Emergency department visits and inpatient stays involving dog bites, 2008. Available at: http://www.hcup-us.ahrq.gov/reports/statbriefs/sb101.pdf (accessed April 8, 2016).

Horowitz, D. (2008). Separation anxiety in dogs. *NAVC Clinician's Brief* pp. 61–62.

HR 3858 (109th Congress) (2006). Pets Evacuation and Transportation Standards Act of 2006. Available at: https://www.congress.gov/bill/109th-congress/house-bill/3858 (accessed May 10, 2016).

Iannuzzi, D. and Rowan, A. (1991). Ethical issues in animal-assisted therapy programs. *Anthrozoos* 4(3), 154–163.

Imanishi, M. et al. (2014). Outbreak of Salmonella enterica serotype Infantis infection in humans linked to dry dog food in the United States and Canada, 2012. *J Am Vet Med Asso. 2014* 244(5), 545–553.

ISDS. One Health Surveillance Workgroup. Available at: http://syndromicmass.nonprofitsoapbox.com/cop/one-health-surveillance (accessed January 31, 2018).

Jelinek, F. and Vozkova, D. (2012). Carcinoma of the trachea in a cat. *J Comp Pathol* 147(2–3), 177–180.

Jones, J., Kruszon-Moran, D., and Wilson, M. (2003). Toxoplasma gondii infection in the United States, 1999-2000. *Emerg Infect Dis* 9(11), 1371–1374.

Ka, D. et al. (2014). Association between passive smoking and atopic dermatitis in dogs. *Food Chem Toxicol* 66, 329–333.

Kozuka, J. (2014). Still a ways to go, but animal welfare in Japan is improving by leaps and bounds. *RocketNews24*, 8 August.

Krahn, L., Tovar, M.D., and Miller, B. (2015). Are pets in the bedroom a problem? *Mayo Clin Proc* 90(12), 1663–1665.

Kressler, R., Burgess, A., Hartman, C., et al. (1986). Murderers who rape and mutilate. *J Interpers Violence* 1(3), 273–287.

Kugeler, K., Farley, G., Forrester, J., and Mead, P. (2015). Geographic distribution and expansion of human Lyme disease, United States. *Emerg Infect Dis* 21(8), 1455–1457.

Kushida, T. and Watanabe, S. (1975). Canine ringworm caused by Trichophyton rubrum; probable transmission from man to animal. *Sabouraudia* 13(1), 30–32.

Kwan, J. and Bain, M. (2013). Owner attachment and problem behaviors related to relinquishment and training techniques of dogs. *J Appl Anim Welf Sci* 16(2), 168–183.

Kwit, N. et al. (2015). Human plague - United States, 2015. *MMWR* 64(33), 918–919.

Laflamme, D. et al. (2008). Pet feeding practices of dog and cat owners in the United States and Australia. *J Am Vet Med Assoc* 232(5), 687–694.

Lambert, K. et al. (2015). A systematic review and meta-analysis of the proportion of dogs surrendered for dog-related and owner-related reasons. *Prev Vet Med* 118(1), 148–160.

Lee, A. et al. (2010). Epidemiologic and zoonotic aspects of ascarid infections in dogs andcats. *Trends Parasitol* 26(4), 155–161.

Lefebvre, S., Reid-Smith, R., Boerlin, P., and Weese, J. (2009a). Evaluation of the risks of shedding Salmonellae and other potential pathogens by therapy dogs fed raw diets in Ontario and Alberta. *Zoonoses Public Hlth* 55(8–10), 470–480.

Lefebvre, S., Reid-Smith, R., Waltner-Toews, D., and Weese, J. (2009b). Incidence of acquisition of methicillin-resistant Staphylococcus aureus, Clostridium difficile, and other health-care-associated pathogens by dogs that participate in animal-assisted interventions. *J Am Vet Med Assoc* 234(11), 1404–1417.

Lefebvre, S. et al. (2013). Effect of age at gonadectomy on the probability of dogs becoming overweight. *J Am Vet Med Assoc* 243(2), 236–243.

Lenth, B. and Knight, R.B.M. (2008). The effects of dogs on wildlife communities. *Natural Areas J* 28(3), 218–227.

Levine, G., Allen, K., Braun, L.T., et al. (2013). Pet ownership and cardiovascular risk: a scientific statement from the American Heart Association. *Circulation* 127, 2353–2363.

Levy, J. et al. (2007). Seroprevalence of Dirofilaria immitis, feline leukemia virus, and feline immunodeficiency virus infection among dogs and cats exported from the 2005 Gulf Coast hurricane disaster area. *J Am Vet Med Assoc* 231(2), 218–225.

Levy, J. et al. (2011). Prevalence of infectious diseases in cats and dogs rescued following Hurricane Katrina. *J Am Vet Med Assoc* 238(3), 311–317.

Lin, D. et al. (2012). Natural and experimental infection of dogs with pandemic H1N1/2009 influenza virus. *J Gen Virol* 93(1), 119–123.

Lloyd, D. (2007). Reservoirs of antimicrobial resistance in pet animals. *Clin Infect Dis* 45(Suppl. 2), S148–152.

Löhr, C. et al. (2010). Pathology and viral antigen distribution of lethal pneumonia in domestic cats due to pandemic (H1N1) 2009 influenza A virus. *Vet Pathol* 47(3), 378–386.

Lonsdale, T. (2001). *Raw meaty bones: promote health.* New South Wales, Australia: Rivetco P/I.

Lopez, A. et al. (2000). Preventing congenital toxoplasmosis. *MMWR* 49(RR02), 57–75.

Loss, S., Will, T., and Marra, P. (2013). The impact of free-ranging domestic cats on wildlife of the United States. *Nat Commun* 4, 1396.

Manning, S.E., Rupprecht, C.E., Fishbein, D., et al. (2008). Human rabies prevention—United States, 2008: recommendations of the Advisory Committee on Immunization Practices. *MMWR Recomm Rep* 57(RR-3), 12.

Mao, J., Xia, Z., Chen, J., and Yu, J. (2013). Prevalence and risk factors for canine obesity surveyed in veterinary practices in Beijing, China. *Prev Vet Med* 112(3–4), 438–442.

Maria Pennisi, et al. Bartonella Species Infection in Cats: ABCD guidelines on prevention and management. *Journal of Feline Medicine and Surgery* 15(7), 563–569. https://doi.org/10.1177/1098612X13489214.

Martin, W. and Anderson, D. (1997). Stealth virus epidemic in the Mohave Valley. I. Initial report of virus isolation. *Pathobiology* 65(1), 51–56.

Mayr, A. (1989). [Infections which humans in the household transmit to dogs and cats.] *Zentralbl Bakteriol Mikrobiol Hyg B* 187(4–6), 508–526.

McDonough, S. et al. (2015). Illuminating dark cases: veterinary forensic pathology emerges. *Vet Pathol* 52(1), 5–6.

McGrath, S. (2014). How to green your pets. *Audubon* Jul–Aug.

McLaughlin, A. and Strunk, A. (2016). Common emergencies in small rodents, hedgehogs, and sugar gliders. *Vet Clin North Am Exot Anim Pract* 19(2), 465–499.

Menor-Campos, D., Molleda-Carbonel, l.J., and López-Rodríguez, R. (2011). Effects of exercise and human contact on animal welfare in a dog shelter. *Vet Rec* 169(15), 388.

Messenger, A., Barnes, A., and Gray, G. (2014). Reverse zoonotic disease transmission (zooanthroponosis): a systematic review of seldom-documented human biological threats to animals. *PLoS One* 9(2), e89055.

Michel, K. (2006). Unconventional diets for dogs and cats. *Vet Clin North Am Small Anim Pract* 36(6), 1269–1281.

Michel, K. et al. (2008). Attitudes of pet owners toward pet foods and feeding management of cats and dogs. *J Am Vet Med Assoc* 233(11), 1699–1703.

Mills, D., Karagiannis, C., and Zulch, H. (2014). Stress––its effects on health and behavior: a guide for practitioners. *Vet Clin North Am Small Anim Pract* 44(3), 525–541.

Monroe, B. et al. (2016). Rabies surveillance in the United States during 2014. *JAVMA* 248(7), 777–788.

Morakova, M. et al. (2011). Human-to-human and human-to-dog Mycobacterium tuberculosis transmission studied by IS6110 RFLP analysis: a case report. *Veterinarni Medicina* 56(6), 314–317.

Morgan, M. and Salit, I. (1996). Human and canine blastomycosis: A common source infection. *Can J Infect Dis* 7(2), 147–151.

Morgan, M., Stout, D., Jones, P., and Barr, D. (2008). An observational study of the potential for human exposures to pet-borne diazinon residues following lawn applications. *Environ Res* 107(3), 336–342.

Morley, P. et al. (2006). Evaluation of the association between feeding raw meat and Salmonella enterica infections at a Greyhound breeding facility. *J Am Vet Med Assoc* 228(10), 1524–1532.

Muller, C. (2015). Dogs can discriminate the emotional expression of human faces. *Curr Biol* 25(5), 601–605.

Müller, K. et al. (2009). Encephalitis in a rabbit caused by human herpesvirus-1. *J Am Vet Med Assoc* 235(1), 66–69.

Nakazawa, Y. et al. (2007). Climate change effects on plague and tularemia in the United States. *Vector Borne Zoonotic Dis* 7(4), 529–540.

National Research Council Ad Hoc Committee on Dog and Cat Nutrition (2006). *Nutrient Requirements of Dogs and Cats.* Washington, DC: National Academies Press.

Nijland, M., Stam, F., and Seidell, J. (2010). Overweight in dogs, but not in cats, is related to overweight in their owners. *Public Health Nutr* 13(1), 102–106.

Noice, F., Bolin, F., and Eveleth, D. (1959). Incidence of viral parotitis in the domestic dog. *AMA Am J Dis Child* 98(3), 350–352.

Olczak, J. et al. (2005). Multivariate analysis of risk factors for feline hyperthyroidism in New Zealand. *N Z Vet J* 53(1), 53–58.

Patrick, G. and O'Rourke, K. (1998). Dog and cat bites: epidemiologic analyses suggest different prevention strategies. *Public Health Rep* 113(3), 252–257.

Patronek, G. (1999). Hoarding of animals: an under-recognized public health problem in a difficult-to-study population. *Public Health Rep* 114(1), 81–87.

Patronek, G. et al. (1996). Risk factors for relinquishment of cats to an animal shelter. *J Am Vet Med Assoc* 209(3), 582–588.

Patz, J., Graczyk, T., Geller, N., and Vittor, A. (2000). Effects of environmental change on emerging parasitic diseases. *Int J Parasitol* 30(12–13), 1395–1405.

Pavlik, I. et al. (2005). Detection of bovine and human tuberculosis in cattle. *Vet Med – Czech*, 50(7), 291–299.

Pedati, C. et al. (2015). Notes from the field: Increase in human cases of tularemia - Colorado, Nebraska, South Dakota, and Wyoming, January– September 2015. *MMWR* 64(47), 1317–1318.

Pennisi, M. (2015). Leishmaniasis of companion animals in Europe: an update. *Vet Parasitol* 208(1–2), 35–47.

People's Dispensary for Sick Animals (2016). PAW PDSA animal wellbeing report 2015. Available at: https://www.pdsa.org.uk/get-involved/our-current-campaigns/pdsa-animal-wellbeing-report (accessed March 5, 2016).

Perna, G., Iannone, G., Alciati, A., and Caldirola, D. (2016). Are anxiety disorders associated with accelerated aging? A focus on neuroprogression. *Neural Plast* 2016, Art. ID 8457612.

Peron, F. and Grosset, T. (2014). The diet of adult psittacids: veterinarian and ethological approaches. *J Anim Physiol Anim Nutr (Berl)* 98(3), 403–416.

Perri, A. (2016). A wolf in dog's clothing: initial dog domestication and Pleistocene wolf variation. *J Archaeol Sci* 68, 1–4.

Pet Food Manufacturers' Association (2015). Pet population 2015. Available at: http://www.pfma.org.uk/pet-population-2015 (accessed March 4, 2016).

Pion, P. et al. (1992). Clinical findings in cats with dilated cardiomyopathy and relationship of findings to taurine deficiency. *J Am Vet Med Assoc* 201(2), 267–274.

Pitout, J. et al. (2003). Association between handling of pet treats and infection with Salmonella enterica serotype newport expressing the AmpC beta-lactamase, CMY-2. *J Clin Microbiol* 41(10), 4578–4583.

Pongrácz, P. et al. (2005). Human Listeners Are Able to Classify Dog (Canis familiaris) Barks Recorded in Different Situations. *J Comp Psychol*, 119(2), 136–144. http://dx.doi.org/10.1037/0735-7036.119.2.136

Public Health Agency of Canada (2016). Pathogen safety data sheets and risk assessment. Available at: http://www.phac-aspc.gc.ca/lab-bio/res/psds-ftss (accessed August 5, 2016).

Raghavan, R. et al. (2015). Geospatial risk factors of canine American trypanosomiasis (Chagas disease) (42 cases: 2000–2012). *Vector Borne Zoonotic Dis* 15(10), 602–610.

Ramsey, D. (1994). Blastomycosis in a veterinarian. *J Am Vet Med Assoc* 205(7), 968.

Reif, J. et al. (1977). Feline urethral obstruction: a case-control study. *J Am Vet Med Assoc* 170(11), 1320–1324.

Reif, J., Dunn, K., Ogilvie, G., and Harris, C. (1992). Passive smoking and canine lung cancer risk. *Am J Epidemiol* 135(3), 234–239.

Reif, J., Bruns, C., and Lower, K. (1998). Cancer of the nasal cavity and paranasal sinuses and exposure to environmental tobacco smoke in pet dogs. *Am J Epidemiol* 147(5), 488–492.

Reinisch, A. (2009). Characteristics of six recent animal hoarding cases in Manitoba. *Can Vet J* 50(10), 1069–1073.

Richards, E. (2016). Does dog walking predict physical activity participation: results from a national survey. *Am J Health Promot* 30(5), 323–30.

Robertson, I. (2003). The association of exercise, diet and other factors with owner-perceived obesity in privately owned dogs from metropolitan Perth, WA. *Prev Vet Med* 58(1–2), 75–83.

Rolls, J. (2013). Rabbits. In: A. Linzey (ed.), *The Global Guide to Animal Protection*. Springfield, IL: University of Illinois Press, p. 123.

Rooney, N. et al. (2014). The current state of welfare, housing and husbandry of the English pet rabbit population. *BMC Res Notes* 7, 942.

Rowe, E. et al. (2015). Risk factors identified for owner-reported feline obesity at around one year of age: Dry diet and indoor lifestyle. *Prev Vet Med* 121(3–4), 273–281.

Roza, M. and Viegas, C. (2007). The dog as a passive smoker: effects of exposure to environmental cigarette smoke on domestic dogs. *Nicotine Tob Res* 9(11), 1171–1176.

Rumbeiha, W. and Morrison, J. (2011). A review of class I and class II pet food recalls involving chemical contaminants from 1996 to 2008. *J Med Toxicol* 7(1), 60–66.

Rupprecht, C. et al. (2010). Use of a reduced (4-dose) vaccine schedule for postexposure prophylaxis to human rabies: recommendations of the Advisory Committee on Immunization Practices. *MMWR* 59(RR02), 1–9.

Rutland, B. et al. (2009). Human-to-dog transmission of methicillin-resistant Staphylococcus aureus. *Emerg Infect Dis* 15(8), 1328–1330.

Sasai, H. et al. (2015). Characteristics of bone fractures and usefulness of micro-computed tomography for fracture detection in rabbits: 210 cases (2007–2013). *J Am Vet Med Assoc* 246(12), 1339–1344.

Scarlett, J., Donoghue, S., Saidla, J., and Wills, J. (1994). Overweight cats: prevalence and risk factors. *Int J Obes Relat Metab Disord* 18(Suppl. 1), S22–28.

Schepers, F., Koene, P., and Beerda, B. (2009). Welfare assessment in pet rabbits. *Anim Welfare* 18(4), 477–485.

Schlesinger, D. and Joffe, D. (2011). Raw food diets in companion animals: a critical review. *Can Vet J* 52(1), 50–54.

Schmidt, V. et al. (2008). Transmission of tuberculosis between men and pet birds: a case report. *Avian Pathol* 37(6), 589–592.

Schneider, R. (1970). Household pets and cancer. *CA Cancer J Clin* 20(4), 234–241.

Schultze, K. (1998). *Natural Nutrition for Dogs and Cats: The Ultimate Diet*. Carlsbad, CA: Hay House Inc.

Schwabe, C. (1984). *Veterinary Medicine and Human Health*, 3rd edn. Baltimore, MD: Williams & Wilkins.

Scott, G., Thomson, R., Malone-Lee, J., and Ridgway, G. (1988). Cross-infection between animals and man: possible feline transmission of Staphylococcus aureus infection in humans? *J Hosp Infect* 12(1), 29–34.

Shore, E., Petersen, C., and Douglas, D. (2003). Moving as a reason for pet relinquishment: a closer look. *J Appl Anim Welf Sci* 6(1), 39–52.

Shute, N. (2016). NPR: He rescued a dog, Then the dog rescued him. Health News From NPR. Available at: http://www.npr.org/sections/health-shots/2016/03/10/469785736/he-rescued-a-dog-then-the-dog-rescued-him (accessed October 4, 2016).

Siegel, J. et al. (1999). AIDS diagnosis and depression in the multicenter AIDS cohort study: the ameliorating impact of pet ownership. *AIDS Care* 11(2), 157–170.

Skoglund P., Ersmark, E., Palkopoulou, E., and Dalén, L. (2015). Ancient wolf genome reveals an early divergence of domestic dog ancestors and admixture into high-latitude breeds. *Curr Biol* 25(11), 1515–1519.

Slizovskiy, I. et al. (2015). Reported health conditions in animals residing near natural gas wells in southwestern Pennsylvania. *J Environ Sci Health A Tox Hazard Subst Environ Eng* 50(5), 473–481.

Smith, B. et al (2014). The prevalence and implication of human-animal co-sleeping in an Australian sample. *Anthrozoos* 27(4), 543–551.

Snyder, L.A. et al. (2004). p53 expression and environmental tobacco smoke exposure in feline oral squamous cell carcinoma. *Vet Pathol* 41(3), 209–215.

Song, S. et al. (2013). Cohabiting family members share microbiota with one another and with their dogs. *Elife* 2, e00458.

Sponseller, B. et al. (2010). Influenza A pandemic (H1N1) 2009 virus infection in domestic cat. *Emerg Infect Dis* 16(3), 534–537.

Stafford, K. (2007). *The Welfare of Dogs*. Dordrecht, The Netherlands: Springer.

Stanley, I., Comwell, Y., Bowen, C., and Van Orden, K. (2014). Pet ownership may attenuate loneliness among older adult primary care patients who live alone. *Aging Ment Health* 18(3), 394–399.

Stärk, K. et al. (2015). One Health surveillance – More than a buzz word? *Prev Vet Med* 120(1), 124–130.

Stevens, J., Teh, S., and Haileyesius, T. (2009). Nonfatal fall-related injuries associated with dogs and cats - United States, 2001-2006. *MMWR* 58(11), 277–281.

St Pierre, L., Kreisle, R., and Beck, A. (1996). *Role of Veterinarians in Educating Immunocompromised Clients on the Risks and Benefits of Pet Ownership*. Ithaca: Dodge Foundation.

Strimple, E. (2003). A history of prison inmate-animal interaction programs. *Am Behav Sci* 70(1), 70–78.

Swainsbury, C., Bengtson, G., and Hill, P. (2016). Babesiosis in dogs. *Vet Rec* 178(7), 172.

Swenson, S. et al. (2010). Natural cases of 2009 pandemic H1N1 Influenza A virus in pet ferret. *J Vet Diagn Invest* 22(5), 784–788.

Sykes, J. et al. (2011). 2010 ACVIM small animal consensus statement on leptospirosis: diagnosis, epidemiology, treatment, and prevention. *J Vet Intern Med* 25(1), 1–13.

Takashima-Uebelhoer, B. et al. (2012). Household chemical exposures and the risk of canine malignant lymphoma, a model for human non-Hodgkin's lymphoma. *Environ Res* 12, 171–176.

Tami, G. et al. (2008). Relationship between management factors and dog behavior in a sample of Argentine Dogos in Italy. *J Vet Beh: Clin Appl Res* 3(2), 59–73.

Taylor, M., Geiger, D., Saker, K., and Larson, M. (2009). Diffuse osteopenia and myelopathy in a puppy fed a diet composed of an organic premix and raw ground beef. *J Am Vet Med Assoc* 234(8), 1041–1048.

The Korea Bizwire (2014). [Kobiz Stats] Pets in South Korea. Available at: http://koreabizwire.com/kobiz-stats-korean-job-seekers-for-employment-tests-2/7970 (accessed March 4, 2016).

Therapy Dogs International (2008). Therapy Dogs International (TDI) testing guidelines. Available at: http://www.tdi-dog.org/HowToJoin.aspx?Page=New+TDI+Test (accessed March 8, 2016).

Thompson, H. et al. (2012). Esophageal foreign bodies in dogs: 34 cases (2004–2009). *J Vet Emerg Crit Care (San Antonio)* 22(2), 254–261.

Tomblyn, M. et al. (2009). Guidelines for preventing infectious complications among hematopoietic cell transplant recipients: a global perpective. *Biol Blood Marrow Transplant* 15(10), 1143–1238.

Tsuchiya, K. (1992). The discovery of the causal agent of Minimata disease. *Am J Ind Med* 21(2), 275–280.

Uchtmann, N., Herrmann, J., Hahn, E., and Beasley, V. (2015). Barriers to, efforts in, and optimization of integrated One Healthsurveillance: a review and synthesis. *Ecohealth* 12(2), 368–384.

Unti, B. (2008). Cruelty indivisible: historical perspectives on the link between cruelty to animals and interpersonal violence. In: Ascione, F. (ed.), *The International Handbook of Animal Abuse and Cruelty: Theory, Research, and Application*. West Lafayette, IN: Purdue University Press, pp. 8–30.

US Dept of Health and Human Services (2015). *Step It UP! The Surgeon General's call to action to promote walking and walkable communities*. Washington, DC: US Dept of Health and Human Services, Office of the Surgeon General.

US Food and Drug Administration (2014). Melamine pet food recall – frequently asked questions. Available at: http://www.fda.gov/AnimalVeterinary/SafetyHealth/RecallsWithdrawals/ucm129932.htm (accessed March 29, 2016).

US Food and Drug Administration (2015). FDA progress report on ongoing investigation into jerky pet treats. Available at: http://www.fda.gov/AnimalVeterinary/SafetyHealth/ProductSafetyInformation/ucm371465.htm (accessed March 31, 2016).

US Food and Drug Administration (2016). Outbreak investigations. Available at: http://www.fda.gov/Food/RecallsOutbreaksEmergencies/Outbreaks/ucm272351.htm (accessed March 27, 2016).

Van Rooij, P., Declercq, J., and Beguin, H. (2012). Canine dermatophytosis caused by Trichophyton rubrum: an example of man-to-dog transmission. *Mycoses* 55(2), e15–17.

Verocaie, G. et al. (2016). Onchocerca lupi nematodes in dogs exported from the United States into Canada. *Emerg Infect Dis* 22(8), 1477–1479.

Veterinary Practice News Editors (2015). New program helps care for pets after owners pass. *Veterinary Practice News* 22 January.

Vigne J.-D., Guilaine, J., Debue, K., Haye, L. and Gérard, P. (2004). Early taming of the cat in Cyprus. *Science* 304(9), 259

Villar, R., Connick, M., Meaney, F., and Davis, M. (1998). Parent and pediatrician knowledge, attitudes, and practices regarding pet-associated hazards. *Arch Pediatr Adolesc Med* 152(10), 1035–1037.

Voith, V., Ingram, E., Mitsouras, K., and Irizarry, K. (2009). Comparison of adoption agency breed identification and DNA breed identification in dogs. *J Appl Anim Welf Sci* 12(3), 253–262.

Volk, J., Thomas, J., Colleran, E., and Siren, C. (2014). Executive summary of phase 3 of the Bayer veterinary care usage study. *J Am Vet Med Assoc* 244(7), 799–802.

Wakeling, J. et al. (2009). Risk factors for feline hyperthyroidism in the UK. *J Small Anim Pract* 50(3), 406–414.

Walker, A. et al. (1977). An epidemiological survey of the feline urological syndrome. *J Small Anim Pract* 18(4), 283–301.

Warner, G. (2010). Increased incidence of domestic animal bites following a disaster due to natural hazards. *Prehosp Disaster Med* 25(2), 188–190.

Weese, J. et al. (2010). Evaluation of Clostridium difficile in dogs and the household environment. *Epidemiol Infect* 138(8), 1100–1104.

Weng, H. and Hart, L. (2012). Impact of the economic recession on companion animal relinquishment, adoption, and euthanasia: a Chicago animal shelter's experience. *J Appl Anim Welfare Sci* 15(1), 80–90.

Westgarth, C. et al. (2012). Is childhood obesity influenced by dog ownership? No cross-sectional or longitudinal evidence. *Obes Facts* 5(6), 833–844.

Williams, M. & Viscusi, J. (2016). Hoarding disorder and a systematic review of treatment with cognitive behavioral therapy. *Cogn Behav Ther* 45(2), 93–110.

World Health Organization (2006). *Constitution of the World Health Organization. Basic documents, 45th edn. Supplement October 2006.* Geneva: WHO.

World Health Organization (2013). WHO Expert Consultation on Rabies. Second Report. Available at: http://apps.who.int/iris/bitstream/10665/85346/1/9789240690943_eng.pdf (accessed April 8, 2016).

World Health Organization (2015). Obesity and overweight. Fact sheet No. 311 (updated January 2015). Available at: http://www.who.int/mediacentre/factsheets/fs311/en/ (accessed March 27, 2016).

World Health Organization (2016a). Questions and answers on melamine. Available at: http://www.who.int/csr/media/faq/QAmelamine/en/ (accessed March 27, 2016).

World Health Organization (2016b). WHO Media Centre fact sheets. Available at: http://www.who.int/mediacentre/factsheets/en (accessed August 25, 2016).

Yabroff, K., Troiano, R., and Berrigan, D. (2008). Walking the dog: is pet ownership associated with physical activity in California? *J Phys Act Health* 5(2), 216–228.

Yamaya, Y., Sugiya, H., and Watari, T. (2014). Tobacco exposure increased airway limitation in dogs with chronic cough. *Vet Rec* 174(1), 18.

Yi, O. et al. (2012). Effect of environmental tobacco smoke on atopic dermatitis among children in Korea. *Environ Res* 113, 0–45.

ZENOAQ (2013). Recent pet statistics for Japan. Available at: http://www.zenoaq.jp/english-test/aij/0804.html (accessed December 5, 2017).

9

Zoological Institutions and One Health

Thomas P. Meehan[1] and Yvonne Nadler[2]

[1] *Brookfield Zoo, University of Illinois at Urbana-Champaign, Brookfield, IL, USA*
[2] *Zoo and Aquarium All Hazards Preparedness, Response, and Recovery Fusion Center, Silver Spring, MD, USA*

9.1 Introduction

Zoos and aquariums function at the intersection of animal, human, and environmental health in two distinct settings: 1) field conservation programs conducted in the natural environment of wildlife species across the globe (in situ); or 2) within the confines of the zoo or aquarium grounds in which staff protect the health and well-being of animals, personnel, and guests. In each of these settings zoos and aquariums function as living laboratories for One Health.

The major goal of zoos and aquariums is to integrate all aspects of their work with conservation activities (WAZA, 2005). Through the protection of species in zoos and in situ, these institutions seek to inspire conservation efforts and their support by connecting the public to nature. While studies show that most people attend zoos for enjoyment or a "family outing" (Reading and Miller, 2007), research shows that key messages about the animals in their care help zoos educate the public about conservation (Adelman et al., 2000; Dierking et al., 2004; Goldowsky, 2009; Kemmerly and Macfarlane, 2009; Falk et al., 2007; Johnson et al., 2016). Respondents' sense of enjoyment and fun were most strongly influenced by their emotional responses to animals, followed by introspection and reflection, cognitive engagement with educational materials, and interactions with zoo and aquarium staff (Luebke and Matiasek, 2013; Sickler and Fraser, 2009). Beyond simply providing information, however, zoos and aquariums provide their public with emotional experiences to help motivate them to conservation action. This interconnection of wildlife, environment, and the public is at the heart of One Health.

9.2 Zoos, Aquariums, and Field Conservation

Field projects encompassing free-ranging wildlife, domestic animal, and human populations are key components of many zoo-based in situ conservation programs. These projects may involve animal rescue, population biology, wildlife ecology, and the assessment of the effects of climate change and environmental toxins on wildlife species. They are natural laboratories for the study of disease ecology and zoonotic pathogen emergence. The Association of Zoos and Aquariums (AZA) developed the Species Survival Plan® (SSP) programs to oversee the population management of select species within member zoos. The SSPs also support field conservation and scientific studies

Beyond One Health: From Recognition to Results, First Edition.
Edited by John A. Herrmann and Yvette J. Johnson-Walker.
© 2018 John Wiley & Sons, Inc. Published 2018 by John Wiley & Sons, Inc.

(AZA, 2017a). They have been instrumental in directing field programs for the conservation of great ape species and the recovery of amphibian species threatened with extinction. The Wildlife Conservation Society, which operates the Bronx, Central Park, Prospect Park, and Queens Zoos in New York, and the New York Aquarium developed a set of principles for government leaders outlining the importance of wildlife health management and research as part of One Health initiatives (WCS, 2004).

9.3 Zoos, Aquariums, and the Care of Animals

Within the zoo setting, a wide variety of species, from domestic animals in petting zoos and free-ranging wildlife encountered locally, to the entire range of zoological species, must be provided with veterinary medical and surgical care. This broad base of experience in clinical medicine puts zoo veterinarians in the forefront of comparative medicine, enabling them to understand and respond to emerging diseases in wildlife, domestic animals, and humans as they team with physicians, public health professionals, and wildlife biologists.

The functional aspects of animal care in a zoological setting are critical components that advance the principles of One Health. These components include routine veterinary medical care, record keeping, diagnostic pathology, and disease surveillance for the animals in human care. Over time, this systematic data collection on diseases affecting zoo animals becomes important beyond the zoo or aquarium itself. Surveillance for zoonotic diseases is important for potential exposures not only for zoo staff but also for the general public.

In the late 1970s, zoos began the use of immersion exhibits. These exhibits recreate ecosystems resembling the wild and minimize barriers separating the public and the animals (Resbach, 2016). This "open" design plan provides patrons with the opportunity to view animals in habitats that better approximate their natural environment. The natural substrates and landscape architecture enrich animal behavior and also relate to the overall zoo surroundings. Zoos often exist in park-like settings in urban areas, complete with native flora and fauna, and may provide opportunities for exposure of collection animals to free ranging wildlife or environmental impacts from weather, terrain, and human activity. The potential interaction of collection animals, native wildlife, and visitors can provide the opportunity to inform zoo visitors about the ecology of their urban or suburban surroundings. Zoonotic disease is also an important consideration when staff and visitors have close contact with zoological animals and native wildlife. Careful monitoring of zoo and aquarium animals can reduce the risk of zoonotic transmission and even identify cases where transmission occurs from the staff or visitors to the zoo animals.

The potential exposure to wildlife, as well as to members of the public, in highly populated areas makes zoo animals potential disease sentinels. As enzootic raccoon rabies advanced across the eastern USA in the 1970s and 1980s, zoos were instrumental in monitoring the spread of the outbreak. The Conservation Research Center of Washington, DC's National Zoo is located 75 miles west of Washington in rural Virginia. Enzootic raccoon rabies was identified there in 1980 in wild raccoons, and zoo staff predicted the spread of the disease to the Washington, DC metro area. The disease was identified at the National Zoo in wild raccoons in May 1983, and the death of a red panda from rabies was attributed to the raccoons (Beck et al., 1987; Kessler, 1983; Schulz, 1986). In New York City, the first reported case was identified in a wild raccoon in the Bronx Zoo. In these cases, wildlife monitoring and disease surveillance in zoo grounds by veterinary pathologists was key to the diagnosis of the disease (Anon., 1992; Strum, 1991; Ramirez, 2000; R. Cook, personal communication, 2002).

Monitoring disease in wildlife, as part of a basic animal care program for collection animals, may occur in a zoo's local surroundings or in remote, on-site conservation programs. In both of these cases, there are benefits to the local communities as a result of active disease surveillance. In the Chicago metropolitan area, a long-term study of wildlife includes surveillance for diseases that may be restricted to animals or may be zoonotic. Organized in 1993, the Environmental Impact Research Group (EIRG) includes wildlife biologists, wildlife ecologists, zoo veterinary clinicians, and veterinary pathologists funded through the Cook County Department of Animal and Rabies Control in metropolitan Chicago, IL (https://www.cookcountyil.gov/service/surveillance-wildlife). This collaboration allows for not just the monitoring of disease within the confines of the zoo, but also monitoring of the ecology of diseases and their wildlife hosts across urban and suburban landscapes. Centering on wildlife within the county forest preserves, the EIRG has studied the prevalence of Lyme disease (Jobe et al., 2007), pathogen dynamics in skunks (Gehrt et al., 2010), and *Baylisascaris* spp. in raccoons (Page et al., 2016). The long-term collection of wildlife blood samples has provided one of the oldest and largest resources of wildlife specimens to the Centers for Disease Control and Prevention (CDC), and was valuable in studying the emergence of West Nile virus and Lyme disease in the area (http://fpdcc.com/conservation/research). Prospective studies of this type provide data on longitudinal patterns of disease in wildlife and may help elucidate the impact of climate change and human activity on ecosystem health in the study areas.

Emerging diseases have also occurred within zoos when animals from different geographic areas were introduced to novel pathogens. One example is a spirurid parasite called *Geopetitia aspiculata*. This parasite was identified as a cause of mortality in nearly 200 individual birds, of a wide range of bird species, in a number of zoos (French et al., 1994; Bartlett et al., 1984). The wild host of the parasite has never been identified and no deaths have been seen in wild birds. The natural host is presumed to be a tropical bird of the order Passeriformes since they are the host group most often infected in zoos (Kinsella and Forrester, 2008).

9.4 Social Aspects of Zoos and Aquariums

Zoos and aquariums are among the most visited public spaces in the USA, with more than 181 million annual visitors (AZA, 2017b). They are also places where people can connect with nature in an urban setting. In a study that polled zoo visitors on their emotional states at one of three different animal exhibits, 279 adults were asked to scale 17 different emotions while viewing the animals. A hidden observer used a pager to signal the respondents to fill out the scales while they were seen watching the animals. The authors found that visitors experienced rich, positive, emotional experiences related to a strong "orientation to animals" and a desire to save the species observed (Myers et al.,2004). In another study of 165 visitors to an aquatic touch tank exhibit, researchers measured heart rate and mood using a psychological survey instrument. These measurements showed that the experience provided relief from mental stress, and that visitors to zoos demonstrated improvement in both psychological and physical measurements on quality of life scales (Sahrmann et al., 2015). In yet another study, in Japan, researchers measured the effect of visiting zoos on physical and mental health. Experiments were run in two different zoos, and participants (70 in one experiment and 163 in the other) completed a generic health-related quality of life evaluation (World Health Organization, 1996) before and after their visit. They also had their blood pressure measured before and after their visits, and steps taken were measured with a pedometer. The results showed a lowering of blood pressure in zoo visitors and over 6000 steps taken during each visit, as well as improvement in quality of life scores (Sakagami and Ohta, 2010). Discussions in the emerging field of conservation psychology suggest that there is a relationship between the emotional connection visitors make with animals and the educational messages supplied by the zoos and aquariums in providing an appreciation of the human-nature relationship (Saunders, 2003). Zoos and aquariums have an important role in fostering this understanding through education, animal interactions, and their pursuit of conservation programs. Understanding the role that humans have in nature is a key component in translating One Health principles into effective public policy.

Beyond experiencing animals in naturalistic settings, zoo visitors are educated through interpretive graphics and classroom presentations. There is also a trend in zoos to increase informal talks and staff "chats." These chats are distributed among the animal exhibits to reach a much larger proportion of visitors, and this staff contact is associated with greater appreciation for the animals and the conservation messaging. Accredited zoos are required to have formal education programs with a conservation theme (AZA, 2017a). Accreditation became a mandatory requirement for AZA membership in 1985. These standards require that education must be a key component of the institution's mission, that the institution must follow a written education plan outlining goals and objectives, and that the plan should include the institution's conservation messages. Many zoos provide means for visitors to donate directly to conservation programs in the form of cash donations or adding them in to purchases on zoo grounds. AZA accredited zoos and aquariums fund over 2500 conservation projects in more than 100 countries and spend, on average, $160 million on conservation initiatives annually.

9.5 Zoonotic Disease Challenges: Protecting Visitors, Staff, and Animals

In addition to caring for a variety of animal species, zoos and aquariums are also responsible for the staff who care for their animals as well as the millions of people who visit their institutions every year. It is important that zoos develop programs to reduce the possibility of zoonotic disease transmission to staff or visitors. Zoo and aquarium staff work closely with animals in their care, and close encounters with "animal ambassadors" are a growing part of the visitor experience in many zoos and aquariums. "Hands-on" interactions present the opportunity for infectious agents to be transferred from animals to humans, and vice versa, and safety programs must be designed to assess and mitigate this risk. These safety programs include medical care, and biosafety and biosecurity protocols. AZA accreditation standards require staff to be trained in the risks from and prevention of zoonotic disease for zoo workers as well as for the visiting public (AZA, 2017a). Whether it is the identification of primate retrovirus exposure in zoo workers (Sandstrom et al., 2000) or prevention of salmonella exposure from reptiles (Friedman et al., 1998) zoo professionals must constantly be alert for the possibility of zoonotic disease transmission.

Procedures to prevent the transmission of zoonotic disease and staff training in zoonosis prevention are required in the over 230 zoos and aquariums accredited by the AZA (2017a). Occupational health programs for staff in zoos are recommended and include monitoring for any signs of zoonotic disease. For example, tuberculosis testing of staff in close contact with susceptible species is routine in zoos. These occupational health programs vary by institution and are designed based on a risk assessment for the types of exposure encountered in different institutions. Additionally, other emerging diseases may pose a threat to visitors and zoo staff such as enterohemorrhagic *Escherichia coli* (EHEC) and methicillin-resistant *Staphylococcus aureus* (MRSA).

E. coli O157:H7 emerged as an important pathogen in humans in 1982. There are a number of strains and serotypes of *E. coli*, which can be identified by their pathological effects. One common strain of EHEC, which causes bloody diarrhea, is the *Shiga* toxin-producing *E. coli* (STEC) of the O157:H7 serotype (Manning et al., 2008; Diamant et al., 2004). It is associated not only with hemorrhagic diarrhea but also with the potentially life-threatening hemolytic uremic syndrome. Initially, cases were associated with contaminated, undercooked beef or produce contaminated with bovine waste (Davis et al., 1993). In 2000, the first cases were identified due to exposure to live animals on dairy farms and in "petting zoos." These cases were a significant change with the concern shifting from a food-borne illness to a zoonotic disease associated with animal contact in a recreational or education

setting. In one of the cases, visitors, mostly pre-school and school-aged children, to a dairy farm could touch cattle, calves, sheep, goats, llamas, chickens, and a pig and could eat and drink while interacting with the animals. Handwashing facilities were few in number; lacked soap and disposable towels, and were out of reach of children. The other case also allowed contact with a variety of species without adequate hand washing and with a dining area near the animal pens (Goode et al., 2001) (Box 9.1).

These outbreaks were the first in the USA associated with direct transmission of *E. coli* O157 from farm animals to humans. Since that time, exposure at agricultural fairs and other animal contact settings has become an important source of transmission. As a result of these outbreaks, the National Association of State Public Health Veterinarians (NASPHV) and the CDC have published the

---

Box 9.1 Two outbreaks of Shiga-toxigenic *E. coli* (STEC) O157:H7

In 2000, two outbreaks of Shiga-toxigenic *E. coli* (STEC) O157:H7 occurred in Washington and Pennsylvania. In the Pennsylvania outbreak 51 persons (median age 4 years) became ill within 10 days after visiting a dairy farm. Eight (16%) of those patients developed hemolytic uremic syndrome (HUS), a potentially fatal complication of STEC infection. The farm in this case encouraged interaction between visitors and animals. While there were 43 species of animals on the farm, the *E. coli* strain implicated in the outbreak was only isolated from the cattle. Most of the visitors to the farm during the outbreak were pre-school or school-aged children at high risk for serious *E. coli* infections. No separate area on the farm was designated for visitor-animal interactions. Visitors could touch cattle, calves, sheep, goats llamas, chickens, and a pig and could eat and drink while interacting with the animals. Handwashing facilities lacked soap and disposable towels, were out of the children's reach, were few in numbers, and were unsupervised.

In the Washington outbreak five persons ranging from 2 to 14 years (median 7 years) with the identical strain of *E. coli* O157 presented with diarrhea and abdominal cramping, four with bloody diarrhea. Four of the patients had been on an elementary school visit to a dairy farm and the fifth child had a sibling who became ill after visiting the farm. An investigation revealed that children were allowed to handle young poultry, rabbits, and goats. Goats, chickens, and a calf were kept in pens and could be touched through a fence. Children brought their own lunches and ate approximately 50 feet from the penned animals. The farm recommended that visitors bring antibacterial wipes to wash their hands and the farm provided a communal wash basin. Five animal stool samples collected from the farm were tested for *E. coli* O157. All were negative. No further illnesses were reported after prevention measures were instituted including the distribution of instructional material and the installation of soap and water hand washing (Goode et al., 2001).

"Compendium of Measures to Prevent Disease Associated with Animals in Public Settings" (National Association of State Public Health Veterinarians, 2013). North Carolina enacted legislation requiring persons displaying animals for public contact at agricultural fairs to obtain a permit from the North Carolina Department of Agriculture and Consumer Services. This permit specifies signage informing of the possibility for zoonotic disease transmission, physical facility design measures, age restrictions for visitors, separation of bedding and manure, staffing and training as well as the provision of hand-washing stations (http://www.ncagr.gov/oep/AnimalContactExhibit.htm). Currently seven states have laws requiring hand-washing stations at animal contact exhibits. The laws differ as to the type of animal exhibits covered by the statute (Hoss et al., 2017). Given the concern about zoonotic disease in an animal contact setting as well as the large number of visitors to zoos, risk reduction in the zoo setting is a primary concern. The AZA (2017a) Accreditation Standards require zoonotic disease training for staff as well as measures to prevent infection in animal contact areas. In part based on public concerns about exposure to contact animals, a study was conducted to determine the prevalence of STEC O157:H7 in contact animals in zoos. The study of nearly 1000 animals in 37 zoos showed a very low prevalence of STEC O157:H7 with only a single positive in an animal that had not yet left quarantine after coming from a commercial farm (Keen et al., 2007). The study suggested fewer new animal introductions, isolation and quarantine of new stock, reduction of transport stress, and improved sanitation and ventilation in a permanent exhibit may account for the decreased prevalence of EHEC compared with animals on farms or traveling "petting zoos."

Antibiotic-resistant bacteria such as MRSA are also an important emerging disease threat. While humans are the primary source of MRSA infections, strains emerged in Europe in the early 2000s that were highly associated with agricultural species, especially swine and cattle. One of these strains, Clonal Complex 398 (CC-398) was identified in 2005 from France and The Netherlands and provided the first evidence of a livestock reservoir of MRSA with transmission to humans (Larsen et al., 2015). After intensive surveillance was implemented in The Netherlands in 2006, it was shown that MRSA was geographically clustered with pig farming. Case-control studies of new MRSA strains showed that human carriers of these strains were more often pig and cattle farmers (Köck et al., 2013). These studies also suggest that spillover has occurred into human populations that do not have direct contact with agricultural animals. For example, in The Netherlands, the MRSA database from the National Institute for Public Health and the Environment (RIVM) was used to identify human MRSA cases from 2003 to 2005 that could not be typed by pulsed-field gel electrophoresis (PFGE) (NT-MRSA). Cases of PFGE-typed MRSA served as controls. A study of 41 cases and 82 controls was followed by molecular typing and identification of CC-398 in the 32 of 35 cases for which molecular typing was done. A subsequent screening of a representative sample of pigs in The Netherlands showed 405 of the animals colonized with a comparable strain of MRSA on 89% of the farms. Comparison with the overall MRSA cases in the database showed that an animal-source MRSA was responsible for 20% of human cases (Van Loo et al., 2007). A study of households with MRSA-infected children examined 29 households where dogs or cats lived with a confirmed MRSA-infected child. The study included 18 dogs and 11 cats, with a total of 149 culture samples. A community-acquired strain of MRSA was isolated from one dog and one cat. This limited study provides evidence for interspecies transmission of MRSA from the child or a contaminated environment. Several cases have been reported in which companion animals were positive for the identical strain of MRSA infecting human household members, suggesting possible human-to-animal transmission (Bender et al., 2016). Based on concerns about the zoonotic threat of MRSA in Belgium, a study was conducted that suggested a very low prevalence in zoo settings (Vercammen et al., 2012). MRSA has been reported in isolated cases in a rhinoceros, a mouflon, and a wild bottle-nosed dolphin (Stewart et al., 2014) and also seen in high prevalence (69%) in a captive chimpanzee colony (Hanley et al., 2015). In another case an elephant receiving intensive care was the source of infection for a number of cases in human caretakers, likely after acquiring the infection from a human carrier (Janssen et al., 2009).

Zoonotic disease transfer from animals to humans or humans to animals may occur in zoo settings. Given the number of visitors and the variety of animal contact opportunities and species, it is important for zoo staff to remain vigilant. MRSA and pathogenic *E. coli* are examples of zoonotic threats that appear to be a lower risk in well-managed zoo settings.

9.6 Case Studies in One Health from Zoological Institutions

9.6.1 West Nile Virus: A Case Study for the One Health Paradigm

9.6.1.1 Emergence of West Nile Virus in North America

The emergence of West Nile virus (WNV) in New York in 1999, highlights the need to adopt a One Health approach for protection of humans, animals, and the environment.

West Nile virus (WNV) is a *Flavivirus* belonging to the same antigenic complex as St Louis, Japanese, and Murray Valley encephalitis viruses. These viruses are commonly spread via mosquito vectors, where various bird species such as robins and European house sparrows serve as competent amplifiers. Certain North American bird species such as corvids and jays are exqui-

sitely sensitive to the virus, often succumbing to infection. (McNamara, 2007). Prior to the summer of 1999, WNV had not been previously detected in North America; however, its global distribution included the Middle East, Africa, and tropical Eurasia. (Rappole et al., 2000).

On August 23, 1999, a New York City hospital reported two case patients with an acute onset of neurologic illness with unknown etiology to the New York City Department of Health. (Peterson and Hayes, 2008) An epidemiologic investigation was conducted, and a cluster of encephalitis patients was identified in a roughly 2 × 2-mile area of Queens, NY. The CDC detected IgM antibody to St Louis encephalitis (CDC, 1999). At that time, this diagnosis was accepted as the cause of the case cluster. It is now known that there is possible cross-reactivity between flavivirus antibodies in the serological screening test methods performed at that time. New York began an adulticide spraying and larvicidal program in northern Queens and the South Bronx on September 3, 1999 (CDC, 1999).

However, beginning in June 1999, prior to the spike in human neurologic illness, wild crows in New York City were dying in unusual numbers, as reported by residents of northern Queens, New York City (Eidson and Komar, 2001). A veterinarian in private practice in Queens had treated birds with neurologic disease, and subsequently released those that had survived (Government Accountability Office, 2002) (Figure 9.1).

It was not until unusual pathology was detected in dead avians in the Wildlife Conservation Society's Bronx Zoo that the connection was made between the human and animal illnesses. The veterinary pathologist at the Bronx Zoo, Dr Tracey McNamara, refused to believe that St Louis encephalitis was the cause of death in those birds, since the mortality patterns and histopathological data did not match what was seen with St Louis encephalitis. After significant initial skepticism on the part of some in the human public health field, virus isolation finally confirmed the emergent pathogen as

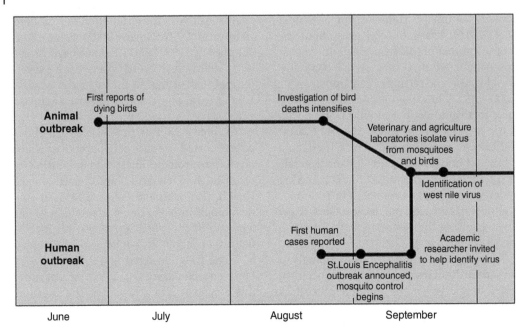

Figure 9.1 Timeline of West Nile virus (WNV) outbreak in New York, 1999. *Source:* Government Accountability Office, 2002.

WNV (T. McNamara, personal communication, May 23, 2017). On September 24, 1999, an announcement was made by the CDC that WNV had been detected for the first time in North America and had caused neurologic disease in humans and avians. Eventually, WNV would spread across the continental USA and cause morbidity and mortality in other species, in addition to human and avian cases.

The discovery of this emerging pathogen prompted sero-survey of the collection at the Bronx Zoo. At the time of the outbreak, it was reported that the collection consisted of between 1079 and 1249 individual avians, and between 935 and 946 mammals (Ludwig et al., 2007). Table 9.1 summarizes serological and clinical data collected from animals during the 1999 outbreak at the zoo.

Much harder to quantify is the true "cost" of the disease outbreak to the Bronx Zoo. In September 1999, the *New York Times* published an article "Exotic Virus Is Identified in 3 Deaths" and it went on to state the following: "New York health officials said they had

found the West Nile virus only in birds that had died in and around the Bronx Zoo" (Jacobs, 1999). Gate receipts at the zoo dropped around 30% (D. Travis, personal communication, November 15, 2016). In addition, diagnostic testing, and extensive medical management of affected birds was necessary in some cases.

9.6.1.2 Centers for Disease Control: ArboNET

To record cases of disease attributable to WNV, the ArboNET database was utilized. ArboNET is a unique system: at the time, it was one of the few databases that captured data from both human and animal reports. The system remains a passive surveillance system, and therefore does not reflect the true burden of disease in humans or animals. For data to be included in ArboNET, laboratory confirmed cases for both humans and animals must be reported to public health authorities. ArboNET reports confirmed cases from humans, mosquitoes, sentinel flocks, dead avians, and veterinary cases,

Table 9.1 Summary of serologic and clinical data from animals sampled during the 1999 West Nile virus (WNV) outbreak at the Bronx Zoo, New York.

Group	No. tested	No. positive	No. with signs[a]	No. dead[b]	Disease:infection ratio	Case fatality rate
Birds	368	125	27	19	0.22	70%
Indoor	32	1	0	0	0	0
Outdoor	336	124	27	19	0.22	70%
Captive	329	113	21	13	0.19	62%
Free ranging	39	12	6	6	0.5	100%
Mammals[c]	117	9	1	0	0.11	0
Captive	116	9	1	0	0.11	0
Free ranging	1	0	0	0	0	0

a)   Number of birds or mammals with clinical signs compatible with or suggestive of, or necropsy findings consistent with WNV infection.
b)   Number of dead birds seropositive for WNV and with clinical and/or necropsy findings consistent with WNV infection.
c)   All outdoors.
Source: Adapted from Ludwig et al., 2007.

Table 9.2 West Nile virus disease cases reported to ArboNET, USA, 2000.

State	Neuroinvasive disease cases[a]	Non-neuroinvasive disease cases	Total cases[b]	Deaths
Connecticut	0	1	1	0
New Jersey	5	1	6	1
New York	14	0	14	1
Total	19	2	21	2

a)   Includes cases reported as meningitis or encephalitis.
b)   Includes confirmed and probable cases.
Source: Centers for Disease Control and Prevention, http://www.cdc.gov/westnile/resources/pdfs/data/2000wnvhum aninfectionsbystate.pdf.

primarily equines (https://www.cdc.gov/westnile/resourcepages/survresources.html).

In 1999, the human toll in the State of New York due to WNV was 59 cases of neuroinvasive disease, and three cases of non-neuroinvasive disease. These counts included confirmed and probable cases. Three deaths were attributed to WNV.

In 2000, the virus had spread to the surrounding states of Connecticut and New Jersey (Table 9.2).

By 2002, the virus had continued to spread across the USA, with human cases being detected across the country (Figure 9.2).

9.6.1.3 A Failure of Early Coordination

In 1999, the investigations of animal disease and mortality (in wild and captive species) and human illness began as very separate investigations. Dead crows were reported 1–2 months prior to human cases. Estimates have hypothesized that several thousand crows and other wild species presumably died in that year of emergence (Rappole et al., 2000). Initially, the link between the avian and human illness was dismissed by a number of agencies involved in the investigation. It is unknown how this delay impacted the

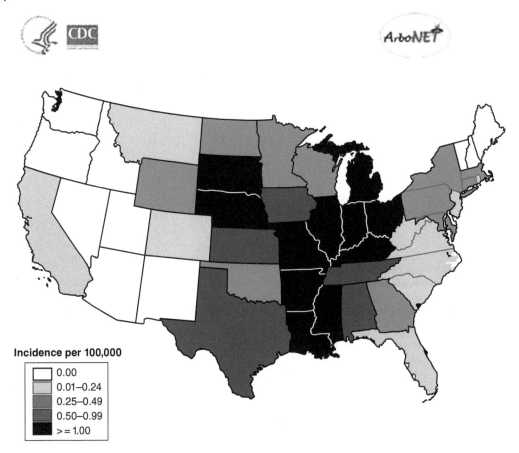

Figure 9.2 West Nile virus neuroinvasive disease incidence reported to ArboNET, by state, USA, 2002. *Source:* Centers for Disease Control and Prevention, http://www.cdc.gov/westnile/resources/pdfs/data/2002stateincidencemap.pdf.

number of human cases of WNV disease, but until this connection was made, the correct diagnosis remained elusive (Government Accountability Office, 2002)

One has to wonder what the outbreak of WNV might have looked like in the summer of 1999 if the connection between human illness and wild bird mortalities had been made sooner.

9.6.1.4 Lessons Learned from the West Nile Virus Outbreak, 1999

Congress requested that the Government Accountability Office (GAO) develop a report to outline the lessons learned from WNV emergence in the USA. Officials recognized,

in retrospect, that the experience of responding to the WNV outbreak was especially relevant when dealing with acts of bioterrorism where interagency coordination is critical. Nearly all of the potential bioterror agents are zoonotic, and animals may be the first victims of an attack (Government Accountability Office, 2002). Some of the lessons learned and reported by the GAO confirms the need for a One Health approach, and include:

1) **Communication with all stakeholders is critical.** During the outbreak, daily conference calls during the outbreak included federal, state, and local public health officials. Veterinary medical health

officials were not always included on these calls.

2) **The zoological community must identify their local public health contacts**. At the time, wildlife and zoological personnel reported that they were uncertain about who from the public health community should be contacted when they suspected an outbreak.

3) **Jurisdictional confusion**. The jurisdictional authority for animal health in the USA was fragmented. The GAO report recognized that domestic companion animal diseases that impact humans often fall under local public health. Livestock diseases are the responsibility of state agricultural agencies and the US Department of Agriculture, and wildlife issues are managed by state wildlife and other federal agencies. Zoological animal health potentially falls under multiple jurisdictions, or none, due to the array of species that are held in these institutions.

4) **Weak relationship between veterinary and human health**. The CDC concluded, "the relationship between public health at the federal, state and local levels and their counterparts in public and private agencies that monitor veterinary health should be strengthened".

9.6.1.5 Zoological Institutions as Forerunners to the 'One Health' Paradigm

It is not surprising to zoological medicine practitioners that one of their colleagues was among the first to recognize a unique disease event. The Bronx Zoo is a member of and accredited by the AZA. These institutions often employ their own staff veterinarians, many whom become board certified by the American College of Zoological Medicine or other specialties. Zoo veterinarians often have extensive training in zoonotic disease. When visitation is part of a zoo's or aquarium's business model, and there may be contact between patrons and various species; these veterinarians must have an advanced understanding of zoonotic disease issues of multiple animal species.

In this instance, Bronx Zoo also had a veterinary pathologist on staff. The AZA institutions are required to determine the cause of death of the species in their care, to prevent illness in conspecifics, and to advance the veterinary medical knowledge base for these species. In general, all animals that die in the institution should be necropsied. However, certain cases (e.g., mortalities of a group of individuals) may only require the examination of a smaller number of representative individuals.

Private practice veterinarians seldom have the opportunity to conduct necropsies on all of their cases, or to submit multiple diagnostic samples to determine the cause of death (Y.N., personal experience). Zoological parks invest significant resources in diagnostics, which is often not the case in other animal healthcare facilities. In the case of the initial outbreak of WNV, it was only when dead birds in the Bronx Zoo collection led to an examination by a highly trained veterinary pathologist, with the budget necessary to submit materials for appropriate diagnostic evaluation, that the cause of the outbreak was correctly identified.

9.6.1.6 Zoological Parks as Sentinels for Human Disease

The zoo's role in detecting the WNV outbreak led to recognition that these facilities are potential partners in public health surveillance. Zoological parks may be ideal sentinels for certain diseases because of the following characteristics:

1) **Animals in zoos are under observation almost constantly**. Unlike their wild counterparts, animal managers observe animals in zoos frequently, and veterinary services are summoned for a rapid diagnosis of disease. Keepers and caretakers become very familiar with the activity levels, food and water consumption, and behaviors of the animals in their care, and they are trained to promptly report

abnormalities. Animals in zoos can be captured and examined more readily than wild species on vast tracts of land.

2) **Zoological specimens are a relatively stationary population**. While moves for breeding recommendations and exhibit changes do occur, these animals can be traced from "birth to death" in terms of location. This information is critical for examining temporal and spatial factors of disease transmission.

3) **Animals in zoos have extensive medical records**. Unlike many domestic or free-ranging wild animals, zoological species have extensive medical records (often including banked biomaterials), which are maintained throughout their lives. This allows for serial surveillance sampling, when warranted, and retrospective epidemiologic analysis when indicated. A number of taxa housed in zoos have specific necropsy and pathology protocols with standardized biomaterial collection processes, which serve to create a repository for tissues for various studies.

4) **Wide variety of susceptible species**: Zoos house a wide variety of species of different taxa. Different zoonotic diseases affect different types of animals in different ways. Depending on the pathogen, different species can be infected, or serve as reservoirs for disease.

5) **Zoos are located throughout the country**. While there are a number of facilities located in rural settings, the majority of these facilities are located in urban and suburban locations, where the human population density is the greatest.

9.6.1.7 A Model for Sentinel Surveillance: The Zoological WNV Surveillance Project

To demonstrate the utility of using zoos for sentinel surveillance, Dr Tracy McNamara of the Bronx Zoo, Dr Dominic Travis of Lincoln Park Zoo in Chicago, and Dr Amy Glaser of Cornell University developed a surveillance project for WNV using submissions from 176 different zoos, aquariums, avian rehabili-

tation centers, universities, and private practitioners. Funding for the project came from several sources such as the CDC, the State of New York, and Lincoln Park Zoo. The project ran for approximately 4 years, from 2001 to 2006.

There were several objectives of the surveillance program. Of paramount importance, can zoos add data to public health surveillance systems for zoonotic disease? And, can WNV diagnostics drive treatment options for ill collection animals?

Samples were submitted from over 12 000 individual animals during that period. Some of the elements of this project that were unique at the time included:

1) The ability to include samples from BOTH zoological collections and true wildlife samples from opportunistic sampling of ill wildlife on zoo grounds.

2) The ability to share results with public health using ArboNET, where data from humans, mosquitoes, dead birds, and veterinary cases could be shared.

9.6.1.8 Lessons Learned from the Zoological WNV Surveillance Project

The zoological community and project managers learned many lessons about conducting a surveillance project of this magnitude. This was the largest, multifacility collaborative surveillance program primarily targeting zoological institutions. The system met several of its objectives; data were provided to ArboNET by some institutions, and the diagnostics drove treatment decisions (D. Travis, personal communication, November 15, 2016). However, lessons learned from that effort continue to challenge advocates of integrated One Health surveillance systems (Uchtmann et al., 2015):

1) **Professional divisions**: Uchtmann et al. (2015) describe some of the barriers to integrated One Health surveillance. While the WNV surveillance system was designed to collaborate with human public health surveillance by encouraging

submission of confirmed case information to local public health departments for inclusion in ArboNET, this did not always occur for a number of reasons.

2) **Incompatible vocabularies**: The lack of consistent use of SNOMED (Systemized Nomenclature of Medicine Clinical Terminology) codes limits data analysis in multispecies surveillance systems. Many of the species sampled during the surveillance period have still not been assigned SNOMED codes. Inconsistent use of terms to define species of a given animal in the zoological WNV data led to analysis issues. An animal may have been serially sampled over time, but submissions may have described the animal using scientific name, common name, or generic descriptor such as "owl." The use of SNOMED codes would have standardized this nomenclature, had they been available.

3) **Sequestration of data**: The sequestration of data is a major obstacle to integrated surveillance. The WNV surveillance project for zoological institutions was established, in part, because of the need for confidentiality on the part of zoos (D. Travis, personal communication, November 15, 2016). As described earlier, when the press reported that the Bronx Zoo had cases of WNV, their gate receipts dropped by 30%. Many zoological institutions would face financial difficulties with a loss of business on this scale. While project managers were privy to individual institutional data, ArboNET allowed the coding of positive birds in zoos by descriptors such as "captive bird" rather than "flamingo," which would have likely resulted in identification of a zoological park as an infected premise. Additionally, while the Zoological WNV Surveillance Project was a system used by a wide number of institutions, other zoos also conducted WNV surveillance on their own, or in conjunction with other agencies. Brookfield Zoo in suburban Chicago has a long-standing disease surveillance program with the Cook County Forest

Preserve District, and those data were not included in the larger Zoological WNV Surveillance Project (T. Meehan, personal communication, January 20, 2017).

The 1999 WNV outbreak led to the largest multifacility collaborative surveillance program developed for zoos and allied institutions. The WNV surveillance project served as an example of how zoos could participate in disease surveillance efforts for emerging diseases, but the system encountered obstacles that continue to vex true One Health practitioners to this day.

9.6.1.9 The Role of Zoological Institutions in Preparing for Pandemics

West Nile virus emergence put the zoological community's interface between the public and exotic animals in a new spotlight. Early in the WNV outbreak period, misconceptions about risk ran wild. Attendance at the Bronx Zoo dropped because patrons were concerned that they could catch the disease merely by attending the zoo. WNV prevented the movement of animals for breeding purposes, and Species Survival Plans were impacted. The WNV experience for zoos is why highly pathogenic avian influenza (HPAI), spreading from Southeast Asia in 1999, quickly caught the attention of the zoological community.

9.6.2 The Emergence of Highly Pathogenic Avian Influenza Virus, 1999

Highly pathogenic avian influenza (HPAI) is a term that is applied to influenza A viruses that have the ability to cause severe morbidity and mortality in gallinaceous birds. Due to the unique ecology of influenza viruses, HPAI viruses are a concern for multiple species and potentially, human public health. HPAI viruses usually arise from mutation or genetic reassortment of the multiple types of influenza viruses that circulate through migratory waterfowl. In addition to the zoonotic potential of some strains, certain types of these viruses, primarily H5 and H7 subtypes, are potentially devastating to agriculture in the USA because of their propensity to cause severe morbidity and mortality in poultry operations. Highly pathogenic H5 and H7 strains are considered Foreign Animal Diseases (FADs) or transboundary diseases because they are not normally found in the USA, because of their extremely negative economic impact upon trade between countries, and because of the significant investment in resources needed for eradication when these strains are detected. It should be noted that vaccination for HPAI to protect birds in the USA is not routinely practiced. Since the lifespan of birds destined for consumption is short, the industry is reluctant to consider vaccination due to trade implications, which could be considerable.

In 1999, emergence of a highly pathogenic H5N1 strain in Southeast Asia caused unusual concern to agriculture and public health. Cases of human disease were reported with the same strain that was affecting poultry, and these human cases had high mortality rates. This was alarming public health officials. Early in the outbreak it was unknown exactly how this virus was being transmitted to people, but most cases of human disease had close contact with sick birds. Because of influenza viruses' propensity to mutate, could this particular strain of influenza become the next great flu pandemic? Would this virus spread to the USA via migratory birds?

Besides the pandemic potential for this H5N1, why was it a concern for zoological institutions? Early outbreaks in zoological parks and sanctuaries caused great angst in zoos across the world. In early December 2002, a small nature preserve in Hong Kong known as Penfold Park experienced a die-off of resident waterfowl and wild egrets that frequented the artificial ponds in the park (Ellis et al., 2004). Thirty-one birds of various species (goose, duck spp., swans) died before the rest of the avian collection was depopulated following confirmation of H5N1. In mid-December 2002, Kowloon Park in Hong

Kong was impacted by H5N1. This large park is located in a densely populated area of the city, and included a fully enclosed (with mesh) aviary, and open ponds for their waterfowl collection. Several birds died of confirmed H5N1 infection. Waterfowl were moved off exhibit, the ponds closed to the public and drained. The remaining birds were managed in a strict isolation/quarantine area, and vaccination was used to try to halt the continued avian infection. The birds that contracted the virus were housed on the ponds, and the meshed aviary was not affected. However, of the birds initially housed on the ponds, 16 of 144 flamingoes, 9 of 20 swans and geese, and 80 of the 179 ducks died due to H5N1. Since many zoological parks manage avian collections on open ponds, these numbers were sobering.

The ability of this virus to infect other animal species was of special concern for zoological veterinarians and managers. In October 2004, a tiger sanctuary in Thailand unknowingly fed infected poultry to a group of their tigers. Within days, some of the animals became extremely ill, and signs of disease included respiratory distress, serosanguinous nasal discharge, and varying degrees of neurologic signs. Despite removing the potentially infected dietary source, the number of ill animals within that group continued to climb, suggesting the possibility of tiger-to-tiger viral transmission. Death due to disease, or euthanasia to halt the spread within the group, resulted in the death of 147 tigers (Thanawongnuwech et al., 2005). These examples led to increased awareness about the potential impact of influenzas in zoological collections in the USA.

9.6.2.1 Consequences of HPAI Detection in a Zoological Institution

There would be multiple consequences of HPAI detection in a zoological institution, including:

1) **Potential depopulation of infected individuals**. Once HPAI is detected in a poultry-producing facility, both ill and unaffected contacts are depopulated to prevent the spread of disease. Depopulation

decreases the possibility of continued environmental contamination and mutation. In the 2014–2015 outbreak of a different HPAI virus in the USA, over 50 million poultry were depopulated to try to halt disease spread of H5N2 and H5N8 strains. This culling is standard practice for poultry, but what about endangered species that reside in zoos? Each State Veterinarian will be highly encouraged to assess the risk on a case-by-case basis to avoid the loss of birds that simply are irreplaceable.

2) **Quarantine could impact revenue streams.** Quarantine is a regulatory action that is taken in response to HPAI detection in poultry. Quarantine measures include the strict control of movement of people, animals, and equipment on and off any infected premises. Zoological institutions often rely on visitation by the public as a significant part of their business model. Infected premises may need to be completely quarantined, resulting in revenue loss, which may affect business viability.

3) **Public health consequences for staff and patrons.** Since H5N1 is a Foreign Animal Disease with agricultural implication AND a zoonotic disease, the CDC would have tremendous control over decision-making to protect the public. While the H5N2 and H5N8 strains that emerged in 2014 in the USA were not zoonotic, public health still closely monitored responders to detect influenza-like illness.

4) **Pandemic potential could lead to decreased staffing.** "Worried well" may not show up for work, thereby compromising ideal staffing levels.

5) **Significant cost of cleaning, depopulation, etc.** It is unclear how much of the cost of cleaning up following an outbreak would have to be borne by the facility. In poultry operations, depopulation and cleanup costs are calculated and compensated by the US Department of Agriculture, but, as of now, it is unclear if the calculation of such reimbursements would be applicable for a zoological institution.

9.6.2.2 The Association of Zoos and Aquariums Prepares for HPAI

Understanding the consequences of HPAI detection in zoological facilities, the Association of Zoos and Aquariums partnered with the US Department of Agriculture (USDA) to prepare zoological facilities for HPAI.

Subject matter experts in USDA and the zoological community developed *The USDA APHIS AZA Management Guidelines for Avian Influenza: Zoological Parks & Exhibitors Surveillance Plan*. A pilot surveillance project was implemented in several institutions to understand the challenge in conducting surveillance in a zoological park for a Foreign Animal Disease, which is significantly different than surveillance in poultry.

The pilot surveillance system ran for one year, 2010–2011, in three zoological institutions. Three hundred forty-five different birds were tested, representing 26 different species. Six hundred eighty-five sampling events (some birds were sampled serially) occurred. Highly pathogenic H5N1 avian influenza virus was not detected in any these samples during the surveillance period.

If surveillance is being conducted for a Foreign Animal Disease such as HPAI, there must be plans in place for what to do if you find it. A complementary HPAI Outbreak Management Plan for HPAI in zoological collections was also developed. This effort kept the zoological community in front of the State and Federal regulatory agencies, who recognized that there would be significant challenges if they needed to manage HPAI in a zoo. Subsequent improvements to that plan have been made following a zoologically based workshop entitled "Flu at the Zoo." This workshop tested the utility of the original Outbreak Management plan, and updated it by including Incident Command System organization (Johnson et al., 2014)

All of the preparedness for pandemic H5N1 helped jump-start the community to increase their readiness for new HPAI strains when they emerged in the USA in 2014.

Fortunately, to date, the H5N1 strain, and the H5N2 and H5N8 strains that emerged in 2014–2015, did NOT directly affect zoological parks or exotic species in the USA. The agricultural community was not as lucky. The emergence of two strains of HPAI (H5N2 and H5N8) in 2014 resulted in the culling of nearly 50 million production birds with a total economic impact to the US economy estimated at $3.3 billion (Greene, 2015).

While zoological institutions were not located in any of the Control Zones established by USDA and State Animal Health officials during the 2014–2015 outbreaks, significant management changes were implemented in facilities near the infected farms to try to protect collections. Tropical birds, which normally would be put in their summer outdoor habitats, were held indoors. Strategies for discouraging wild waterfowl on zoo grounds (the suspected reservoirs of disease) were implemented. Zoological personnel, the Association of Zoos and Aquariums, American Association of Zoo Veterinarians, and State Veterinarians dedicated a significant amount of time to develop prevention and mitigation strategies for HPAI (Y. Nadler, personal communication with zoological veterinarians, AAZV Annual Conference, September 28, 2015).

9.6.2.3 Lessons Learned from HPAI Surveillance System

Not surprisingly, some of the lessons learned from the WNV experience in zoos were again experienced, but outcomes improved with this surveillance effort. Upon examination of the notable lessons learned from WNV, here are the improvements noted with the HPAI surveillance system managers:

1) **Communication with all stakeholders is critical.** Communication channels between State and Federal regulatory officials and zoological animal health experts were greatly improved. While zoos did not have a case of HPAI during the surveillance period, subject matter experts at USDA provided guidance for stakeholders. When the 2014–2015 outbreaks occurred, the zoological industry held specific conference calls with these experts, which included regulatory agencies and public health.

The Association of Zoos and Aquariums ZAHP Fusion Center, and the University of Illinois College of Veterinary Medicine's Zoo Ready project have become conduits of communication about emerging and foreign animal disease for the exotic animal industries. Their communication workshops are designed to share the lessons learned about communication by hosting critical stakeholders to discuss the issues and to enhance relationships critical in disease events.

2) **Sequestration of data**, a barrier to One Health surveillance, remained an issue in the HPAI surveillance project. Generally speaking, HPAI surveillance diagnostic results reside in databases within the National Animal Health Laboratory Network (NAHLN) systems. HPAI surveillance data for wild birds may exist in several databases, such as National Wildlife Health Center (Madison, WI). Due to the concern about access to diagnostic test results and the potential negative impact on zoological collections, the zoo HPAI surveillance project developed their own database to house diagnostic and epidemiologic data associated with the samples. Data standards used by national and international HPAI surveillance systems were used to ensure data compatibility, should this need to be shared. However, the system would have been more economical if the participants had consented to using these larger, preestablished systems.

3) **The zoological community must identify their local public health contacts.** Based upon recommendations made following WNV, the HPAI Outbreak Management Plan recommended that local public health contacts be made PRIOR to detection in the facility, whether

the facility was conducting surveillance or not. While the authors cannot know that each facility actually identified their local public health contacts, that message was shared with the community on many conference calls and presentations during the HPAI outbreak.

4) **Jurisdictional confusion**. The jurisdictional authority for animal health in the USA remains fragmented. This is more evident in the zoological community, because of the variety of species that are held in these institutions. However, because HPAI is a Foreign Animal Disease, there are protocols in place for managing this disease by enforcement of the Animal Health Protection Act. In an *emerging* disease, such as WNV in 1999, the path for response and jurisdictional authority often takes time to establish. Since HPAI is primarily considered a disease of livestock, the responsibility of State agricultural agencies and the US Department of Agriculture is clear. Since there is concern that HPAI viruses could mutate into strains that could infect humans, the CDC and local public health are involved at many levels. The threat of the emergence of a potential pandemic could shift authority from animal health regulatory officials to public health.

5) **Weak relationship between veterinary and human health**. The WNV experience highlighted the nearly total lack of communication between public health and veterinary medical practitioners. With emergence of the H5N2 and H5N8 strains in North America, there was much greater integration and oversight of an "agricultural" disease by public health to try to prevent human disease. This greater degree of communication may be due in part to decades of work with seasonal influenza (and its consequences) by the public health community. Greater collaboration between animal and human influenzas may be key to combating that next major human pandemic of flu, which is considered "overdue."

9.7 Conclusion

Modern zoological institutions are so much more than a menagerie of animals, seemingly gathered for exhibition purposes. In addition to providing high-quality habitats for their animals, modern zoos are committed to spreading the message of conservation; this includes embracing the One Health/Ecosystem health model. Modern zoological institutions often have highly specialized medical programs for their animals, which includes veterinarians who are Board certified by the American College of Zoological Medicine. Veterinary pathologists are on the staff of some of the larger zoos in the USA, and zoological referral laboratories are available for other institutions. When visitation or animal contact is part of their business model, these veterinarians are well trained in zoonotic disease prevention and detection.

The advances in medicine and care for these animals, and the commitment of funding for diagnostics often leads to definitive diagnosis of disease, which is not always the case in companion animal or production animal medicine. Animal health is a top priority, with comprehensive wellness programs, and observational surveillance for health and welfare. Continuous observation and sample collection during wellness exams provides opportunities for surveillance of these animals not always afforded to those who study in situ populations of wildlife.

Because of these attributes, zoological institutions can be vitally important contributors to public health systems. The interface of local wildlife, collection animals, and humans is a unique opportunity for convergence of environment, host, and pathogen. Zoos and public health must continue to collaborate with urban planning professionals and policy makers to advocate for funding of mutually beneficial surveillance programs.

References

Adelman, L.M., Falk, J.H., and James, S. (2000). Impact of National Aquarium in Baltimore on visitors' conservation attitudes, behavior, and knowledge. *Curator* 43(1), 33–61.

Anon. (1992). Bronx Zoo kills two raccoons after a rabid one intrudes. *The Schenectady Daily Gazette*, 29 July.

AZA (Association of Zoos and Aquariums) (2017a). Accreditation Standards for education. Available at: https://www.aza.org/assets/2332/aza-accreditation-standards.pdf (accessed June 19, 2017).

AZA (Association of Zoos and Aquariums) (2017b). Zoo and Aquarium Statistics. Available at: https://www.aza.org/zoo-and-aquarium-statistics (accessed June 18, 2017).

Bartlett, C.M., Crawshaw, G.J., and Appy, R.G. (1984). Epizootiology, development, and pathology of *Geopetitia aspiculata* Webster, 1971 (Nematoda: Habronematoidea) in tropical birds at the Assiniboine Park Zoo, Winnipeg, Canada. *Journal of Wildlife Diseases* 20(4), 289–299.

Beck, A.M., Fesler, S.R., and Glickman, L.T. (1987). An epizootic of rabies in Maryland, 1982-84. *American Journal of Public Health* 77(1), 42–44.

Bender, B.J., Waters, K.C., Nerby, J., Olsen, K.E., and Jawahir, S. (2016). Methicillin-resistant *Staphylococcus aureus* (MRSA) isolated from pets living in households with MRSA-infected children. *Clinical Infectious Diseases* 54(3), 449–450.

Centers for Disease Control (1999). Outbreak of West Nile-like viral encephalitis– New York, 1999. *Morbidity and Mortality Weekly Review* 48(38), 845–849.

Davis, M., Osaki, C., Gordon, D., et al. (1993). Update: Multistate outbreak of Escherichia coli O157:H7 infections from hamburgers – Western United States, 1992-1993. *Morbidity and Mortality Weekly Report* 42(14), 258–263.

Diamant, E., Palti, Y., Gur-Arie, R., Cohen, H., Hallerman, E.M., and Kashi, Y. (2004). Phylogeny and strain typing of *Escherichia coli*, inferred from variation at mononucleotide repeat loci. *Applied Environmental Microbiology* 70(4), 2464–2473.

Dierking, L.D., Adelman, L.M., Ogden, J., Lehnhardt, K., Miller, L., and Mellen, J.D. (2004). Using a behavior change model to document the impact of visits to Disney's Animal Kingdom: A study investigating intended conservation action. *Curator* 47(3), 322–343.

Eidson, M. and Komar, N. (2001). Crow deaths as a sentinel surveillance system for West Nile virus in the Northeastern United States, 1999. *Emerging Infectious Diseases* 7(4), 615–620.

Ellis, T.M., Bousfield R.B., and Bissett, L.A. (2004). Investigation of outbreaks of highly pathogenic H5N1 avian influenza in waterfowl and wild birds in Hong Kong in late 2002. *Avian Pathology.* 33(5), 492–505.

Falk, J.H., Reinhard, E.M., Vernon, C.L., Bronnenkant, K., Deans, N.L., and Heimlich, J.E. (2007). Why Zoos and Aquariums Matter: Assessing the Impact of a Visit to a Zoo or Aquarium. Silver Springs, MD: Association of Zoos and Aquariums.

French, R.A., Todd, K.S., Meehan, T.P., and Zachary, J.F. (1994). Parasitology and pathogenesis of *Geopetitia aspiculata* (Nematoda: Spirurida) in zebra finches (*Taeniopygia guttata*): experimental infection and new host records. *Journal of Zoo and Wildlife Medicine* 25(3), 403–422.

Friedman, C.R., Torigian, C., Shillam, P.J., et al. (1998). An outbreak of salmonellosis among children attending a reptile exhibit at a zoo. *Journal of Pediatrics* 132(5), 802–807.

Gehrt, S.J., Kinsel, M.J., and Anchor, C. (2010). Pathogen dynamics and morbidity of striped skunks in the absence of rabies. *Journal of Wildlife Diseases* 46(2), 335–347.

Goldowsky, A. (2009). Connecting and interacting–a trip to the new zoo. *Museums and Social Issues* 4(2), 187–205.

Goode, B., O'Reilly, C., Dunn, J., et al. (2001). Outbreaks of *Escherichia coli* O157:H7 infections among children associated with farm visits–Pennsylvania and Washington, 2000. *Morbidity and Mortality Weekly Report* 50(15), 293–297.

Government Accountability Office (2002). West Nile Virus Outbreak: Lessons for Public Health Preparedness. Report to Congressional Requesters. GAO/HEHS-00-180.

Greene, J.L. (2015). Update on the Highly Pathogenic Avian Influenza Outbreak of 2014-2015. Washington, DC: Congressional Research Service.

Hanley, P.W., Barnhart, K.F., Abee, C.R., Lambeth, S.P., and Weese, J.S. (2015). Methicillin-resistant Staphylococcus aureus prevalence among captive chimpanzees, Texas, USA, 2012. *Emerging Infectious Diseases* 21(12), 2158–2160.

Hoss, A., Basler, C., Stevenson, L., Gambino-Shirley, K., Robyn, M.P., and Nichols, M. (2017). State laws requiring hand sanitation stations at animal contact exhibits. *Morbidity and Mortality Weekly Report* 66(1), 16–18.

Jacobs, A. (1999). Exotic virus is identified in 3 deaths. *The New York Times* 26 September.

Janssen, D., Lamberski, N., Dunne, G., et al. (2009). Methicillin-resistant Staphylococcus aureus skin infections from an elephant calf – San Diego, California, 2008. *Morbidity and Mortality Weekly Report* 58(8), 194–198.

Jobe, D.A., Nelson, J.A., Adam, M.D., and Martin, S.A. (2007). Lyme disease in urban areas, Chicago. *Emerging Infectious Diseases* 13(11), 1799–1800.

Johnson, B., Thomas, S., Ardoin, N., and Saunders, M. (2016). Investigating the long-term effects of informal science learning at zoos and aquariums - Final briefing report. New York, NY: Wildlife Conservation Society.

Johnson, Y.J., Nadler, Y., Field, E., et al. (2014). Flu at the zoo: emergency management training for the nation's zoos and aquariums. *Homeland Security & Emergency Management* 11(3), 415–435.

Kazacos, K.R., Gavin, P.J., Shulman, S.T., et al. (2002). Raccoon roundworm encephalitis – Chicago, Illinois, and Los Angeles, California, 2000. *Morbidity and Mortality Weekly Report* 50(51), 1153–1155.

Keen, E.J., Durso, L.M., and Meehan, T.P. (2007). Isolation of *Salmonella enterica* and Shiga-toxigenic *Escherichia coli* O157 from feces of animals in public contact areas of United States zoological parks. *Applied Environmental Microbiology* 73(1), 362–365.

Kemmerly, J.D. and Macfarlane, V. (2009). The elements of a consumer-based initiative in contributing to positive environmental change: Monterey Bay Aquarium's Seafood Watch program. *Zoo Biology* 28(5), 1–14.

Kessler, R. (1983). Rabies epidemic spreads to National Zoo, kills red panda. *Washington Post*, 8 November.

Kinsella, J.M. and Forrester, D.J. (2008). Tetrameridosis. In: Atkinson, C.T., Thomas, N.J., and Hunter, D.B. (eds), *Parasitic Disease of Wild Birds*. Ames, IA: Wiley-Blackwell, pp. 376–384.

Köck, R., Schaumburg, F., Mellmann, A., et al. (2013). Livestock-associated methicillin-resistant Staphylococcus aureus (MRSA) as causes of human infection and colonization in Germany. *PLoS One* 8(2), 1–6.

Larsen, J., Petersen, A., Sørum, M., et al. (2015). Methicillin-resistant *Staphylococcus aureus* CC398 is an increasing cause of disease in people with no livestock contact in Denmark, 1999 to 2011. *European Surveillance* 20(37), 1–17.

Ludwig, G.V., Calle, P.P., Mangiafico, J.A., et al. (2007). An outbreak of West Nile virus in a New York City captive wildlife population. *American Journal of Tropical Medicine and Hygiene* 67(1), 67–75.

Luebke, J.F. and Matiasek, J. (2013). Exploratory study of zoo visitors' exhibit experiences and reactions. *Zoo Biology* 32, 407–416.

Manning, D.S., Motiwala, A.S., Springman, A.C., et al. (2008). Variation in virulence among clades of Escherichia coli O157:H7 associated with disease outbreaks.

Proceedings of the National Academies of Science pf the USA 105(12), 4868–4873.

McNamara, T. (2007). The role of zoos in biosurveillance. *International Zoo Yearbook* 41, 12–15.

Myers, O.E., Saunders, C.D., and Bijulin, A.A. (2004). Emotional dimensions of watching zoo animals: an experience sampling study building on insights from psychology. *Curator* 47(3), 299–321.

National Association of State Public Health Veterinarians, Animal Contact Compendium Committee (2013). Compendium of Measures to Prevent Disease Associated with Animals in Public Settings. *Journal of the American Veterinary Medical Association* 243(9), 1270–1288.

Page, L.K., Delzell, D.A.P., Gehrt, S.D., et al. (2016). The structure and seasonality of Baylisascaris procyonis populations in raccoons (Procyon lotor). *Journal of Wildlife Disease* 52(2), 286–292.

Peterson, L.R. and Hayes, E.B. (2008). West Nile Virus in the Americas. *Medical Clinics of North America* 92, 1307–1322.

Ramirez, A. (2000). Albany: Rabies case Metro Briefing. *The New York Times* 20 June.

Rappole, J.H., Derrickson, S.R., and Hubalek, Z. (2000). Migratory birds and spread of West Nile virus in the Western Hemisphere. *Emerging Infectious Diseases* 6(4), 319–328.

Reading, R.P. and Miller, B.J. (2007). Attitudes and attitude change among zoo visitors. In: Zimmerman, A., Hatchwell, M., Dickie, L., and West, C. (eds), *Zoos in the 21st Century: Catalysts for Conservation?* Cambridge, UK: Cambridge University Press, pp. 63–91.

Resbach, P. (2016). Zoo and aquarium design: Yesterday, today and (the day after) tomorrow. *WAZA Magazine* 17, 3–8.

Sahrmann, J.M., Niedbalski, A., Bradshaw, I., Johnson, R., and Deem, S.L. (2015). Changes in human health parameters associated with a touch tank experience at a zoological institution. *Zoo Biology* 35(1), 4–13.

Sakagami, T. and Ohta, M. (2010). The effect of visiting zoos on human health and quality of life. *Journal of Animal Science* 81, 129–134.

Sandstrom, P.A., Phan, K.O., Switzer, W.M., et al. (2000). Simian foamy virus infection among zoo keepers. *Lancet* 355, 551–552.

Saunders, C.D. (2003). The emerging field of conservation psychology. *Human Ecology* 10(2), 137–149.

Schulz, W.G. (1986). Keeping Zoo's Wild Kingdom Physically Fit. *Chicago Tribune*, 20 July.

Sickler, J. and Fraser, F. (2009). Enjoyment in zoos. *Leisure Studies* 28(3), 313–331

Stewart, J.R., Townsend, F.I., Lane, S.M., et al. (2014). Survey of antibiotic-resistant bacteria isolated from bottlenose dolphins *Tursiops truncatus* in the southeastern USA. *Disease of Aquatic Organisms* 108, 91–102.

Strum, C. (1991). Outbreak of rabies is spreading North. *The New York Times* 15 November.

Thanawongnuwech, R., Amonsin, A., Tantilertcharoen, R., et al. (2005). Probable tiger-to-tiger transmission of avian influenza H5N1. *Emerging Infectious Diseases* 11(5), 699–701.

Uchtmann, N., Herrmann, J.A., Hahn, E.C., and Beasley, V.R. (2015). Barriers to, efforts in, and optimization of integrated One Health surveillance: a review and synthesis. *EcoHealth* doi: 10.1007/s10393-015-1022-7.

Van Loo, I., Huijsdens, X., Tiemersma, E., et al. (2007). Emergence of methicillin-resistant *Staphylococcus aureus* of animal origin in humans. *Emerging Infectious Diseases* 13(12), 1834–1839.

Vercammen, F., Bauwens, L., Deken, R.D., and Brandt, J. (2012). Prevalence of methicillin-resistant *Staphylococcus aureus* in mammals of the Royal Zoological Society of Antwerp, Belgium. *Journal of Zoo and Wildlife Medicine* 43(1), 159–161.

WAZA (World Association of Zoos and Aquariums) (2005). Building a Future for Wildlife: The World Zoo and Aquarium Conservation Strategy. Berne, Switzerland: WAZA.

WCS (Wildlife Conservation Society) (2004). The Manhattan Principles, as defined during a meeting entitled Building Interdisciplinary Bridges to Health in a "Globalized World." Available at http://www. cdc.gov/onehealth/pdfs/manhattan/twelve_ manhattan_principles.pdf (accessed December 20, 2017).

World Health Organization (1996). WHOQOL-BREF Introduction, Administration, Scoring and Generic Version of the Assessment. Available at: http://www.who.int/mental_health/ media/en/76.pdf (accessed June 18, 2017).

Section 2

Four Perspectives on One Health Policy

10

One Health Leadership and Policy

William D. Hueston[1], Ed G.M. van Klink[2], and Innocent B. Rwego[3]

[1] *University of Minnesota, Minneapolis, MN, USA*
[2] *University of Bristol, Lower Langford, Bristol, UK*
[3] *University of Minnesota-Makerere University Uganda Hub, Kampala, Uganda*

10.1 Introduction and Definitions

Leadership is the process of catalyzing action. Leadership differs from "leader," a term that refers to a position or the person in that position such as the Dean of a university faculty, the Director General of an international organization, or the Chief Executive Officer of a company.

Policy means a course of action. Policy can be expressed in many ways: a strategic plan describing a long-term vision and mission, an operational plan that outlines the objectives for the short term such as the next year, or even a standard operating procedure that describes how to respond in a specific situation. Policies are developed by government bodies, the private sector, and nonprofit organizations.

One Health recognizes the interconnectedness of human, animal, and environmental health. By extension, One Health also recognizes the interrelationship of biological systems with societal and economic systems. Health policy is less likely to be effective if it doesn't deal with economic aspects, gender, and other contributors. One Health approaches address the social determinants of disease as well as the agent, host, and environmental determinants. The One Health approach increases the likelihood of making positive incremental progress by drawing from multiple disciplines, organizations, and sectors (public, private, academic) to address the grand challenges in health.

This chapter looks at leadership in the context of One Health and the resulting implications for development of shared policy to address grand challenges in health.

10.2 Grand Challenges in Health (aka "Wicked Problems")

Today's emphasis on One Health grew out of the renewed realization that few of the complex health issues we face today have easy solutions. Unlike a physician or veterinarian who fixes a broken leg or gives a vaccination to prevent tetanus, there is no simple technical solution to antimicrobial resistance or emerging infectious diseases or climate change or global food insecurity. There is no single right answer, just better or worse answers. These are complex issues with many interdependent parts. In fact, they are so complex that no single individual or discipline, think tank or private company, government agency or intergovernmental organization

Beyond One Health: From Recognition to Results, First Edition.
Edited by John A. Herrmann and Yvette J. Johnson-Walker.
© 2018 John Wiley & Sons, Inc. Published 2018 by John Wiley & Sons, Inc.

fully understands them. Nevertheless, these issues are compelling and demand action.

Determining and agreeing on appropriate action is difficult since there is no single or simple "solution." Food insecurity provides an example of the difficulty. Food insecurity – the lack of access to and availability of safe, affordable, and nutritious food – exists around the world in various situations from impoverished inner cities in the USA to arid regions in rural sub-Saharan Africa The same actions taken in different locations may have very different consequences since food insecurity is a manifestation of a complex set of systems including weather, culture, politics, and economics. Indeed, well-intentioned actions may lead to consequences worse than the original problem itself. Shipping large quantities of "food aid" to poor countries has destabilized domestic food systems in some countries, putting local farmers out of business and decreasing sustainable food security in the long run.

These complex problems are called "grand challenges," "social messes," complex adaptive challenges, or "wicked" problems (in contrast to tame problems). The One Health approach is uniquely suited and indispensable for addressing these grand challenges so as to make incremental progress while minimizing unintended negative consequences of actions.

10.3 Implications of Grand Challenges for One Health Leadership

Grand challenges are difficult in part because no single individual or organization has the authority, resources, or even a complete understanding of all facets of the issues necessary to address them successfully. One Health leadership differs from leadership in a hierarchical organization where there is a single leader, or "boss." While the boss can order employees to do something, progress on grand challenges requires shared leadership involving multiple individuals, organizations, and sectors (public, private, academic, civil society). Consequently, One Health leadership involves cooperation and the formation of coalitions committed to shared goals and objectives. Even when everyone can agree that a problem exists and that action is needed, both separate and collective actions are necessary. Therefore, One Health leadership is a shared responsibility.

It is human nature to seek explanations for the problems we encounter. Collectively this often becomes a search for someone or something to "blame." We also seek simple solutions because they're easier to understand and compelling to advocate. Grand challenges often evoke the same behavior, with individuals or organizations pointing fingers at each other and proclaiming the merits of their own favorite policy proposal. The One Health leadership approach recognizes the powerful human feelings that underlie these natural tendencies and works with those who have a stake in the issue (i.e., stakeholders) to move beyond the heated rhetoric.

The foundation of One Health leadership is active stakeholder engagement and the development of transdisciplinary teams. Relevant disciplinary experts working together with a wide spectrum of stakeholders gain better understanding of the complexity of the challenge than experts working alone. Actions are more carefully designed and their consequences to other components of the system are more likely to be anticipated and addressed. While individual leaders may arise to address certain aspects of the challenge, the overall process of One Health leadership is a shared activity. Therefore, One Health leadership can be described as the process of catalyzing collective action for the public good using a One Health approach.

10.4 Critical Competencies for One Health Leadership

Teamwork:

- One Health leadership is a team approach that leverages the knowledge, skills, and abilities of all team members.

- Teams benefit from the leaderly actions of team members while embracing shared decision-making and initiatives.
- Teams achieve synergy where the collective results are greater than the sum of individual efforts alone.

Interpersonal skills:

- *Self-awareness*: an understanding of one's abilities and limitations. Appreciating one's social style and strengths helps one better to relate to others. Self-awareness also supports reflection on what has happened or will happen in specific situations.
- *Emotional intelligence*: the ability to interpret the nonverbal emotional interplay among people. Emotional intelligence supports empathy for others' feelings and adds to the richness of interactions.
- *Communications*: the two-way exchange of information and opinions that characterize human relations. Key communications skills include active listening, the ability to summarize key themes during a conversation, and both speaking and written approaches to sharing of information.
- *Facilitation*: the ability to help the group dynamics. Key facilitation skills include navigating initial introductions and the process of getting to know one another; encouraging active participation of all involved; dealing with disruptive or counterproductive behavior; and helping individuals (and organizations) identify shared interests (as opposed to their contrasting "positions"). Facilitators focus on "both/and" approaches to dealing with polarity and paradox rather than "either/or."

Critical thinking:

- *Systems thinking*: recognition of the interdependency of various contributors to an issue or problem. The interconnectedness of different elements also means that pressure on any single element in a system will influence the other elements as well. Systems thinking helps to identify these consequences before taking action.
- *Strategic thinking*: future-oriented big-picture conceptualization that helps to identify

where an individual or organization wants to be in the future and various trajectories by which to get there.

Key knowledge:

- Understanding of terminology and concepts from multiple disciplines including medicine, ecology, economics, ethics, and engineering.
- Analytical skills such as epidemiology, risk analysis, cost-benefit analysis, and modeling.

Note: no single individual will embody all of these interpersonal skills, critical thinking, and key knowledge competencies, which is why a team approach is fundamental to One Health leadership.

10.5 Policy-Making with One Health in Mind

Policy-making is a continual process (Box 10.1). One Health policy-making represents a collective plan of action that encompasses the many perspectives needed to identify the best approaches for addressing the specific grand challenge. Since grand challenges have no simple technical solutions, One Health policy-making occurs on many levels concurrently and is continually revised as new scientific information and feedback are gathered. The One Health approach suggests that a portfolio of policy initiatives has a greater likelihood of creating positive change than any single action, regardless of how good it sounds.

While examples in developing countries often are cited, the One Health approach works even in countries with many resources. Working together toward shared goals has obvious benefit for a wide range of health challenges around the world.

Change is the norm in biological, social, and economic systems, so that the grand challenges of health also are constantly changing. Change requires adaptation so that policies must change to keep pace. The One Health concept recognizes the need for policies to evolve to suit the changing conditions.

Box 10.1 A bit of policy theory

The Cambridge Online Dictionary defines policy as a set of ideas or a plan of what to do in particular situations that has been agreed by a group of people, a business organization, a government, or a political party. The policy process can be represented as a cycle. The numbers in brackets refer to the explanations in the text below.

a variety of sources will be considered including political opinions, stakeholder interests, scientific information, public opinion, commercial and economic interests.

3) Policy development is the process of reaching agreement on the course of action.

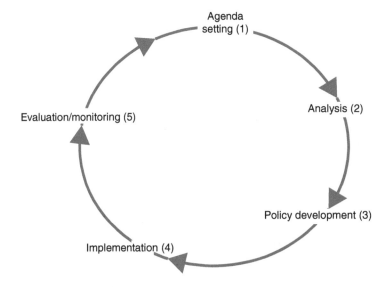

1) Agenda setting is the start of the policy process, when a problem or an issue is recognized and it is decided that something will need to be done.

2) The next step is the analysis, in which the policy-makers endeavor to learn as much as possible about the issue and potential approaches to deal with it. Information from

4) Implementation is translation of the plan to action, i.e., making it happen.

5) Evaluation and monitoring help ensure that the policy actually has the desired effect. The results of the evaluation and monitoring provide feedback to inform necessary policy adjustments which brings the cycle back to agenda setting.

10.6 Integrating One Health Leadership Approaches in Hierarchical Organizations

Most organizations operate with hierarchical leadership – there is a person in charge, someone "at the top" who is the final authority for decisions. This applies to government

agencies, most private sector companies, and most nonprofits. Hierarchical leadership also is used for incident command in emergency response such as fire-fighting and catastrophic animal disease outbreaks, whether they originate from natural, accidental, or intentional exposures. One Health shared leadership can make a valuable contribution in these situations, through influence up the chain of command and influence across organizations. The key to effective "leading up" and "leading across" is providing valuable information to empower leaders to make the best solutions. Influence does not need to be officially recognized and rewarded in order to be effective. Mastery of the One Health leadership competencies described earlier can increase influence effectiveness.

10.7 Demonstrating One Health Leadership and Policy in Action

The One Health concept itself sounds idealistic and can be difficult to explain. Creating One Health approaches is difficult if everything appears to be working well. Grand challenges also often appear intractable: little change is immediately seen regardless of the actions taken.

Crises such as the emergence of a new or re-emerging disease threat present a window of opportunity for promoting One Health leadership and policy-making. Current events are real, people are affected, mistakes are recognized, and policy-makers want to do something to make a positive difference. In crises, One Health approaches can demonstrate immediate benefits through coordinated action and more efficient utilization of resources to successfully address the issues.

Small successes need to be recognized and celebrated in order to build momentum. Demonstrating benefits and helping organizations to be more successful increases the commitment to One Health approaches.

Several case studies follow to illustrate One Health leadership and policy in action:

- The emergence of national One Health strategies in Africa in the face of multiple emerging disease threats with some painful lessons learned from insufficient previous approaches.
- The global coalescence of international organizations, non-governmental charities, and national governments in launching a joint campaign to eliminate dog-mediated rabies in humans.

- The evolution of joint action to address simultaneous (and related) outbreaks of Q fever in humans and dairy goats in The Netherlands.
- The convergence of disparate groups in the USA (government agencies, private sector pharmaceutical and healthcare companies, professional organizations, and food animal producer groups) in developing a portfolio of policies to address the stubborn challenge of antimicrobial resistance.

These case studies show that applying the leadership principles described for the One Health approach is generally triggered by a crisis. While the start is often focused on a specific disease or problem, as illustrated by our case studies, other grand challenges, such as climate change or global food security, don't involve a disease per se. The structures and working relationships that emerge to address a single issue using the One Health approach often have broader applicability for other issues. In The Netherlands the outbreak of Q fever and the resulting cooperation between the health and agricultural ministries has led to a structure whereby representatives of all relevant disciplines regularly meet and discuss threats. This has already proven its worth in relation to Zika virus risk analysis.

The case studies also show the benefit of involving stakeholders at the local, regional, national, or supranational levels. The worldwide control of rabies is instigated by large supranational organizations that have the recognized authority to foster the multicountry collaboration needed for the program, but they cannot go it alone. The campaign will have to rely on national governments to make the decisions, allocate resources, and develop conducive policies, and on local partners to implement the required activities. The same applies to antimicrobial resistance: initiatives are employed at all levels, and coordination among sectors and disciplines is the challenge. The antimicrobial resistance case also shows that progress can be gained once individual representatives of organizations involved, from all different sides of the issue, are prepared to identify shared interests and explore solutions rather than focusing on their differences and getting stuck in a blame game.

In all cases, current scientific information and a wide variety of social, economic, and political data are essential. Very often an enormous amount of information already exists, even though there are gaps. More importantly, data often are not shared between the different organizations involved. Managing relationships and overcoming distrust is a major prerequisite of data sharing. This is another critical component of One Health leadership – the ability to build trust amongst key stakeholders involved in addressing a particular grand challenge.

10.8   Case Study 1: National One Health Policy Development in Cameroon and Rwanda

Highly publicized outbreaks of zoonotic disease spurred the development of national One Health policies in Africa early in the twenty-first century. Complex challenges like anthrax disease in gorillas (Leendertz et al., 2006), pigs cross-reacting with pandemic A/H1N1/2009 influenza virus isolated from humans (Njabo et al., 2012), and the spread of H5N1 highly pathogenic avian influenza (HPAI) (Njouom et al., 2008) fueled initial discussions of the need for broader One Health approaches. Two countries demonstrated the role that national governments can play in promoting national One Health policies (Box 10.2).

10.8.1   Cameroon

Fear of HPAI in the poultry industry led to initial discussions among technical experts on how to use a multisectoral approach to respond to and control disease outbreaks. A National Integrated Plan for Avian Influenza control through the Common Fund Project

> **Box 10.2 Case study 1: Key messages about One Health leadership and policy**
>
> 1) Emerging disease outbreaks often create "windows of opportunity" for development of national One Health policy frameworks that promote multisectoral and multidisciplinary collaboration and partnership.
> 2) One Health strategies often begin with a focus on animal and human health surveillance, disease detection and response, and prevention.
> 3) An independent mechanism such as a cross-sectoral coordinating committee that promotes shared leadership and reports to a neutral entity can promote more effective and efficient implementation of One Health activities.

(PFC) was created and the Cameroonian prime minister signed a decree setting up a multisectoral committee for the prevention and control of emerging and re-emerging zoonotic diseases.

The involvement of the Prime Minister's office and the establishment of an inter-ministerial committee comprised of Directors from relevant ministries made implementation of the One Health policy easier. Implementation also was promoted by interested funders such as the US Agency for International Development (USAID), committed partners such as the US Centers for Disease Control and Prevention (CDC), and the global encouragement resulting from the Global Health Security Agenda, to which Cameroon was a signatory (https://www.ghsagenda.org/where-ghsa). The Cameroonian One Health Strategy has evolved over time after a joint situation analysis and needs assessment conducted by the Ministry of Environment and Natural Protection and the Ministry of Public Health (Ouli-Ndongo et al., 2012). The National Program for Emerging and re-emerging Zoonotic Diseases (NPFEZD) was created with participation from more than 12 government ministers under the leadership of the Prime Minister's office. The NPFEZD was tasked to manage and implement the One Health strategy in Cameroon with five focus areas: 1) development of a One Health institutional framework; 2) training and sharing of knowledge; 3) development of research topics on emerging and re-emerging infectious diseases; 4) strengthening of surveillance systems for environmental health, animal health, and human health; and 5) communication and sensitization on the One Health Concept.

10.8.2 Rwanda

The risk of hemorrhagic disease outbreaks spreading from neighboring countries and the lessons learned from HPAI H5N1 preparedness and response exercises in Rwanda set the stage for a country-wide situation analysis. Rwanda has one of the highest population densities in the world at 415.5 people per square kilometer in 2011 (United Nations, 2013). Emerging disease outbreaks are recognized as a threat to the social, economic, and societal health of the country (Changula et al., 2014; https://www.cdc.gov/vhf/ebola/outbreaks/history/chronology.html). The analysis identified weak prioritization of disease risks and a lack of collaboration within and between government institutions on zoonotic disease surveillance, outbreak investigation, and response despite strong political will, the presence of necessary infrastructure and some opportunities for early successes like integration of e-surveillance systems for human and animal health. Appointment of a One Health Steering Committee (OHSC) in 2011 by government was the first step, with members from the Ministry of Health, the Ministry of Agriculture – Rwanda Agricultural Board, the Rwanda Development Board – Tourism and Conservation, the University of Rwanda, and the Rwanda Environment Management Authority. The OHSC led the development of a One Health National Strategic plan (MOH, 2013), the main goals of which

include: 1) building disease detection, response, and applied research capacity within the country; 2) strengthening animal and human disease surveillance; and 3) improving disease detection and outbreak response. Last but not least, the goal is to promote interdisciplinary One Health collaboration and partnerships in Rwanda.

10.9 Case Study 2: The Campaign for Global Elimination of Dog-Mediated Human Rabies

Rabies continues to kill tens of thousands of people in the developing world, whereas the public health consequences in North America, Europe, and Australia/New Zealand are minimal. Rabies in humans is almost always fatal. More than 95% of rabies cases in humans are the result of bites by dogs infected with rabies. Dog-mediated rabies is considerably more common in rural areas, among children, and in socially and economically disadvantaged areas in Asia and Africa. The problem in many of these areas is compounded by endemic canine rabies, a lack of awareness of the disease, and a lack of access to post-exposure prophylaxis (PEP) for people who have been bitten by suspected rabid dogs (WHO-OIE-FAO, 2015).

Historically, rabies in animals was a veterinary medical issue and rabies in humans was a public health issue, each handled by separate government agencies with separate budgets and personnel. Despite the existence of effective vaccines and the demonstrated success of vaccination campaigns in eliminating dog-mediated rabies, support for PEP of exposed humans was seen as a higher priority. Paradoxically, if only 10% of the funding currently spent on human post-exposure treatments was used for mass vaccination of dogs in endemic areas, dog-mediated rabies in humans could be prevented and the transmission cycle effectively broken.

The successful eradication of smallpox in humans and progress toward polio and guinea worm eradication increased the interest of public health agencies for identifying additional eradication targets. Simultaneously, development of an international vaccine bank by the World Organization for Animal Health (OIE) offered a means for large-scale purchase and distribution of rabies vaccines to countries committed to mass vaccination campaigns.

Through the facilitation and advocacy of a non-governmental organization, the Global Alliance for Rabies Control (GARC), and the influence exerted by One Health champions working for global intergovernmental organizations and nonprofit funders, the global elimination of dog-mediated human rabies was identified as one of the top One Health priorities for the World Health Organization of the United Nations (WHO), the OIE, and the Food and Agriculture Organization of the United Nations (FAO) (WHO-OIE-FAO-GARC, 2016).

The multifaceted campaign that emerged from this partnership exemplifies key principles of the One Health approach in addressing the determinants of disease as well as its

---

Box 10.3 Case study 2: Key messages about One Health leadership and policy

1) Facilitation and advocacy by non-governmental organizations can catalyze effective One Health efforts when shared interests are identified and the value of partnership is recognized by all interested parties.
2) Addressing socioeconomic determinants of disease along with disease prevention and control is a hallmark of effective One Health approaches.
3) Successful One Health campaigns require both technical feasibility (effective vaccine) and organizational capacity (global vaccine bank and infrastructure and cooperation within targeted communities) as well as funding sources and political will of government leaders.

---

prevention and control (Box 10.3). The elimination campaign focuses not only on vaccinating dogs and improving access to post-exposure treatment, but also on dog bite prevention, bite management, increasing public awareness, and gaining political support for the program in endemic areas.

10.10 Case Study 3: Antimicrobial Resistance – USA

While there is universal scientific agreement that the use of antibiotics creates selective pressure for the development of resistance, agreement on how to address antimicrobial resistance (AMR) has been elusive. Increasing human illness and fatalities associated with AMR led to finger-pointing between human medicine and veterinary medicine. Fueled by advocacy groups, both sides adopted strident arguments that popularized gross exaggerations such as: "US agriculture feeds tons of antibiotics indiscriminately and veterinarians contribute to the problem" versus "the real problem is physicians' overuse of antibiotics and poor control of hospital acquired infections." Understandably, both sides felt a bit righteously indignant, even though the polemics included a modicum of truth. For example, US veterinarians have worked with food animal organizations, like the National Pork Board, for years to develop antibiotic stewardship guidelines, and veterinarians commonly use antibiotic susceptibility testing in making treatment choices. Meanwhile, physicians acknowledged the widespread and generally unnecessary use broad-spectrum antibiotics to treat otitis media in children and the pernicious impact of nosocomial disease. Producers, patients, and the press all weighed in with their opinions and recommendations for seemingly simple solutions like "ban antibiotic use in animals," "put more regulations on drug companies," or "restrict physician haphazard use of antibiotics."

The One Health breakthrough emerged slowly as stakeholders recognized common ground: we all want to be able to use antibiotics that work when they are indicated and we all fear emergence of "superbugs" resistant to every treatment option. Through active engagement of public health, veterinary, and human medicine associations, animal producer organizations, nonprofit organizations, and even drug companies, some concrete steps have emerged:

- Drug companies began voluntarily withdrawing their label indications for the use of antibiotics for growth promotion in animals.
- Veterinary medical associations working with the US Food and Drug Administration formulated more stringent guidelines for the use of antibiotics in animal feed.

- The American Academy of Family Physicians and the American Academy of Pediatrics jointly issued guidelines for diagnosis and treatment of otitis media in children, including the use of aggressive pain management and observation as the first option for non-severe cases.
- The US Affordable Care Act signed into law in 2010 required healthcare facilities to meet certain standards of care and increased reporting requirements, focusing more attention on hospital-acquired infections (nosocomial disease) and encouraging better communication among care providers to reduce unnecessary or duplicative prescriptions.

Antimicrobial resistance is a global grand challenge (Figure 10.1). While the situation

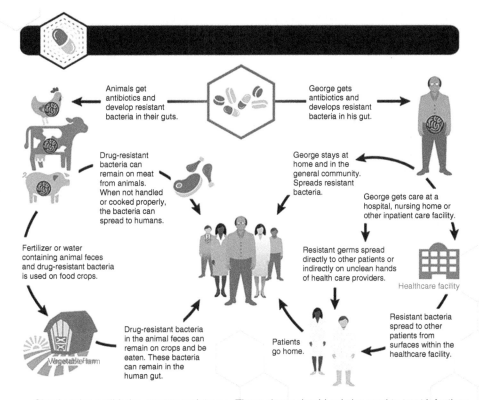

Animals get antibiotics and develop resistant bacteria in their guts.

George gets antibiotics and develops resistant bacteria in his gut.

Drug-resistant bacteria can remain on meat from animals. When not handled or cooked properly, the bacteria can spread to humans.

George stays at home and in the general community. Spreads resistant bacteria.

George gets care at a hospital, nursing home or other inpatient care facility.

Fertilizer or water containing animal feces and drug-resistant bacteria is used on food crops.

Resistant germs spread directly to other patients or indirectly on unclean hands of health care providers.

Healthcare facility

Vegetable Farm

Drug-resistant bacteria in the animal feces can remain on crops and be eaten. These bacteria can remain in the human gut.

Patients go home.

Resistant bacteria spread to other patients from surfaces within the healthcare facility.

Simply using antibiotics creates resistance. These drugs should only be used to treat infections.

Figure 10.1 Examples of how antibiotic resistance spreads. *Source:* Centers for Disease Control and Prevention (https://www.cdc.gov/drugresistance/threat-report-2013/pdf/ar-threats-2013-508.pdf#page=11).

Box 10.4 Case study 3: Key messages about One Health leadership and policy

1) One Health leadership brings stakeholders together to identify shared interests and reach consensus about actions to address grand challenges.
2) Grand challenges like antimicrobial resistance (AMR) don't have simple technical solutions; to make progress requires a portfolio of policies across the spectrum of stakeholders, including public and private sectors.
3) Progress on global grand challenges like AMR takes patience and determination; AND progress IS possible (Note: even slow progress IS progress!).

---

may be different in every country and region of the world, the need for One Health leadership is apparent (Box 10.4). Everyone has a stake in the AMR issue, and the more engagement of and collaboration between relevant parties, the better the strategies that emerge from their deliberations and the broader the public support for their implementation.

References

Changula, K., Kajihara, M., Mweene, A.S., and Takada, A. (2014). Ebola and Marburg virus diseases in Africa: Increased risk of outbreaks in previously unaffected areas? *Microbiology and Immunology* 58(9), 483–491.

Leendertz, F.H., Lankester, F., Guislain, P., et al. (2006). Anthrax in Western and Central African great apes. *American Journal of Primatology* 68, 928–933.

MOH (Ministry of Health) (2013). One Health Strategic Plan (2014-2018). Republic of Rwanda, Ministry of Health, Rwanda Biomedical Center. Available at: http://www.rbc.gov.rw/IMG/pdf/one_health.pdf (accessed December 11, 2017).

Njabo, K.Y., Trevon, L., Fuller, T.L., et al. (2012). Pandemic A/H1N1/2009 influenza virus in swine, Cameroon, 2010. *Veterinary Microbiology* 156(1-2), 189–192.

Njouom, R., Aubin, J.T., x Bella, A.L., et al. (2008). Highly pathogenic avian influenza virus subtype H5N1 in ducks in the Northern part of Cameroon. *Veterinary Microbiology* 130(3-4), 380–384.

Ouli-Ndongo, M., Koulagna, K.D., Baschirou, D.M., et al. (2012). Cameroon "One Health" National Strategy. Republic of Cameroon.

United Nations (2013). *World Statistics Pocketbook*. New York: United Nations Department of Economics and Social Affairs, Statistics Division; United Nations Publications, Series V, No. 37.

WHO-OIE-FAO (2015). Rationale for investing in the global elimination of dog-mediated human rabies. Available at: http://apps.who.int/iris/bitstream/10665/185195/1/9789241509558_eng.pdf (accessed December 15, 2017).

WHO-OIE-FAO-GARC (2016). Global elimination of dog-mediated human rabies. Report of the Rabies Global Conference 10-11 December 2015, Geneva, Switzerland. Available at: http://www.who.int/rabies/resources/who_htm_ntd_nzd_2016.02/en/(accessed on December 15, 2017).

11

Implementing One Health

Laura H. Kahn

Woodrow Wilson School of Public and International Affairs Princeton University, Princeton, NJ, USA

11.1 Financing One Health Initiatives

Implementing One Health at the national and international levels will be challenging. Organizational structures, pertaining to human, animal, and environmental health, are typically spread across different departments and agencies with disparate missions and budgets. In the USA, the President proposes budgets for Executive branch departments and agencies, but Congress ultimately decides how much funding they receive through the appropriations process. In general, human health receives vastly more funding than animal or environmental health even though the latter two greatly impact human health.

The mission of the US Department of Health and Human Services is to protect the health of all Americans. The President's proposed fiscal year 2018 budget is approximately US$1112.9 billion, a 3% decrease from the FY 2017 budget, (USDHHS, 2017a, 2017b). Ninety percent of the DHHS budget would go to Medicare and Medicaid, the two major federal government healthcare programs, which cover approximately 17% and 20% of the US population, respectively. The remaining 10% would go to various mandatory and discretionary programs as well as children's entitlement programs.

In the FY 2017 DHHS budget, antimicrobial resistance, a critical One Health-related issue, had been targeted to receive US$877 million dollars (USDHHS, 2017a). However, the FY 2018 budget did not mention any funding dedicated to it (USDHHS, 2017b). In the proposed FY 2018 DHHS budget, the Centers for Disease Control and Prevention (CDC) is slated to receive US$514 million for the National Center for Emerging and Zoonotic Infectious Diseases, a decrease of approximately 18% from the previous year's budget. In FY 2018, the Food and Drug Administration (FDA) would receive US$1.3 billion for food safety, a 13% decrease from the previous budget. Also in the FY 2018 budget, the CDC is proposed to receive US$51 million to monitor, conduct surveillance, analyze data, and disseminate technical guidance, training, and technology to state health departments on food safety, (USDHHS, 2017b). But even with the proposed FY 2018 budget cuts, DHHS remains better funded than agriculture, animal health, or environmental health.

A number of different federal departments oversee animal health even though none has animal health as part of their primary missions.

Beyond One Health: From Recognition to Results, First Edition.
Edited by John A. Herrmann and Yvette J. Johnson-Walker.
© 2018 John Wiley & Sons, Inc. Published 2018 by John Wiley & Sons, Inc.

The mission of the US Department of Agriculture (USDA) is to "provide leadership on food, agriculture, natural resources, rural development, nutrition, and related issues based on public policy, the best available science, and effective management" (USDA, 2017a). Its proposed fiscal year 2018 budget is US$137 billon dollars, a 12% decrease from the 2017 USDA budget (USDA, 2017b).

In FY 2017, the USDA's budget constituted only about 3% of the US$4.2 trillion dollar total federal budget – this was before the proposed FY 2018 cuts. The National Institute of Food and Agriculture (NIFA), the USDA's equivalent to the National Institutes of Health (NIH), has a proposed fiscal year 2018 budget of approximately US$1.4 billion dollars, a decrease of 24% from the previous year, (USDA, 2017a, 2017b). The NIH's proposed FY 2018 budget of US$25.9 billion dollars (a 22% decrease from the FY 2017 budget), is almost 19 times greater than NIFA's budget. Within NIFA, the Agriculture and Food Research Initiative, the primary funding source for animal agriculture research, is proposed to receive US$349 million research in the FY 2018 budget, an amount unchanged from the previous year's budget (USDA. 2017c).

Wildlife health receives minimal funding. The US Fish and Wildlife Service, part of the Department of the Interior, has a mission to "work with others to conserve, protect and enhance fish, wildlife and plants and their habitats for the continuing benefit of the American people" (USFWS, 2017). The proposed budget for FY 2018 was US$2.8 billion, an 8% decrease from the FY 2017 budget of US$3.03 billion (USDI, 2017, 2018). Wildlife health efforts are not explicitly listed in the budget; however, wildlife health is affected by conservation and restoration efforts. The proposed fiscal year 2018 budget for conservation and restoration, a subsection of ecological services, is US$29.8 million dollars, almost a 14% decrease from the FY 2017 budget (USFWS, 2017).

The US Environmental Protection Agency's mission is to protect human health and the environment. It regulates industry to diminish environmental contamination, and it conducts research on environmental issues. It works to improve air quality, promote clean water, unpolluted land, and to ensure the safety of manufactured chemicals. The proposed FY 2018 EPA budget is US$5.7 billion, a 31% decrease from the FY 2017 budget of $8.1 billion (USEPA, 2017a, 2017b, 2017c). Policy-makers must understand that a contaminated environment jeopardizes the health of humans and animals.

At the international level, large funding disparities between human, animal, and environmental health also exist. The United Nations' World Health Organization (WHO) has over 7000 employees working at its international headquarters in Geneva, Switzerland, in its 150 country offices, and in six regional offices. Its mission is "…to build a better, healthier future for people all over the world." To accomplish this goal, their proposed budget for the 2018–2019 fiscal year is approximately US$4.4 billion (WHO, 2017).

The United Nations' Food and Agriculture Organization's mission consists of three parts: eliminating hunger, food insecurity, and malnutrition; eliminating poverty and ensuring economic and social progress; and sustainably using and managing natural resources. It employs almost 3250 professional and support staff in its headquarters in Rome, Italy, in five regional, nine subregional, and 80 country offices. Its budget for 2016–2017 is US$2.6 billion (FAO, 2017a, 2017b, 2017c).

The World Organization for Animal Health (OIE) is the only international entity whose mission includes control of animal diseases and animal welfare. It is not under the umbrella of the United Nations, but rather is overseen by an independent World Assembly of OIE Delegates of 180 member countries. Its overall budget in 2015, the most recent budget available, was €25.7 million (approximately US$28.5 million) (OIE, 2017a, 2017b). Fewer than 100 people staff the OIE's headquarters in Paris, France. Twelve regional representatives are based in

Africa (Mali, Botswana, Tunisia, Kenya), South America (Argentina, Panama), Eurasia (Japan, Thailand, Russia), Europe (Belgium, Kazakhstan), and the Middle East (Lebanon). Compared to WHO and FAO, the OIE is tiny (OIE, 2017c).

There is no international organization for the environment. The United Nations has an Environment Programme (UNEP) established in 1972 with the mission of promoting wise use of the environment. Its 2016 budget was US$683.6 million plus an additional US$90.2 million of funding carried over from previous years. Most of the funding is allocated to climate change and ecosystem management. Other areas of support include: chemicals and waste, resource efficiency, and disasters and conflicts (UNEP, 2017a).

To improve ecosystem conservation and management, the UNEP produces a World Database on Protected Areas, supports the design and establishment of ecosystem health monitoring systems, and supports the

development of biodiversity and conservation strategies through efforts such as the National Biodiversity Strategies and Action Plan Forum, which helps countries develop biodiversity conservation programs. It is unclear how many countries are implementing effective biodiversity conservation programs (UNEP, 2017b).

11.2 Conclusion

Ultimately, political leaders will be responsible for preserving a habitable planet for humans and all other species. Funding primarily human health misses the key point that human health depends on healthy animals, healthy environments, and healthy ecosystems. Vast funding disparities between these areas hinders the implementation of the One Health concept. Policy-makers and the public need to be educated on why One Health is vital for global health and sustainability.

References

FAO (Food and Agriculture Organization of the United Nations) (2017a). About FAO. Rome: FAO. Available at: http://www.fao.org/about/en/(accessed July 1, 2017).

FAO (Food and Agriculture Organization of the United Nations) (2017b). Strategic planning. How is FAO funded? Rome: FAO. Available at: http://www.fao.org/about/strategic-planning/en/(accessed December 11, 2017).

FAO (Food and Agriculture Organization of the United Nations) (2017c). Who we are. Structure and finance. Rome: FAO. Available at: http://www.fao.org/about/who-we-are/en/(accessed December 11, 2017).

OIE (World Organisation for Animal Health) (2017a). Annual Report 2015. Geneva: OIE. Available at: http://www.oie.int/fileadmin/home/eng/Media_Center/docs/pdf/Key_Documents/EN_RA2015_LR.pdf (accessed July 10, 2017).

OIE (World Organisation for Animal Health) (2017b). Headquarters. Geneva: OIE. Available at: http://www.oie.int/en/about-us/wo/headquarters/(accessed July 10, 2017).

OIE (World Organisation for Animal Health) (2017c). Our Missions. Objectives. Geneva: OIE. Available at: http://www.oie.int/about-us/our-missions/(accessed July 20, 2017).

UNEP (United Nations Environment Programme) (2017a). Annual Report 2016. New York: UNEP. Available at: http://web.unep.org/annualreport/2016/index.php (accessed July 10, 2017).

UNEP (United Nations Environment Programme) (2017b). Ecosystem Management. Preserving our Ecosystems. What we do. New York: UNEP. Available at: http://web.unep.org/ecosystems/what-we-do/preserving-our-ecosystems (accessed 10 July 2017).

USDA (United States Department of Agriculture) (2017a). About the U.S. Department of Agriculture. What We Do. Washington, DC: USDA. Available at: https://www.usda.gov/our-agency/about-usda (accessed July 6, 2017).

USDA (United States Department of Agriculture) (2017b). FY 2017 Budget Summary. Washington, DC: USDA, p. 1. Available at: https://www.obpa.usda.gov/budsum/fy17budsum.pdf (accessed July 10, 2017).

USDA (United States Department of Agriculture) (2017c). FY 2018 Budget Summary. Washington, DC: USDA, p. 1. Available at: https://www.usda.gov/sites/default/files/documents/USDA-Budget-Summary-2018.pdf (accessed July 6, 2017).

USDHHS (United States Department of Health and Human Services) (2017a). FY 2017 Budget in Brief. Washington, DC: USDHHS, pp. 4–5, 15. Available at: https://www.hhs.gov/sites/default/files/fy2017-budget-in-brief.pdf (accessed July 10, 2017).

USDHHS (United States Department of Health and Human Services) (2017b). FY 2018 Budget in Brief. Washington, DC: USDHHS, p. 10. Available at: https://www.hhs.gov/sites/default/files/Consolidated%20BIB_ONLINE_remediated.pdf?language=es (accessed July 12, 2017).

USDI (United States Department of the Interior) (2017). Budget Justifications and Performance Information Fiscal Year 2017, U.S. Fish and Wildlife Service. Washington, DC: USDI, p. 57. Available at: https://www.fws.gov/budget/2016/FY2017_FWS_Greenbook.pdf (accessed July 15, 2017).

USDI (United States Department of the Interior) (2018). Budget Justifications and Performance Information Fiscal Year 2018, U.S. Fish and Wildlife Service. Page 45, Washington, DC: USDI, p. 45. Available at: https://www.fws.gov/budget/2018/FY2018-FWS-Greenbook.pdf (accessed July 15, 2017).

USEPA (United States Environmental Protection Agency) (2017a). EPA's Budget and Spending. Washington, DC: USEPA. Available at: https://www.epa.gov/planandbudget/budget (accessed July 10, 2017).

USEPA (United States Environmental Protection Agency) (2017b). FY 2018. EPA Budget in Brief. Washington, DC: USEPA, p. 7. Available at: https://www.epa.gov/sites/production/files/2017-05/documents/fy-2018-budget-in-brief.pdf (accessed July 10, 2017).

USEPA (United States Environmental Protection Agency) (2017c). Our Mission and What We Do. Washington, DC: USEPA. Available at: https://www.epa.gov/aboutepa/our-mission-and-what-we-do (accessed July 10, 2017).

USFWS (United States Fish and Wildlife Service) (2017). About the U.S. Fish and Wildlife Service. Washington, DC: USEPA. Available at: https://www.fws.gov/help/about_us.html (accessed July 10, 2017).

WHO (World Health Organization) (2017). Seventieth World Health Assembly. Proposed Programme Budget 2018-2019. Geneva: WHO, p. 5. Available at: http://apps.who.int/gb/ebwha/pdf_files/WHA70/A70_7-en.pdf (accessed April 10, 2017).

12

The Social Cost of Carbon

William J. Craven

California State Senate, Sacramento, CA, USA

Disclaimer: The views expressed are the author's own and should not be attributed to the California State Senate.

12.1 Introduction

How do we calculate, in today's dollars, estimates of the future economic, social, and public health costs of greenhouse gas emissions that are causing global climate change? How much is it worth, in today's dollars, to reduce the future negative effects of climate change? Underlying these questions is a broader inquiry: what is to be done about a lack of acceptance, in many political sectors, of widely known scientific research regarding climate change and the multiple costs to society of continuing to use fossil fuels for energy production?

Several US agencies have developed a metric called the "social cost of carbon" (SCC) to get a handle on the first two questions. This metric is essentially a pricing strategy to consider the economic externalities caused by carbon dioxide emissions that can be reflected in regulations dealing with any number of topics in which energy consumption or fuel efficiency may be an issue. The latter question represents one of the most polarizing reversals in US political history that has confounded many in the USA as well

as its international partners. The storyline caused by the political turmoil of the US administration will reverberate for years to come.

The SCC is a complicated amalgam of economic, scientific, and ethical considerations. While it has received significant attention in the US media, similar pricing strategies have been developed internationally and many more are in process. In the USA the SCC has been used many times to inform federal regulations on numerous topics in which greenhouse gas emissions are involved. The US federal government was criticized in litigation for not having a numeric scheme to underpin its climate-related regulations. Now that it has developed a numeric approach, challenges to the metric have been rejected by a handful of courts. In 2007, a Federal circuit court held that certain fuel efficiency standards for vehicles that excluded monetizing reductions in greenhouse gas emissions constituted an unlawful "arbitrary and capricious" regulation (*Center for Biological Diversity vs. National Highway Transportation Safety Administration*, 2007). Cost-benefit analyses are a customary part of regulatory rule-making in the USA. In 2016, for example, the SCC was upheld in the Seventh Circuit US Court of Appeals in a case dealing with refrigerator energy standards. The decision clearly ratified the effort to place a cost

Beyond One Health: From Recognition to Results, First Edition.
Edited by John A. Herrmann and Yvette J. Johnson-Walker.

on carbon dioxide emissions and to measure the social costs of climate change on a global basis, both outcomes that have now been rejected under the current administration (*Zero Zone, Inc. vs. United States Department of Energy*, 2016; Roston, 2016).

The SCC traces its origin to the administration of George W. Bush. As suggested earlier, a court invalidated that administration's fuel economy standard because it did not adequately address the issue of costs associated with carbon dioxide emissions. In 2009, under President Obama, an interagency working group was convened to consider how to assess the effects, both positive and negative, of carbon dioxide emissions and to develop a measure that could be used by multiple federal agencies. This approach allowed regulators to coordinate across agencies and to develop a unified approach (Revesz, 2017). In addition to providing consistency, the working group wanted federal agencies to use the best available information in their regulatory impact analyses that are required for new regulations. The interagency group was comprised of scientific and economic experts from the White House and a wide array of federal agencies including: Council on Environmental Quality, National Economic Council, Office of Energy and Climate Change, and Office of Science and Technology Policy, Environmental Protection Agency (EPA), and the Departments of Agriculture, Commerce, Energy, Transportation, and Treasury. Prior to the current administration, the SCC has been updated twice through peer-reviewed studies (EPA, 2015). It has also been expanded to include additional greenhouse gases other than carbon dioxide.

12.2 Some Context on Cost-Benefit Analyses

Some context for the concept of cost-benefit analyses is perhaps useful: it used to be the case that conservatives and liberals generally agreed that the social and economic costs of regulations should be evaluated in advance of implementation. That notion, although somewhat controversial 40 years ago when proposed in the administration of Ronald Reagan, is now commonplace. It became firmly ingrained in the federal government under President Clinton through an executive order and it remains in place today. Many believe that such cost-benefit analyses enhance public confidence that new regulations will achieve the intended results more efficiently and effectively. The original concern of some progressive groups was that many environmental and public health benefits were difficult to quantify and would not be accounted for in the analyses. That concern has somewhat diminished. At the same time, the science for assessing the costs of regulations continued to improve and those developments, many of which have been peer-reviewed, are now reflected in analyses of the costs of climate change. The requirement for cost-benefit analyses is a triumph for conservative, often Republican, leaders at both the federal and state level, and has now become accepted even by Democratic administrations. But it is very inconvenient when it comes to climate change. Advocates who reject the anthropogenic aspects of climate change and its deleterious effects on humans, animals, and ecosystems want to eliminate the metric. Many fossil fuel industry executives and lobbyists from industries with high greenhouse gas emissions want to cripple it so that the regulatory costs of reducing greenhouse gas emissions are drastically reduced.

12.3 The Social Cost of Carbon (SCC)

The SCC is a cost-benefit approach that attempts to estimate "the net damages incurred by society from a one metric ton increase in carbon dioxide emissions in a given year" (EPA, 2015). While still evolving, the SCC is based primarily on three economic models that estimate changes in agricultural productivity, human health, elevated mortality rates, property damage from increased flood risks, changes in energy costs, and more. As the US EPA observed, however, the models do not take into account all of the benefits associated with emission reductions (EPA, 2015). According to the General Accounting Office, the SCC has been used in more than 150 regulatory actions since 2008 and has been updated three times. It played a key role in the approach of federal agencies under the Obama administration's climate-related regulations, such as capping the emissions of power plants (Clean Power Plan), improving vehicle efficiency, and improving energy efficiency in many consumer products.

In its most recent iteration, the SCC estimates a cost of US$36/ton of carbon dioxide emitted into the atmosphere with projected increases to US$50/ton in 2030 and almost US$70/ton in 2050. A recent and important National Academy of Sciences report recommends further refinements (National Academies of Sciences, 2017) but, in the early days of the current US administration, a key question, discussed later, is whether the SCC will survive at all, or if it does, in what form.

Here is an example of the SCC as applied: The US EPA and the US Department of Transportation concluded a cost-benefit analysis for light-duty vehicles. Increasing fuel efficiency standards was said to cost industry US$350 billion over 40 years. Benefits to society were calculated at US$280 million (including reduced pollution and congestion, and more energy security). As noted by one commentator, "So higher fuel efficiency standards don't pass muster: They are US$70 million in the 'red.' Yet once the social costs of carbon are taken into account, the cost-benefit analyses showed net benefits of more than US$100 billion," thus justifying the fuel efficiency standards (Wihbey, 2015). This snapshot of the fuel efficiency standards encapsulates the debate: Critics claim the SCC can be used to justify regulations that would not otherwise pass muster in traditional cost-benefit analyses. Supporters argue

that the SCC is an important tool to monetize the future effects of carbon pollution.

The most recent review of the SCC by the prestigious National Academy of Sciences (NAS), a nonprofit organization whose members are elected by their peers and who comprise much of the scientific leadership across the USA, is particularly important. Among other things, the NAS recommended that the SCC be updated to include the valuation of more benefits that will occur as climate pollution is reduced. It confirmed that the SCC is based on the latest peer-reviewed literature, and it made recommendations to ensure that this remains the case going forward. It may well be that the NAS recommendations could result in a higher valuation of the benefits of emission reductions. As recently noted by the Natural Resources Defense Council, this could mean that the economic benefits of reducing emissions are greater than the SCC currently estimates (Yeh, 2017).

12.3.1 Looking at Costs

Considering that the USA emitted 5.4 billion tons of carbon dioxide in 2015, and using the cost of $36/ton, the unmitigated damage to the US economy is roughly US$205 billion annually, which can also be thought of as a subsidy to those who are making those emissions (Than, 2015). This estimate may be conservative because not all economic sectors are included and costs associated with some emergencies, such as drought and some other extreme weather events, are excluded from the SCC. The Natural Resources Defense Council (NRDC) and a group of scientists analyzed health data to consider the economic costs of specific vectors, usually insects that transmit diseases or parasites to humans and other animals, likely to worsen with climate change-related events, including ozone and smog pollution, heatwaves, hurricanes, wildfires, mosquito-borne diseases, and river flooding, and calculated total damages of US$14.1 billion from 2002 to 2009 (NRDC, 2011).

Other estimates of the per ton cost of carbon dioxide emissions are much higher. Some environmental groups and economists have speculated that the motives of those who lobby against the SCC may be influenced by the fact that this US$200 billion is a windfall to US fossil fuel-based industries (Jina, 2017). A 2017 study recommended a price on carbon of between US$40 and US$80 per ton by 2020, and from US$50 to US$100 per ton by 2030. That conclusion comes from the High-Level Commission on Carbon Prices headed by Nobel Laureate Joseph Stiglitz and Lord Nicholas Stern. The report recognizes that carbon prices and mechanisms will differ across countries, depending on the national context. It notes that the slower the global efforts to reduce carbon emissions the higher the costs will become. And the report acknowledges that poorer nations should pay less (Carbon Pricing Leadership Coalition, 2017).

Both the World Bank (WB) and the International Monetary Fund (IMF) are increasingly focused on investments to reduce emissions and to develop regulatory mechanisms that can be adopted in individual nations to reduce emissions (Davenport, 2016). The World Bank recognizes that climate change's role in exacerbating global poverty will only increase over time. The IMF sees carbon pricing as a revenue source. There are numerous examples of science and economically based national actions taken to reduce emissions globally and far too many to mention, but examples include:

- China has begun a limited cap and trade system in seven cities and provinces with plans to expand it nationwide.
- Mexico has a national climate change law and a greenhouse gas reduction target.
- South Korea's cap and trade system covers two-thirds of its national emissions and supports a target to reduce emissions to 30% below business as usual by 2020.
- The European Union (EU) has the largest carbon emissions trading system in the world, but it has been hampered by a low price on carbon; however, the EU is actively engaged in exploring remedies.
- Colombia and Chile have introduced carbon taxes in 2017 (Carbon Pricing Leadership Coalition, 2017).

The overall goal of the WB and IMF regarding carbon emissions is to have carbon pricing cover 25% of the world's carbon emissions by 2020, and 50% by 2030. As noted in a recent paper, the estimated cost of climate change is in the range of 0.2–2% of global income (Fan et al., 2016). The authors state that "if the SCC were around $120 per ton, then the cost of carbon dioxide emissions in 2013 would be about 1% of world income. $120 per ton, although high, is well within the range of available estimates [citations omitted]."

The business community is, of course, not silent, although its role is complicated by the machinations of some in the fossil fuel industries and their well-funded and omnipresent lobbying efforts. However, at least 70 companies have already internalized a price on carbon, some in the US$50–60/ton range, although the goal of the United Nations Global Compact is to establish a price of $100/ton by 2020 (Kingo, 2016). Many businesses are deeply interested in obtaining accurate information concerning climate change to ensure that its effects are correctly priced in markets so that investors can make informed decisions. This is becoming especially important for insurers, who must accurately anticipate these risks. For example, the 2011 floods in Thailand disrupted supply chains of 14 500 companies with worldwide costs of US$20 billion, but with only US$12 billion covered by insurance. Government and business leaders from China, the UK, Canada, Australia, The Netherlands, and the USA are collaborating on policy options. Some contend, perhaps somewhat cynically, that setting the correct price for carbon will ultimately do more to change human behavior regarding climate change than environmental activism (Aldrick, 2017).

Without diving too deep into the SCC underbrush, two additional concepts that need at least brief mention are vulnerable to manipulation by opponents of the SCC. The first pertains to the discount rate and the second to the global distribution of greenhouse gasses. It is indeed challenging to estimate the costs of climate change regulations in today's dollars that will pay future dividends many decades, if not centuries, from today. To help with such calculations, economists use the concept of a discount rate to compare present costs with future benefits. A quick summary: the higher the discount rate, the lower the estimate of harm. One need not be an elected official to know that the public is often more preoccupied with day-to-day concerns than with problems that may materialize in the distant future. The costs incurred by burning carbon may be seen as future problems, while the benefits (heat, electricity, fuel) are realized today. Carbon dioxide persists in the atmosphere over many years and its effects will not be seen for decades (Baron, 2017b). Many fear that politicians may favor policies that will increase the discount rate in order to reduce the SCC, which would "imply that many current regulations appear to have costs that exceed their benefits" (Baron, 2017b). For example, a change in the discount rate from 2.5% to 5% would reduce the cost of a ton of carbon dioxide to $12. Yet, whatever the discount rate, the argument of the fossil fuel industry is that the social cost of carbon metric increases the ostensible costs of regulations, which can then be framed, for political reasons, as creating unnecessary regulations that are an impediment to economic growth.

Obviously, the choice of discount rate has major consequences. The models used by the federal government use discount rates of 5%, 3%, and 2.5% to account for various uncertainties and different objectives of the federal agencies that served on the original interagency working group. The discount rate used by federal agencies, prior to 2017, is the mid-range 3%.

Because carbon dioxide emissions and climate change are global in their impacts (the effects of a ton of emissions are global, not limited to the place where the emissions originated), the SCC is based on worldwide impacts of carbon dioxide emissions. Despite the Seventh Circuit decision mentioned earlier, a second way that politicians may do a favor to major carbon-polluting industries is to limit the application of the SCC to greenhouse gasses produced just by, and affecting only, the USA. However, if the SCC were to focus only on the USA, our regulations would no longer consider the global effects of our emissions. They would no longer include impacts in poorer nations, or those near sea level, or other vulnerable populations. The world would suffer, but certain US industries would benefit (Baron, 2017a). Such a move could lower the SCC by 70% or more. And, of course, while the beneficiaries of a lower price would include the fossil fuel industries, such an effort also ignores the compelling reality that climate change is global. Researchers at the IMF concluded in 2015 that worldwide subsidies to energy, chiefly fossil fuel energy sources, total $5.2 trillion per year. This figure includes the externalities of carbon pollution that are paid by society, and not the firms that produce or sell the energy (IMF, 2015).

12.3.2 Getting the SCC as Good as it Can Get

As noted earlier, the SCC models may actually undervalue the cost of carbon dioxide pollution. The US$37/ton price may be low, as stated in the recent report from the National Academy of Sciences. A report in *Nature Climate Change* by researchers at Stanford University estimated a cost of US$220/ton (Burke et al., 2015). Assuming the price of carbon pollution does increase (whether or not this is acknowledged by carbon-based energy advocates), the vast majority of climate scientists agree that delays in reducing emissions of greenhouse gases will only increase the expense of environmental and public health damages and make those impacts more expensive to mitigate.

What is remarkable about the hostility to the SCC by many politicians and many industry groups is that it may be completely misdirected. As noted in the Yale paper (Wibhey, 2015), a 2014 study for the Brookings Institution looked at 53 regulations using the SCC. It concluded that only about 14% of the net benefits from those regulations were from reducing carbon dioxide, and "weighing the social cost of carbon tipped the scales in favor of a different policy in only about one in every eight rule-making scenarios." The study concluded that the SCC will need to be much higher for it to have much effect. "It has nowhere near the power of a carbon tax, a cap-and-trade scheme, or any other true, systematic "price on carbon." (Wihbey, 2015). A *cap-and-trade system* caps the total amount of greenhouse gas emissions and allows industries with lower emissions to sell their extra credits to larger emitters. It is often considered a market-based mechanism to reduce emissions. In contrast, a *carbon tax* sets a price on carbon directed on the carbon content of fossil fuels. In other words, cap-and-trade focuses on quantifying emission reductions, while a carbon tax focuses on price with the goal of driving a decrease in emissions. Both are macro policies to reduce emissions largely regardless of source.

In contrast, SCC models are more indirect tools that are designed to analyze the costs and benefits of proposed regulations that focus on a specific source of emissions. The SCC models are not designed to reduce emissions directly, or to establish a price for emissions, although either may be a welcome co-benefit. At the same time, in countries that pride themselves on the implementation of regulations or pricing strategies that are cost-effective, the SCC metrics, when accurate, are indispensable in dealing with an array of topics such as power plant efficiency or fuel efficiency or any number of other technologies where choices can be made about regulatory approaches to cost-effective greenhouse gas emissions. Even if carbon taxes were imposed or a cap-and-trade

system adopted, there would still be a need for sector-specific regulations on energy efficiency or similar topics to assure the public that the regulations are pragmatic and efficient and likely to make a difference in reducing greenhouse gas emissions.

A leading effort to update the SCC calculations comes from one of its originators in the Obama administration, the economist Michael Greenstone, who is now the director of both the Becker-Friedman Institute for Research in Economics and the Energy Policy Institute of Chicago, and works with Climate Impact Lab, a recent multi-university collaborative. Climate Impact Lab is leading an effort to improve the SCC by using detailed data from 25 000 regions of the world through measuring climate impacts on mortality, labor, energy demand, crop yields, migration, and crime. Along with many others, Greenstone believes that data-driven numbers can inform better regulatory decisions and policy outcomes (McMahon, 2017).

Unlike the current US administration, most of the rest of the world is committed to implementing the Paris Agreement, which is an agreement within the United Nations Framework Convention on Climate Change (UNFCCC) proposed to become effective in 2020. The Paris Agreement deals with greenhouse gas emissions, climate adaptation, and financing. It proposes to limit global warming to 2°C this century. Nearly 200 nations participated in the negotiations and the agreement was adopted by consensus in late 2015. The Agreement provides that each country determine its own greenhouse gas reductions in order to mitigate global warming. While critics argue that the Agreement is not enforceable or aggressive enough, defenders point to the fact that it is another tangible step forward on a global basis to address climate change (Kingo, 2016). Although the USA has officially and unilaterally announced its intention to withdraw from the Agreement, the other 19 countries of the Group of 20 (G20) reiterated their support at the July, 2017, meeting in Hamburg, Germany. Many industrialized nations have adopted carbon pricing strategies of their own, and many have reduced emissions on a per capita basis more than the USA. In fact, according to the Carbon Dioxide Information Analysis Center, the primary climate change data analysis of the US Department of Energy, the USA trailed Germany, Sweden, Italy, France, and the UK in decreasing emissions from 1990 to 2014 (Drum, 2017). Altogether, more than 40 nations already use some form of carbon pricing, with more planning to implement them in the future. These carbon pricing mechanisms cover about 50% of the emissions from these nations, or about 13% of annual global greenhouse gas emissions (World Bank, 2017)

12.4 Current Challenges to Reducing and Mitigating the Effects of Climate Change

The two most important dates in the early months of the new US administration on the topic of climate change were March 28, 2017, and June 2, 2017. On March 28, the White House issued an executive order that seeks to unravel years of progress in federal climate policies and could have immediate effects on federal agencies and the social cost of carbon approach to developing regulations. The executive order, *Promoting Energy Independence and Economic Growth*, disbands the Interagency Working Group that developed the SCC for use in developing federal regulations. It also withdrew all of the technical reports related to the SCC. Instead, the executive order replaces the SCC with a former cost-benefit approach used during the administration of George W. Bush, which is more of a guidance document that allows agencies to develop their own metrics to assess the climate impacts of proposed regulations and far less specific in requiring a uniform analytical metric as did the SCC. The order does not completely eliminate cost-benefit analyses, but it could lead to the use

of a greater discount rate (to reduce the future value of emission reductions), and it could also lead to focusing on the effects of emissions only in the USA, as if such emissions do not have a global effect. The Clinton-era executive order requiring cost-benefit analyses remains in place. Then, on June 2, the White House announced that the USA would withdraw from the Paris climate agreements, a declaration that has left much of the world astonished and appalled. Experts are debating the technical issues involved in such a "withdrawal" since the prescribed process for withdrawing could take most of the remainder of the current four-year term of office. Even if the withdrawal does not have immediate effect, and is yet another in a long series of anti-climate change bromides from the current administration, it effectively removes the USA from its global leadership role in environmental protection with potential negative effects, not only for the planet, but for the US economy as well.

It is worth noting that the administration's efforts to unravel most of the previous work on climate change, including eroding the social cost of carbon calculations, has raised questions about the overall cost-benefit analysis of that ongoing effort. A very recent report by Columbia University's Sabin Center for Climate Change Law concluded that the benefits of the Obama-era rules to reduce greenhouse gas emissions would greatly exceed any costs, and result in close to $300 billion in net benefits per year that the current administration is abandoning (Rahman and Wentz, 2017). As a consequence of these two recent actions of the US government, many objective leaders in the international community and in the USA are struggling to understand the consequences and the best courses of action to further reduce greenhouse gas emissions. As of now, the international community seems to recognize that the USA has abdicated a leadership role in climate change policy and it seems clear that other nations, including the European Union and China, will try to fill the vacuum. Within the USA, states such as California, New York, and many others, as well as several major cities, will continue their efforts to reduce emissions. Recently, for example, the states of Colorado, Minnesota, and Illinois increased their regulatory costs of carbon in the context of their public utilities (Bade, 2017). Following successful litigation by environmental interests, Minnesota's price will be $43.06 by 2020 (Bade, 2017). Also, California extended its cap-and-trade program with super-majority votes in both houses.

However, there is no mistaking the fact that the current US administration has dealt the cause of climate change two major setbacks and set the tone for many others to come. It is also clearly the case that new and better information about climate change will become available, and that our ability to measure the economic impacts of these changes will also improve. Not everything can be quantified – that is not news. Moreover, climate scientists are the first to say that there is much about the full magnitude of climate change that we do not yet know. But on August 7, 2017, a final draft report from 13 federal agencies as part of the National Climate Assessment that was obtained by the *New York Times* concluded that even if emissions of greenhouse gases somehow stopped completely, the world would experience additional temperature increases ranging from 0.30 to 2.0°C in this century. The report also restated the scientific consensus that human activities are primarily responsible for "recently observed climate change," including more than half of the global mean temperature increase since 1951, and it reviewed the significant improvements that have been made in attributing some extreme weather events to climate change. It recommended not exceeding the limit in the Paris Agreement of a 2°C increase in global mean temperature (Friedman, 2017)

It may not be likely, but it is worth hoping that the current administration will channel its professed adherence to conservative economics and take a closer look at the benefits of a cost-benefit approach to climate change regulations. It is possible that the military's apparent influence in the current administration may represent a glimmer of hope since it has recognized the impacts of climate change on its mission for many years. Additionally, some federal courts have issued rulings that prohibit federal agencies from ignoring climate impacts of federally approved projects that may exceed the economic benefits of those projects. As reported by the Los Angeles Times, several coal mines and pipelines have been snagged in these lawsuits (Halper, 2017). Regulatory agencies need to act with intellectual rigor. Unless the present administration's plan is to jettison completely concerns about climate change, the appropriate federal agencies must comprehensively confront the totality of impacts and costs of what can be done in the USA to reduce emissions. In addition, they must do so transparently, in full view of Congress and the public. Lastly, the cost-benefit approach to climate change must be improved over time and must always be based on the best available science and economics. Is it wishful thinking to suggest that even conservatives and market adherents may want to know exactly how much carbon pollution harms the economy?

References

Aldrick, P. (2017). Global environment is heating up for fossil fuels and their producers. *The Times [London]* 15 July.

Bade, G. (2017). Minnesota regulators boost carbon cost estimates for utility planning. *Utility Dive* 28 July.

Baron, J. (2017a). How geographic boundaries determine the social costs of carbon. *The Regulatory Review* 17 January.

Baron, J. (2017b). The discount rate for the social cost of carbon. *The Regulatory Review* 18 January.

Burke, M., Hsiang, S.M., and Miguel, E. (2015). Global non-linear effect of temperature on economic production. *Nature* 527, 235–239.

Carbon Pricing Leadership Coalition (2017). *Report of the High Level Commission on Carbon Pricing*. Paris: CPLC, p. 3.

Center for Biological Diversity vs. National Highway Transportation Safety Administration (2007). 538 F. 2nd 1172, 9th Circuit.

Davenport, C. (2016). Carbon pricing becomes a cause for the World Bank and I.M.F. *The New York Times* 23 April.

Drum, K. (2017). The US brings up the rear when it comes to reducing carbon emissions. *Mother Jones* 1 June.

EPA (Environmental Protection Agency) (2015). *Fact Sheet, The Social Cost of Carbon*. Washington, DC: EPA.

Fan, V.Y., Jamison, D.T., and Summers, L.H. (2016). The inclusive cost of pandemic influenza risk. Working Paper 22137. Cambridge, MA: National Bureau of Economic Research. Available at: http://www.nber.org/papers/w22137 (accessed July 15, 2017).

Friedman, L. (2017). Scientists fear Trump will dismiss blunt climate report. *New York Times* 7 August.

Halper, E. (2017). Trump's push to ignore climate costs generates a backlash in court, slowing some projects. *Los Angeles Times* 4 October.

IMF (International Monetary Fund) (2015). How large are global energy subsidies? IMF Working Paper. Washington, DC: IMF.

Jina, A. (2017). The $200 billion fossil fuel subsidy you've never heard of. *Forbes* 1 February.

Kingo, L. (2016). Executive Update: Setting a $100 price on carbon. United Nations Global Compact News. Available at: https://www.unglobalcompact.org/

news/3361-04-22-2016 (accessed May 10, 2017).

McMahon, J. (2017). How markets beat other policies at tackling the energy-climate change problem. *Forbes* 3 August.

National Academy of Sciences (2017). *Valuing Climate Damages: Updating Estimation of the Social Cost of Carbon Dioxide*. Washington, DC: National Academy of Sciences.

NRDC (Natural Resources Defense Council) (2011). Health and climate change, accounting for costs. *Health Facts* November.

Rahman, N. and Wentz, J. (2017). The price of climate deregulation: adding up the costs and benefits of Federal greenhouse gas emission standards. Sabin Center for Climate Change Law, Columbia Law School, pp. 1–14.

Revesz, R. (2017). Structural reforms to improve cost-benefit analyses of financial regulation. *The Regulatory Review* 7 August.

Roston, E. (2016). Climate change may be doubted by some, but now it's the law. *Bloomberg* 11 August.

Than, K. (2015). Estimated social costs of climate change not accurate, Stanford scientists say. *Stanford News* 12 January.

Wihbey, J. (2015). Understanding the social cost of carbon and connecting it to our lives. *Yale Climate Connection* 12 February.

World Bank (2017). *Pricing Carbon*. Washington, DC: World Bank.

Yeh, S. (2017). Top scientists validate approach to climate policy-making. Natural Resources Defense Council. Available at: https://www.nrdc.org/experts/starla-yeh/top-scientists-validate-approach-climate-policy-making (accessed March 10, 2017).

Zero Zone, Inc. vs. United States Department of Energy (2016). 832 F. 3rd 654, 677, 7th Circuit.

13

Complex Problems, Progressive Policy Solutions, and One Health

John A. Herrmann

University of Illinois at Urbana-Champaign, Urbana, IL, USA

13.1 One Health as Prevention

For decades, we have known that prevention of disease, or of natural and man-made disasters, promotes and maintains health and saves societies financial and material resources (United States Surgeon General, 2011; World Bank, 1993; Horton and Lo, 2013). The Lancet Commission on Investing in Health predicted that the global investments required to reduce the mortality rates of poor countries to levels approximating those of rich countries in one generation will generate a return on investment in the range of US$9 to US$20 per dollar spent during the period from 2016 to 2035 (Jamison et al., 2013). When the intrinsic value of health is added to the calculation of the return on investment for preventive services, the total return is even higher (Clark, 2013). However, One Health is very complex, as can be seen in the chapters of this book, and diverse societies across the globe are not adept at policy-making that focuses on tackling difficult problems through prevention strategies. Responding to actual circumstances as they develop is less abstract, and easier to sell politically, than anticipating and deterring potential harmful outcomes. Societies, whether they are members of the Organization

for Economic Cooperation (OECD) or represent developing countries, have trouble allocating resources to prevention plans because there is, often, no obvious correlation between a prevention policy and that which *did not* occur due to that prevention policy. Response, mitigation, and recovery expenses can be readily cost-accounted; the calculus of ascribing *costs saved* to an event that never happened, less so. How much cost savings accrue to a community due a reduction in tobacco use? Can we monetize the value of biodiversity to agriculture? How can policy-makers connect a tax on sugared drinks to future healthcare costs? What are the true physical, social, mental, and economic costs of manufacturing consumer products, from automobiles to the smallest trinkets? Should economic growth be a goal for rich, developed countries or should economic sustainability and income equality supplant the economics of consumerism?

13.1.1 Successes

There have been some impressive successes from policies that recognize the One Health concept and are designed to conserve resources while improving health. Over the 15 years that the United Nations Millennium Development Goals (MDGs) of 2000 were

Beyond One Health: From Recognition to Results, First Edition.
Edited by John A. Herrmann and Yvette J. Johnson-Walker.

the overarching development framework for the world, much progress on many critical issues of human and environmental health was achieved (United Nations, 2015c). Some highlights are:

- The proportion of undernourished people in the developing regions has fallen by almost half since 1990, from 23.3% in 1990–1992 to 12.9% in 2014–2016.
- The literacy rate among youth aged 15 to 24 has increased globally from 83% to 91% between 1990 and 2015. The gap between women and men has narrowed.
- Many more girls are now in school compared to 15 years ago. The developing regions as a whole have achieved the target to eliminate gender disparity in primary, secondary, and tertiary education.
- Measles vaccination helped prevent nearly 15.6 million deaths between 2000 and 2013. The number of globally reported measles cases declined by 67% for the same period.
- Contraceptive prevalence among women aged 15 to 49, married or in a union, increased from 55% in 1990 worldwide to 64% in 2015.
- Between 2000 and 2013, tuberculosis prevention, diagnosis, and treatment interventions saved an estimated 37 million lives. The tuberculosis mortality rate fell by 45% and the prevalence rate by 41% between 1990 and 2013.
- Of the 2.6 billion people who have gained access to improved drinking water since 1990, 1.9 billion gained access to piped drinking water on premises. Over half of the global population (58%) now enjoys this higher level of service.
- Worldwide, 2.1 billion people have gained access to improved sanitation. The proportion of people practicing open defecation has fallen almost by half since 1990.

Improvement in nutrition, increased vaccination rates, decreased prevalence of tuberculosis, and more access to clean water and sanitation, are all One Health issues. Capitalizing on this progress, the United

Nations (UN), in late 2015, established the 17 Sustainable Development Goals (SDGs), the "next steps" on the path to ending poverty while protecting the planet. In a Resolution adopted by the UN General Assembly on September 25, 2015, the SDGs were formalized, to begin on January 1, 2016, under the banner, "Transforming our world: the 2030 Agenda for Sustainable Development" (United Nations, 2015a).

The focus of the 17 SDGs on "meeting the needs of the present without compromising the ability of future generations to meet their own needs," is essential One Health thinking. Although it can be argued that not all of the SDGs reflect the One Health concept, a number are striking in their alignment with the human:animal:ecosystem health triad:

- Zero hunger.
- Good health and well-being.
- Clean water and sanitation.
- Affordable and clean energy.
- Sustainable cities and communities.
- Responsible consumption and production.
- Climate action.
- Life below water.
- Life on land.

Implied within the SDGs is a focus on food safety and security, another example of a global success story and covered in Chapter 3. Food safety policy is an example of international cooperation: effective surveillance systems and market forces work in concert to prevent food-borne illnesses while not running counter to the economic viability of food-producing or food-importing countries (United Nations, 2015b).

13.1.2 Failures

On the other hand, the multi-decade attempt to reform the USA's healthcare system is a good example of a failure of using One Health principles in policymaking. The USA is the only OECD country that does not have an integrated and universal healthcare access and payment system. The US healthcare system is based mostly on fee-for-service specialist providers and for-profit payers, usually healthcare insurance companies, and it spends almost two-and-a-half times more on healthcare than the OECD member country mean, with average or below average population health outcomes (OECD, 2017; Squires and Anderson, 2015). When looking at spending for prevention, the USA fares no better. Comparing healthcare spending to social service outlay, broadly defined, the USA is the only OECD country that spends more on healthcare than on social services. Indeed, as Bradley and Taylor (2013) state, "The academic literature is unequivocal about the importance of what is referred to as the 'social determinants of health', such as housing, education, income, occupation, environmental contacts, lifestyle and other similar exposures." In other words, allocating resources to prevention programs now lessens the need for healthcare expenditures later, with improved health along the way.

If prevention, in the form of policies designed to address social, biological, chemical, and physical determinants of health, is recognized as essential to improving human health outcomes while making more efficient use of resources, then why does the USA continue to lag behind its peer countries on social service spending? The reasons for the inability of the USA to improve the access and quality of its healthcare system, while containing costs, are myriad and too complicated to address in this chapter. But among them are the country's foundational beliefs, such as self-reliance and individualism; the belief that disease, and health, are individual choices that are best addressed in a one-to-one relationship with a healthcare provider; a staunch mistrust of a central government and "socialized" medicine; and the mistaken belief that the current healthcare system is consistent with free market philosophies. In describing the consequences of these attitudes, Bradley et al. (2016) suggested that, "There seems to be something uniquely American about spending more on health care and getting less health." Too often, the US healthcare system devolves into what Schneider and Squires

(2017) describe as "very expensive acute care 'rescue' services." Adopting such a narrow view of health, and the way to promote and recover it, is the antithesis of the One Health concept. Although human healthcare appears to be a particularly human endeavor, it remains part of the triad of One Health. The ecosystem, including both the natural world and the built environment, in which most humans reside is made up of multiple risks and determinants that affect human and animal health and that must be understood in their relationship to each other. Only when those One Health principles are recognized will US policy-makers appreciate that the true conservative approach to healthcare is to realize that health is a basic human right and that universal access to affordable, quality healthcare will, in the long term, save lives, improve quality of life, and conserve essential resources.

13.2 Translating Science: Risk Communication and Science Literacy

The successes of the UN MDGs and other initiatives, the eradication of smallpox and rinderpest, the near eradication of poliomyelitis, the dramatic decrease in mortality due to HIV/AIDS, and the improvement in the prevention of human rabies cases stand in stark contrast to the failure of healthcare reform in the USA, the pernicious persistency of the anti-vaccine movement, and the obstinacy of those who put carbon-based energy generation profits over clean energy innovation. Successes reflect progressive thinking based on critical evaluation of data and a recognition of the primacy of prevention strategies in improving the physical, social, mental, and economic health of communities. Many failures indicate fossilized attitudes based on ideology and short-term economic self-interest taking precedence over careful consideration of evidence and a disregard for the need to conserve resources to promote health and alleviate suffering. Successes in global health represent effective public policy drawn from collaborations between informed individuals, community focused non-governmental entities, and governments that recognize that they work for the people rather than for their own interests and are willing to work cooperatively across boundaries of geography, subject matter, species, politics, philosophy, and perspective. How do societies foster such collaborations?

There seem to be three areas that might promote effective public health policy:

- Communication of science findings, especially health science, to the public in an accurate, readily accessible, and understandable form.
- A liberal education for all, beginning in primary grades, that puts science literacy as one of the centerpieces of curricula ("liberal education" meaning broad based – including sciences, critical thinking, intellectual traditions, art, music, history, literature, ethics, etc.).
- Community empowerment and participatory democracy.

13.2.1 Communication of Science

It is not uncommon, when confronted with conflicting findings from multiple studies, for nonscientists to believe that science is equivocal and that scientific "truth" is malleable and elusive. This is not surprising: unless individuals are broadly educated in the liberal arts and trained in science, technology, engineering, or mathematics (STEM) disciplines, few understand the iterative nature of scientific inquiry. In attempting to explain to community groups over the past decades why, for example, one study will conclude that coffee consumption is beneficial to health, to be contradicted a short time later by another study that reports the opposite, the author has described a pendulum, driven by the knowledge acquired from science research. Early in the process of science,

when preliminary studies are published, the amplitude of the pendulum is very long, with conflicting results driving the arc 90 degrees in each direction, tracing a semicircle. Subsequent studies attempt to answer the questions that arise from previous work and each iteration serves as a basis for new questions to be generated, and answered, by even more studies. As the repetitive process of science proceeds, the amplitude of the pendulum's swing decreases with successive studies, until the pendulum describes an arc that is very short and centered on the equilibrium point of what can be considered scientific certainty.

Another analogy that has been used is that of a scale, similar to the scale of justice, with the weight of evidence on both sides of a question equilibrating with subsequent studies on a specific topic until balance, in the form of a reasonable degree of scientific certainty, is achieved. Often that balance can be achieved through a systematic review of the literature or through the process of meta-analyses.

Compounding the public's frustration with early, often disparate results on many topics is the expeditious availability, through internet publication, of journal articles that were previously accessible only by subscribers to science journals. Journal articles are often reviewed by traditional and nontraditional news outlets alike, with varying degrees of competence. Often the results are presented as "science lite," with no context of the nature of the study design, the quality of the methodology, the listing of limitations, or a discussion of the external validity of the findings. Schoenfeld and Ioannidis (2013) found, in their review of nutritional epidemiology, that although implausibly strong associations have been claimed for most food ingredients and cancer risk, the evidence was weak and the effect size shrunk through meta-analyses. Access to science research in an open format, as on the internet, is a boon to transparency but most readers need a guide, a public educator, to help them understand the significance of published findings.

Julia Belluz, a former Knight Science Journalism Fellow at the Massachusetts Institute of Technology and a National Magazine Award-winning journalist covering medicine and public health, explained a number of reasons why science is difficult to cover and translate into sensible reading for the public:

1) The sheer volume of science research is difficult to evaluate. From 1985 to 2010 there was a 300% increase in the number of published medical studies.
2) Journalists often don't put the latest studies into context, suggesting that the most recent research holds definitive answers.
3) Media "hype" in science is on the rise and journalists are pressured to produce internet "hits" that are measurable in online newsrooms.
4) Research is often difficult to interpret and it takes time to do so, which puts writers up against deadlines.
5) Health science evolves slowly (the iterative process) and breakthroughs are rare; talking about the methodical accretion of evidence is not news (Belluz, 2016).

Among her many suggestions to achieve better communication of science to the public, she suggests that journalists need better training in study design and research methods. Others have made a compelling case for teaching science literacy, specifically an understanding of One Health concepts, across university curricula and promoting collaborations among seemingly disparate professions to improve overall health.

13.2.2 Liberal Education and the Sciences

Among the many definitions of liberal education, some common themes emerge: empowerment of individuals to learn; preparation to deal with complexity, diversity, and change; development of a broad knowledge base (of science, culture, history, etc.) underpinning specific areas of study; recognition of social responsibility; and acquisition of skills, such as communication, analytical thinking, and problem solving, transferable to real-world settings. These are wide-ranging goals that were described by the Association of American Colleges and Universities (AACU) when they launched their Liberal Education and America's Promise (LEAP) program in 2005. The program recognized the need for broadly educated students to contribute, and compete, in a rapidly changing world, one that is dependent on technological innovations and scientific advances, faced with a changing nature of work, and reliant upon democratic vitality (https://aacu.org/leap/what-is-a-liberal-education). Rowe (2017) recently wrote that "Citizens need training in skills beyond those that will enable them to earn a living. Widespread availability of liberal education is an essential component of any society that seeks to sustain democratic institutions."

Schneider (2004) includes citizenship as integral to a liberal education, structuring it around three major themes: inquiry and intellectual judgment; social responsibility and civic engagement; and integrative and culminating learning. Additionally, Caryn Tighe Musil of the Association of American Colleges and Universities states that "educating for democratic citizenship is understood not simply as an extra-curricular option, but as a fundamental goal of a twenty-first century liberal education" (Musil, 2003).

Another take on liberal education is the concept of "confluent education," which Brown described as the dynamic process that is required to solve complex problems in real life, capitalizing on the confluence of knowledge, attitudes, behaviors, and experiences that animate inquiry and intentional action (Brown, 1971; Peloquin, 2002; Hackbarth, 1997). The focus is not only on knowledge gleaned from formal, often didactic, education, but also on the individuals' abilities to self-discover and construct knowledge, and the interaction of the two.

It follows that scientific literacy, specifically, is more about the ideas behind hard facts rather than the facts themselves, more about processes that generated, and can generate, new facts instead of facts that are simply remembered, or looked up, and restated for exams. In the supporting documents for LEAP, the former Chairman and CEO of Lockheed-Martin, Norman Augustine, is quoted, "So what does business need from our educational system? One answer is that it needs more employees who excel in science and engineering and the remainder of a workforce that is exposed to enough science and mathematics to function in the rapidly evolving high-tech world. And who wants a technology driven economy when those who drive it are not grounded in such fields as ethics?" (https://aacu.org/leap/what-is-a-liberal-education). Real, lifelong scientific literacy comes from being able to think critically about data, assemble a broad base of knowledge, recognize the interrelatedness of seemingly disparate topics, and put that knowledge into an ethical framework.

In 2003, the Institutes of Medicine (IOM) produced their pivotal report "Who Will Keep the Public Healthy? Educating Public Health Professionals for the 21st Century" (IOM, 2003). Among the report's conclusions were:

- "A variety of forces – among them globalization, technologic and scientific advances, and rapid demographic shifts – are hastening the need to refocus attention and resources away from traditional biomedical efforts toward those of population health."
- "The ecological model recognizes accumulating evidence that the health of individuals and the community is determined relatively little by health care per se and far more by multiple other factors, and by their interactions."
- "Clearly demonstrated was the need for public health and health care sectors to be better able to characterize and communicate risk and uncertainty."
- "Public health professionals will need to apply new approaches to research, approaches that involve practitioners, researchers, and the community in joint efforts to improve health and to understand global health issues that increasingly transcend national boundaries."
- "All undergraduates should have access to education in public health."

Over the past decade, there has been a significant increase in the number of undergraduate programs in public health. Many have embraced One Health as an integral part of their curriculum. One in particular, at the University of Illinois at Chicago, School of Public Health, has incorporated One Health as one of the six "Curricular Themes" that bring core content into confluence, "promoting coherence within and across courses along the entire educational sequence." Karin Opacich, the visionary Director and lead developer of the program, advocated for seven "Overarching Curricular Goals," which were later adopted, and which guide the program (Box 13.1).

Key words and phrases embedded in these goals are "nuanced," "world view," "expansive view of health," "informed," "critical and analytical thinking," "communicate," "astute," and "educated consumers of health information." The principles of epidemiology, recognized as the first science of public health, serve as the basis for not only an introductory course in epidemiology but also a two-course sequence in critical thinking. Within those two courses are extensive, student-centered instruction on study design, survey development, the hierarchy of evidence, analysis of selected public health journal articles, Bloom's taxonomy of educational objectives, and the logical fallacies commonly employed in argumentation, especially in discussion of public policy. The curriculum is designed to help students recognize the strengths and limitations of study design and methodology, assess the quality of data, evaluate the significance of results and their applicability to real world populations, and communicate findings in an effective manner to a community audience.

A recommendation has been made to extend training in epidemiology and public

---

Box 13.1 Overarching curricular goals in public health education at the University of Illinois at Chicago

The overarching goals of the University of Illinois at Chicago baccalaureate curriculum in public health are to produce citizens who will:

1) Rise to the challenge of understanding the world in a nuanced way expressing a broad world view and an expansive view of health.
2) Be informed, attuned, and energized advocates of health accepting individual responsibility to effect positive change.
3) Demonstrate skill in critical and analytical thinking.

4) Communicate effectively both orally and in writing with a variety of audiences.
5) Be sensitive and astute observers.
6) Commit to being educated consumers of health information.
7) Apply skills and tools acquired to an array of roles in the realm of employment contributing directly or indirectly to public health.

Source: http://publichealth.uic.edu/bachelor-of-arts/curricular-goals-and-themes

---

health beyond those students who elect to major in public health. In their report, "The Educated Citizen and Public Health: A Consensus Report on Public Health and Undergraduate Education," the Council of Colleges of Arts and Sciences (CCAS) (Riegelman et al, 2007) commented on the intellectual value of integrating training in public health across undergraduate majors: it involves critical thinking and decision-making; it gives students a methodology for understanding populations; and it demonstrates that population-scale thinking relies on multiple disciplines. Similarly, the CCAS recommended that epidemiology "has evolved into a discipline that can and should be viewed as an integral part of a general and liberal education." Among the many benefits that the CCAS anticipates with such training are: critical thinking based on the application of statistical theory and quantitative literacy; understanding of the scientific method and using that understanding to inform evidence-based arguments of public policy; recognizing risk factors and being able to assess underlying causes of communicable and noncommunicable diseases of the individual and of populations.

Public health and epidemiology courses and minors invite students to take socially responsible steps and to provide valuable

direction for career choices. Considering the magnitude of world health problems and the diversity of societies and cultures, public health minors help students to focus on solutions, to be sensitive to differences and aware of vulnerable populations, and to be optimistic about world affairs. Through such programs, colleges and universities address critical needs for an educated citizenry and foster leadership development.

Riegelman et al., 2007.

Chaddock, recognizing that One Health principles are based on the population focus of public health and that epidemiology is the first science of One Health, issued a call to action for universities to incorporate One Health principles across disciplines long thought to be unrelated, from agriculture and architecture to urban planning and water security (Box 13.2).

Communicating science findings in an effective and efficient manner, to the widest and most broadly educated audience possible, and educating undergraduate students in the principles of public health and epidemiology, and by association, One Health, would set the stage for operationalizing One Health thinking into public policy. However, another missing piece is empowered communities that can engage in participatory democracy.

Box 13.2 One Health and an educated citizenry

Now is the time for academic institutions to step forward in leading new One Health initiatives to create impactful, relevant research-driven solutions and train the next generation of innovative leaders. One Health concepts are ideally suited to provide robust, system-wide health-related solutions that the global society will need and expect. There is an enormous unrealized potential for all schools/colleges on a campus or amongst campuses to collaborate and leverage their strengths to solve many of society's most important One Health issues, such as prevention and treatment of obesity in humans and animals, infectious and zoonotic diseases that threaten global peace and security, healthcare costs and the need to adopt wellness programs, and safe and nutritious food and water for the world's growing population –to name just a few.

Universities with transdisciplinary programs have opportunities to take leadership positions by being at the forefront of One Health education. Educational "business as usual" will be for followers; an action-oriented sense of urgency will be created by futuristic educational leaders. One Health concepts fit easily in the curricula of health-related professions; although, it may be a bit more challenging to incorporate these concepts into the curricula of other schools/colleges because they are not thought of in an intuitive manner. This is a challenge, but once conquered it yields so many benefits for students and society.

One Health concepts and case studies could effectively be incorporated into current curricula, with examples and impacts discussed in teaching models, assignments, and high-impact projects throughout many disciplines including those outside the traditional health sectors. Unique opportunities exist for the integration and incorporation of One Health-related concepts throughout the undergraduate, graduate, and professional programs; in other words integrate One Health concepts throughout the University curriculum, where appropriate.

At the heart of the One Health initiative is the role of engaging students in educational opportunities around a team concept. It is important to identify opportunities whereby teaching students from various disciplines and colleges can form teams. Team approaches involving people with different, yet complementary skills and experiences provide synergy in addressing complex, important societal needs. It is essential that students learn how to work collaboratively with colleagues across professions to address important societal issues involving health and well-being.

One Health transdisciplinary, high-impact education, experiential plans are ambitious and innovative, and may include: a certificate program; undergraduate learning community; new curricula for master's and doctorate degrees with students from varying disciplines learning together; "core" One Health fundamentals online course; university-wide seminars; summer research exchange programs; externships with highly regarded research faculty members; federal government summer transdisciplinary team externships; international transdisciplinary programs and teams with global partners; and One Health/one classroom with students from various disciplines learning together. Students are keen to explore not only new knowledge, but also new models of learning and collaboration.

Faculty ask if they are going to be recognized and rewarded for working in transdisciplinary collaborative teams. They indicate that this is not the culture for the University. However, given the right encouragement, recognition, and academic credit, faculties are poised to deliver.

Mike Chaddock, Michigan State University

13.2.3   Community Empowerment and Participatory Democracy

The value of science to a republican people, the security it gives to liberty by enlightening the minds of its citizens, the protection it affords against foreign power, the virtue it inculcates, the just emulation of the distinction it confers on nations foremost in it; in short, its identification with power, morals, order and happiness (which merits to it premiums of encouragement rather than repressive taxes), are considerations [that should] always [be] present and [bear] with their just weight.

Thomas Jefferson, on the book duty, 1821

In his address to the American Psychological Society in 1980, Rappaport (1981) described the conceptual paradox of prevention and empowerment: *prevention*, he claimed, is an extension of a "needs model" in which a community becomes a client for those with expertise who define community deficiencies and formulate programmatic solutions; *empowerment*, instead, implies that many competencies are already present within communities and may be operationalized to solve community issues if resources are available. In his view, prevention implies doing something "to" a community from outside, whereas empowerment allows a community to develop their own solutions from within. However, this view puts health educators and health promotion planners in an awkward position. How can a community become fully empowered when the knowledge base of what works to improve the health, as broadly defined previously, of a community is unavailable to them except through consultation with those with experience and expertise from outside of the community?

Wallerstein and Bernstein (1994) expanded upon the concept of empowerment by asking what the role of health educators is within the prevention-empowerment dialectic. They suggested that health educators serve a "resource and help create favorable conditions and opportunities for people to share in community dialogue and change efforts" and to "engage in the empowerment process as partners in the learning process."

From 1997 to 2001, the National Association of County and City Health Officials (NACCHO), in collaboration with the Centers for Disease Control and Prevention (CDC), used this expanded concept of community empowerment as the basis for the development of the Mobilizing for Action through Planning and Partnerships (MAPP), a community-wide strategic planning framework for improving public health. The MAPP model acknowledges that a community's health is a "what we as a society do collectively to assure the conditions in which people can be healthy" (NACCHO, 2008). MAPP is based on collective community participation and decision-making, the understanding that community solutions to challenges best come from within the community, and that many entities, from police and fire services to health providers and social agencies, provides public health services within a community.

Through the MAPP process, communities can create and implement a well-coordinated plan that uses resources efficiency and effectively. Community involvement throughout the creation and the implementation of a health improvement plan results in creative solutions to public health problems. Moreover, continuous community involvement leads to community ownership of the process. Community ownership, in turn, increases the credibility and sustainability of health improvement effort.

NACCHO, 2008.

Horton and Lo (2013) captured the potential tension between outside experts, funding agencies, and community partners in developing nations: "What a country wants is not a series of new donor-driven initiatives. It wants development partners to invest in a plan that has been devised by the country itself, one that meets the country's unique needs. Too many partners pay only lip service to the wishes of the countries, launching initiatives that do not put countries and their peoples at the centre of each stage of discussion and planning." The authors describe six institutional functions that must be satisfied to assure that investments are used efficiently and effectively to achieve the goals set by the community; institutions for: information; policy deliberation; finance; stewardship; normative standards and best practices; and independent assessment.

Implied within the community empowerment models and their practical application is the idea that all individuals have a right to education, access to information, autonomy and self-determination, and that the strength of a community lies within the recognition of those rights. And to fully consider the One Health aspects and implications of policy decisions, people must have a chance for self-determination through, among other opportunities, education, property rights, suffrage, and reproductive autonomy. In 1948, in the aftermath of two World Wars, the United Nations issued the Universal Declaration of Human Rights (United Nations, 1948) as a common standard for fundamental human rights to be universally protected. Among them are equal dignity and rights of men and women; the right to own property; freedom of thought and expression; a right to a standard of living adequate to well-being; and the right to education. Although progress has been made, the World Bank (2013) delineated five policy priorities needed to ensure gender equality, economic benefit, and community development:

- Reduce the excess mortality of girls and women.
- Shrink education gaps.
- Broaden women's access to economic opportunity.
- Diminish gender differences in household and societal environments.
- Limit intergenerational inequality over time.

Similarly, Revenga and Shetty (2012) reported that improving gender equality has broad economic impact, leading to more women in the workforce, higher wages for girls and women, greater educational attainment, lower adolescent and adult pregnancy, and lower maternal and childhood mortality. The University of Wisconsin, through their "Women and One Health" program, recognized the critical roles in many cultures that women and girls play in food and water security, their family economics, and the overall well-being of their communities (https://4w. wisc.edu/project/women-and-one-health/). Healthy communities with a vibrant, participatory civil society depend on the empowerment of women and One Health approaches that make agriculture more sustainable and promote the health of humans, animals, and the ecosystem.

In their 2008 report, "Contributing to One World, One Health," the Food and Agriculture Organization of the UN reiterated the key role of women in maintaining the health of family and animals. Since women in many developing nations are commonly marginalized from support services, a community-based, bottoms-up approach is necessary for effective infectious disease surveillance for humans and animals (FAO, 2008). A recent study, using data from 173 countries and covering the period from 1990 to 2012, suggested that a country can only achieve a high functioning participatory democracy through the guarantee of equal rights, in all aspects of society, to both men and women (Wang et al., 2017).

13.3 The Economics of One Health

One Health is a conceptual framework to ensure that interdisciplinary collaboration and communication occurs among the private and public sectors concerned with human, animal, and ecosystem health. One Health, based on a holistic assessment of the conditions that determine the health of individuals and communities, should be the basis of disease prevention efforts and should inform policy at local, national, and international levels. But how does the cost-benefit analysis (CBA) play out?

The World Bank developed an extensive assessment of the economics of One Health, focusing on human, animal, and wildlife services and tasks such as surveillance, biosecurity, diagnostics, control (vaccination, hygiene), culling/compensation, training, and communication. Drawing primarily on public domain data from countries in sub-Saharan Africa, southern and eastern Asia, and Latin America, they calculated that the cost of a global, integrated One Health surveillance designed to bring the zoonotic disease prevention and control systems up to World Organization for Animal Health (OIE) and World Health Organization (WHO) standards ranged from US$1.9 billion per year to US$3.4 billion (World Bank, 2012). Although the costs for prevention and control strategies are significant, they are much less than the losses incurred in response to extensive outbreaks. The same World Bank study reported that the economic losses from six major outbreaks of zoonotic diseases from 1997 to 2009 totaled, at a minimum, US$80 billion. The costs, in 2015, of the recent Ebola epidemic, in Guinea, Sierra Leone, and Liberia have been estimated at US$2.2 billion in lost GDP for the three countries most affected, which is 17% of their combined 2015 GDP (Guinea, US$6.7 billion; Sierra Leone, US$4.2 billion; Liberia, US$2.1 billion) (https://data.worldbank.org/data-catalog/GDP-ranking-table). Additional costs for the global response to the crisis totaled another US$3.611 billion, bringing the total direct costs to over US$5.8 billion (United States Agency for International Development, 2015). And those costs do not account for losses in food security and increases in poverty rates due to loss of livestock and healthcare costs.

The devastating economic impact of epidemics is not confined to human contagion. The actual and estimated costs of the 2001 foot-and-mouth disease (FMD) in the UK totaled £1.4 billion in direct compensation to livestock owners, £1.3 billion for eradication efforts, £0.3 billion in other public expenses, £0.6 billion in private sector costs such as interruptions in the human food chain, and approximately £5.0 billion losses in the hospitality and tourism industries (National Audit Office, 2002). Although the zoonotic potential of FMD virus is minimal, its human health impact was reflected in an increase in psychological morbidity, primarily among livestock farmers directly affected and other rural workers in high FMD prevalence areas (Peck, 2005).

The World Bank study (2012) also estimated the annual expected return on investment for prevention activities, for 20%, 50%, and 100% reductions in outbreak impact, as ranging from 14% to 123%. The estimated percent savings for investment and recurring costs per activity ranged from 5% to 40 % for surveillance, biosecurity, and diagnostic and control measures.

As detailed in the chapters of this book on climate change, epidemiology, and emerging and infectious diseases, and in a large canon of peer-reviewed journal articles, the impact of climate change on infectious diseases, mostly through the expansion of vector ranges and changes in the vector-pathogen-host dynamic, has caused considerable concern. Altitudinal, latitudinal, seasonal, and inter-annual associations between climate change and infectious disease have been described (Patz et al., 2005; McMichael et al., 2006; Lafferty, 2009; Altizer et al., 2013). The long-term annual cost of climate change alone has been estimated to be in the range of 0.2–2% of global income. The annual cost of a pandemic, taking into account its impact on income (premature deaths to reduce the labor force, absenteeism, reduced productivity, trade and travel restrictions, social distancing) and the intrinsic value of lives prematurely lost and of illnesses suffered, has been estimated at US$570 billion, or 0.7% of global income (Fan et al., 2016). If indeed climate change and extreme weather events are and will be associated with an increase in large-scale infectious outbreaks, affecting humans or animals or both, the costs to respond, mitigate, and recover will be compounded.

13.4 From Here to There

Some years ago, in 1996, Hillary Clinton entitled her book, "It Takes a Village and Other Lessons that Children Teach Us." Despite the uncertain origins of the proverb that informed the title of the book, the recognition that community is often needed to solve difficult problems was welcomed by many workers and thinkers in public health. It takes a community to decrease the percentage of our populations that are overweight and obese; simplifying the issue to one of too many calories in and too

few calories out, is not only ineffective but also denies the strong associations of many social determinants and environmental exposures to the problem. It takes a community to provide a burgeoning global population an adequate supply of safe, wholesome, nutritious food, produced in a sustainable manner, at a reasonable cost to consumers and a reasonable return to producers in an environmentally safe, energy sustainable, and humane manner. It takes a community to recognize that we don't get to pollute the environment for our own financial gain; we borrow it from our children and grandchildren for its safekeeping. It takes a community to move from the recognition that we are all part of the One Health triad to the development of creative, evidence based, policy-driven results.

References

Altizer, S., Ostfeld, R.S., Johnson, P.T., Kutz, S., and Harvell, C.D. (2013). Climate change and infectious diseases: from evidence to a predictive framework. *Science* 341, 514–519.

Belluz, J. (2016). Health journalism has a serious evidence problem. Here's a plan to save it. *VOX* weblog post. Available at: https://www.vox.com/2016/6/21/11962568/health-journalism-evidence-based-medicine?curator=MediaREDEF (accessed June 13, 2017).

Bradley, E.H. and Taylor, L.A. (2013). *The American Health Care Paradox: Why Spending More Is Getting Us Less*. New York, NY: Public Affairs.

Bradley, E.H., Sipsma, H., and Taylor L.A. (2016). American health care paradox—high spending on health care and poor health. *QJM* 110(2), 61–65.

Brown, G.I. (1971). *Human Teaching for Human Learning: An Introduction to Confluent Education*. New York, NY: Viking.

Clark, H. (2013). Towards a more robust investment framework for health. *Lancet* 382, E36–37.

Fan, V.Y., Jamison, D.T., and Summers, L.H. (2016). The inclusive cost of pandemic influenza risk. Working Paper 22137. Cambridge, MA: National Bureau of Economic Research. Available at: http://www.nber.org/papers/w22137 (accessed December 14, 2017).

FAO (UN Food and Agriculture Organization) (2008). Contributing to One World, One Health. United Nations. Available at: http://www.fao.org/docrep/011/aj137e/aj137e00.htm (accessed 26 June, 2017).

Hackbarth, S. (1997). Reflections on confluent education as discipline-based inquiry. Paper presented at the Annual Meeting of the American Educational Research Association, Chicago, IL.

Horton, R. and Lo, S. (2013). Investing in health: why, what and three reflections. *Lancet* 382, 1859–1861.

IOM (Institute of Medicine, Committee for the Study of the Future of Public Health) (2003). *Who Will Keep the Public Healthy?* Washington, DC: National Academy Press.

Jamison, D.T., Summers, L.H., Alleyne, G., et al. (2013). Global health 2035: a world converging in a generation. *Lancet* 382, 1898–1955.

Lafferty, K.D. (2009). The ecology of climate change and infectious diseases. *Ecology* 90(4), 888–900.

McMichael, A.J., Woodruff, R.E., and Hales, S. (2006). Climate change and human health: present and future risks. *Lancet* 367, 859–869.

Musil, C.M. (2003). Educating for citizenship. *Peer Review* 5(3), 5.

NACCHO (National Association of County and City Health Officials) (2008). Mobilizing for Action through Planning and Partnerships. NACCHO Fact Sheet. Available at: http://www.naccho.org/uploads/downloadable-resources/Programs/Public-Health-Infrastructure/MAPP-factsheet-system-partners.pdf (accessed June 16, 2017).

National Audit Office (2002). *The 2001 Outbreak of Foot and Mouth Disease.* London: NAO. Available at: https://www.nao.org.uk/report/the-2001-outbreak-of-foot-and-mouth-disease/(accessed June 27, 2017).

OECD (Organization for Economic Cooperation and Development) (2017). OECD Health Statistics 2017. Available at: http://www.oecd.org/els/health-systems/health-data.htm (accessed May 15, 2017).

Patz, J.A., Campbell-Lendrum, D., Holloway, T., and Foley, J.A. (2005). Impact of regional climate change on human health. *Nature* 438, 310–317.

Peck, D.F. (2005). Foot and mouth outbreak: lessons for mental health services. *Advances in Psychiatric Treatment* 11, 270–276.

Peloquin, S.M. (2002). Confluence: Moving toward with affective strength. *American Journal of Occupational Therapy* 56, 69–77.

Rappaport, J. (1981). In praise of paradox: a social policy of empowerment over prevention. *American Journal of Community Psychology* 9(1), 1.

Revenga, A. and Shetty, S. (2012). Empowering women is smart economics. *Finance and Development* 49(1), 40–43.

Riegelman, R.K., Albertine, S., and Persily, N.A. (2007). The Educated Citizen and Public Health: A Consensus Report on Public Health and Undergraduate Education. Williamsburg, VA: Council of Colleges of Arts and Sciences. Available at: http://www.ccas.net/files/public/Publications/Public_Health_and_Undergraduate_Education.pdf (accessed June 15, 2017).

Rowe, S.C. (2017). Liberal education: cornerstone of democracy. *American Journal of Economic Sociology* 76, 579–617.

Schneider, C.G. (2004). Practicing liberal education: Formative themes in the re-invention of liberal learning. *Liberal Education* 90(2). Available at: https://aacu.org/publications-research/periodicals/practicing-liberal-education-formative-themes-re-invention-liberal (accessed May 15, 2017).

Schneider, E.C. and Squires, D. (2017). From last to first – Could the US health care system become the best in the world? *New England Journal of Medicine* 377, 901–904.

Schoenfeld, J.D. and Ioannidis, J.P.A. (2013). Is everything we eat associated with cancer? A systematic cookbook review. *American Journal of Clinical Nutrition* 97(1), 127–134.

Schultz, M. (2008). Rudolph Virchow. *Emerging Infectious Diseases* 14(9), 1480–1481.

Squires, D. and Anderson, C. (2015). US Healthcare from a global perspective: spending, use of services, prices and health in 13 countries. *Issue Brief (Commonwealth Fund)* 15, 1–15.

United Nations (1948). Universal Declaration of Human Rights. New York, NY: United Nations. Available at: http://www.un.org/en/universal-declaration-human-rights/(accessed June 25, 2017).

United Nations (2015a). Sustainable Development Goals. New York: United Nations. Available at: http://www.un.org/sustainabledevelopment/sustainable-development-goals/(accessed May 30, 2017).

United Nations (2015b). Resolution adopted by the General Assembly on 25 September 2015. New York: United Nations. Available at: http://www.un.org/ga/search/view_doc.asp?symbol=A/RES/70/1&Lang=E (accessed May 30, 2017).

United Nations (2015c). The Millennium Development Goals Report. New York: United Nations. Available at: http://www.un.org/millenniumgoals/2015_MDG_Report/pdf/MDG%202015%20rev%20(July%201).pdf (accessed May 30, 2017).

United States Agency for International Development (2015). West Africa – Ebola Outbreak: Fact Sheet #6, Fiscal Year (FY) 2016. Washington, DC: USAID. Available at: https://www.usaid.gov/sites/default/files/documents/1866/west_africa_fs07_01-21-2016.pdf (accessed June 27, 2017).

United States Surgeon General (2011). National Prevention Strategy. Washington, DC: National Prevention Council. Available at: https://www.surgeongeneral.gov/priorities/prevention/strategy/report.pdf (accessed May 15, 2017).

World Bank (1993). *World Development Report 1993: Investing in Health*. Washington, DC: World Bank and Oxford University Press.

World Bank (2012). People, Pathogens and Our Planet: The Economics of One Health. Washington, DC: World Bank. Available at: https://openknowledge.worldbank.org/handle/10986/11892 (accessed June 26, 2017).

World Bank (2013). Economic Development = Equal Rights for Women? Washington, DC: World Bank. Available at: http://www.worldbank.org/en/news/feature/2013/09/24/Economic-Development-Equal-Rights-for-Women (accessed June 25, 2017).

Wallerstein, N. and Bernstein, E. (1994). Introduction to community empowerment, participatory education and health. *Health Education Quarterly* 21(2), 141–148.

Wang, Y.T., Lindenfors, P., Sundström, A., Jansson, F., Paxton, P., and Lindberg, S.L. (2017). Women's rights in democratic transitions: A global sequence analysis, 1900–2012. *European Journal of Political Research* doi:10.1111/1475-6765.12201.

Section 3

Conclusion

14

The Long and Winding Road

John A. Herrmann and Yvette J. Johnson-Walker

University of Illinois at Urbana-Champaign, Urbana, IL, USA

14.1 One Health: Many Facets, All Interrelated

The concept of One Health is not simply about infectious diseases spilling over from animals to humans. It is about the understanding that all "health" – physical, emotional, social, financial, mental – is related to our natural and built environments, whether those environments are pristine, sparsely populated, "wild" areas or crowded urban communities. This holistic view of health and its determinants was captured by Gaylord Nelson, the US Senator who led the Earth Day movement in the USA, in 1970:

> Some people who talk about the environment talk about it as though it involved only a question of clean air and clean water. The environment involves the whole broad spectrum of man's relationship to all other living creatures, including other human beings. It involves the environment in its broadest and deepest sense. It involves the environment of the ghetto which is the worst environment, where the worst pollution, the worst noise, the worst housing, the worst situation in this country – that has to be a critical part of our concern and consideration in talking and cleaning up the environment.
>
> *Gaylord Nelson, April 19, 1970.*

In the preceding chapters of this book, authors presented the scientific consensus on many different topics and offered several general policy ideas to resolve some of the "sticky" problems that we, as global citizens, face.

The chapters on climate change (Chapter 2) and the social cost of carbon (Chapter 12) recognized the anthropogenic nature of climate change and the health impacts already seen, especially within the most vulnerable of communities, associated with the global rise in temperatures and the resultant extreme weather events. Policy designs to mitigate the health and economic costs of climate change reflect technological innovation (alternative energy, smart grids, micro grids, improvements in energy efficiency of consumer durables), development of economic incentives (carbon taxes and cap and trade programs), incorporation of externalized costs of energy production into federal and state policy (social costs of carbon), and participation in international agreements that prioritize all of the above (Paris Agreement). Essential to all of these policy plans is the need to work with market forces to achieve desired ends. The creation of environmental-economic "win-win" situations is the most effective and most rapid way to change corporate, community, and

Beyond One Health: From Recognition to Results, First Edition.
Edited by John A. Herrmann and Yvette J. Johnson-Walker.

individual behaviors and to protect our environments from further harm, create meaningful work for people, mitigate existing damage, and provide the conditions in which all people can be healthy.

The chapters on epidemiology (Chapter 1), emerging infectious diseases (Chapter 7), the health impacts of companion animal ownership (Chapter 8), and financing health agencies (Chapter 11) support the need for an enhanced, integrated One Health surveillance system: one that collects, correlates, and analyzes real-time data from human, domestic animal, and wild animal populations, while incorporating environmental data such as weather, geography, and potential chemical and physical exposures. This will be difficult to accomplish but those challenges should not be insurmountable. We need not only increased funding for surveillance but also improved communication about the value of surveillance, its analysis and its findings, to the most vulnerable populations and to policy-makers. In 2015, Uchtmann et al. wrote:

For the future, we propose using needed outcomes for health and sustainability to set priorities for One Health programs of education, surveillance, and stewardship. Professionals and paraprofessionals should gather, interpret, and widely communicate the implications of data, not only on infectious diseases, but also on toxic agents, malnutrition, ecological damage, the grave impacts of warfare, societal drivers underlying these problems, and the effectiveness of specific countermeasures.

The same authors recommended nine policies to enhance One Health surveillance:

1) Unify vocabularies – across ecosystems, etiologic agents, health outcomes, social and economic determinants, political drivers and countermeasures employed.
2) Establish mandated reporting of complex One Health stressors.
3) Provide accessible laboratory capabilities, especially gaining access to private laboratory accessions and results.
4) Establish disease surveillance, disease reporting, and best management practices in animal healthcare as prerequisites for insurance, indemnity, and trade in animals/animal products.
5) Expand surveillance to underserved communities.
6) Evaluate multiple sources of diagnostic and syndromic data in real time, using supercomputers when necessary with automated reporting to individuals responsible for health protection.
7) Include in One Health surveillance expert assessments of regional drivers, probabilities, impacts, and economic costs of defense preparedness, terrorism, conventional warfare, and nuclear warfare.
8) Co-train students preparing for careers in human and veterinary medicine, public health, conservation, agriculture, engineering, business, law, military service, international relations, and communications in core components of One Health, and assign One Health responsibilities to interdisciplinary teams of recent graduates.
9) Increase public recognition of One Health problems and solutions.

Similarly, the chapters on ecosystems (Chapter 6) and managed wildlife/zoos/aquariums (Chapter 9) stressed the importance of biodiversity and conservation education. Travis et al. (Chapter 6) described biodiversity as necessary "for the delivery of ecosystem services that are essential for human health." He and his co-authors described the need for characterizing relationships between universal patterns of system stressors and health outcomes. These themes were introduced by the authors of Chapter 5, which dealt with the One Health aspects of environmental toxicants. In their conclusion, the authors argued that the vast, but quickly diminishing, biodiversity of the Earth needs to be sustained to regulate our atmosphere and climate, as well as to produce soil, purify the land and water, regulate human and animal pests and pathogens, and provide the sense of awe in the majesty of nature.

Since the development of carbon-based polymers over 100 years ago, people, animals, and the environment have been exposed to many chemicals, most of which have never been tested for toxicity individually or in combination with other toxicants or natural exposures. Chapter 5 described an expanding body of evidence that links chemical exposures, especially those compounds that can be classified as endocrine-disrupting toxicants, to an expanding list of maladies, from cancers and obesity to developmental delays and anatomic abnormalities. Because of the pervasive exposure to plastic-based consumer products, it is impractical, if not impossible, to invoke the Precautionary Principle for every product on the market. However, the best strategy, quite possibly, is to avoid plastics as much as possible, especially in the preparation and serving of heated foods and beverages. The authors recommended that current renewable energy technologies must be promoted and even greater efficiencies pursued, that integrated pest management strategies must be employed to reduce the use of agricultural and residential pesticides, that further pollution controls must be enacted on the transportation sector while promoting "clean" technologies for vehicles, and finally, that the use of GPS-based conservation tillage techniques, cover crops, and vegetative buffer strips to prevent run-off of herbicides and pesticides into ground water becomes standard practice for agriculture. These approaches will require the collaboration of toxicologists, engineers, agronomists, urban planners, the public and politicians, as well as experts in architecture, public health, transportation, and communications.

With a world population projected to reach 9.8 billion in 2050, and 11.2 billion in 2100, (United Nations, 2017) having enough safe, nutritious food and potable water may be one of the greatest global challenges ever faced. Chapter 3 recognized the gains made in food safety through technological advances (genetic "fingerprinting" of pathogens, sharing of outbreak data across the globe) and through the efforts of the Food and Agricultural Organization of the United Nations, the World Health Organization, and the Global Food Safety Initiative, a non-governmental organization of private sector food safety experts designed to benchmark food supply efficiencies, information exchange, public awareness campaigns, and current food safety practices. However, challenges remain, and the authors recommend even greater surveillance and communication, across the entire food chain – production, harvest, processing, distribution, preparation, and consumption – and in the areas of foodborne illness, zoonotic diseases, and antimicrobial resistance. Among other topics, the chapter on water security (Chapter 4) described the risks to water security associated with climate change. Since water security is dependent not only on drinking water usage but also on diversion of water resources for energy and food production, drought and extreme weather events, already strongly associated with climate change, will challenge access to both sufficient quantity and acceptable quality of water for human usages. Indeed, as the authors conclude, balancing the demands of each component of the water/energy/food nexus will require a reduction in water and food waste, followed quickly by improvements in countries' abilities to reuse, recycle, and/or recover both food and water. Regional level solutions are most efficient but must be coordinated across utility and market sectors. The failure to do, the authors predict, can result in not only reduction in economic growth and quality of life but also civil unrest.

The skills, knowledge, and attitudes of leadership required to advance One Health thinking across countries and health issues were advocated in Chapter 10. The authors listed teamwork; interpersonal skills (including self-awareness, emotional intelligence, communications, and facilitation); critical thinking including systems and strategic thinking; and key knowledge as essential skills needed to effectively confront the "wicked problems" in One Health that we see today. Correspondingly, Chapter 13 suggested that we must do a better job of educating citizens in not only science, technology, engineering, and math (STEM) disciplines, but broadly in art, literature, history, civics, and other traditional subject areas that make up the classical "liberal" education. The author also suggested that we must improve our ability to communicate science findings and the iterative nature of the scientific method to the public. Lastly, the chapter supported community empowerment and participatory democracy as the sociopolitical structure that allows communities and individuals the level of self-determination necessary to live healthy and productive lives. The theme of Chapter 13 could be summarized as "educate, communicate, participate."

Even the casual reader should recognize that each of these chapters is interrelated, representing a sort of textual microcosm of the One Health concept. Climate change (Chapter 2) affects the ecosystem services (Chapters 6 and 9), which in turn affect food (Chapter 3) and water (Chapter 4), safety, and security. Incursions into previously undeveloped ecosystems to accommodate the increased demands of food production, and changing patterns of vector and pathogen distribution by latitude and altitude, determine exposures of humans and animals to novel infectious diseases (Chapters 7 and 8). Ecosystem services, as well as human and animal health, are diminished by long-term exposures to environmental toxicants (Chapter 5). Epidemiology (Chapter 1), and its sister, Critical Thinking (Chapter 13), are the approaches, along with the scientific method, used to study the associations between the exposures, detailed in Chapters 2 through 9, related to One Health challenges. Our ability to study, prevent, mitigate, respond, and recover from these challenges (e.g., accounting for the externalized costs of carbon-based energy production (Chapter 12)) depends upon the development of leadership skills (Chapter 10) and funding (Chapter 11) necessary to develop the surveillance data needed to study the epidemiology of acute and chronic diseases.

14.2 One Health Policy Development

Recognizing the rapid pace of technological advances, and of discovery in biological, chemical, and physical sciences, the American Association for the Advancement of Science, in the USA, inaugurated its first class of Science and Technology Policy Fellows in 1973 to "connect science with policy and foster a network of science and engineering leaders who understand government and policymaking, and are prepared to develop and execute solutions to address societal challenges" (AAAS, 2017). More than 3600 alumni have completed the program and many are still engaged in the public policy-making process. The need for individuals with science and technology training in policy work has never been more critical, as the science base and technological innovations increasingly provide fuel for the socioeconomic engine, to the extent that the study of public policy should be looked upon as a cognate subject with STEM disciplines. This is especially true for those problems that might best be resolved by incorporating One Health thinking.

14.2.1 Policy Basics and Challenges to Enacting One Health-based Policies

How does one operationalize the One Health concept? How do we move from "recognition to results?" This book has offered some real world examples of policies enacted in response to contemporary health challenges. Failure to adequately consider the impact of a policy on all three components of the One Health triad can result in unintended consequences for the forgotten components. So, what does One Health policy look like and how do we facilitate the development of policies and programs that embrace the One Health perspective? What obstacles must be overcome before One Health-focused policies and programs can become the norm rather than the exception?

Serious, meaningful policies are introduced for many reasons but, in the authors' experience, generally fall into three categories:

- Obvious need – for basic services such as water and sanitation, emergency services, food safety, infectious disease control, public safety.
- Public outcry – concern over product safety, social inequities, lack of basic services, violence, environmental contamination.
- Emergencies – immediate threats like natural and man-made disasters, civil strife, forced immigration, disease outbreaks.

Once the size and seriousness of a problem are identified and are thought amenable to policy intervention, the sponsors of a proposal must consider the three pillars of public policy:

- Content – what the proposed policy will and won't do and its short- and long-term consequences; its relevance to the community; its potential effectiveness and efficiency in accomplishing its goals; its inclusion of metrics to assess if its goals are attained in a reasonable time frame, if at all; its economic feasibility; its legality.
- Context – the social, economic, and political forces that support or oppose a policy proposal; the hurdles that may exist if the policy is adopted.
- Characters – the leadership, champions, advocates and lobbying groups for and against policy proposals.

Kingdon (1984) described the "policy window" that is only open to passage of new policy when three "streams" or "currents" are running together in the same direction: the *problem stream*, the *policy stream*, and the *politics stream*. A given public health issue, once recognized as important by advocates, may not gain any policy traction unless the problem is framed in a way that stimulates, among legislators and/or the citizenry, a sense of obvious need or public outrage (or at least significant interest), or approaches emergency status. The policy itself must be written with clarity and concision, with a background narrative that "grabs" its audience. It must be self-explanatory and easy to grasp. The proposal must be socially and culturally acceptable, and preferably revenue neutral, with any costs offset by short- or long-term savings. A policy proposal, especially one that is potentially contentious, needs a champion, preferably one who is charismatic and a gifted speaker. And, lastly, it is important to remember that when it comes to policy-making, inertia is a far more powerful force than consensus.

14.2.2 Microeconomic One Health Dilemmas

Effective implementation of the principles of One Health requires action at both the microeconomic and macroeconomic level. The microeconomic level takes place within our households and is determined by our personal spending power. The personal decisions we make drive the economy. We have the power to determine which products are available in the market and how they are produced, distributed, and recycled, reused, or land-filled.

Many readers are familiar with the concept of "carrots and sticks" in policy proposal writing: "carrots" are used to change behavior through incentives (tax credits or lower prices or some other reward) and "sticks" are used as disincentives (additional fees, higher prices, civil or criminal prosecution). In science policy, evidence developed over years of research often is not enough to push policy-makers and the public to support policy change that coincides with best available evidence. Ideological beliefs can persuade individuals to ignore best evidence to preserve preset biases, no matter how much evidence exists to the contrary. Often, policy advisers who have academic and experiential credentials in science, as well as science-based organizations, become frustrated with the policy-making process because so many issues for which the science is clear are value laden and fraught with ethical, social, and economic considerations at odds with the evidence.

An example is the widespread use of bottled water, and more specifically, water bottled in plastic containers. At least two One Health concerns emerge from their use: 1) the life cycle analysis of the plastic bottles, from manufacturing (carbon footprint) to disposal (land fill capacity, marine and ground water contamination, very low percentage recycled) clearly indicates the egregious environmental impacts of the product; and 2) the human and animal health impacts are no longer hypothetical (potential endocrine-disrupting chemical (EDC) and heavy metal exposure). Despite evidence that bottled water costs exponentially more than tap water, that much of bottled water is sourced from municipal tap water supplies, that taste tests show no advantage over bottled water, that bottled water is subject to a leachate of EDCs and heavy metals from the plastic containers, that plastic bottles take up significant land-fill space, and that only 9% of plastics have been recycled since the 1950s (Geyer et al., 2017), the public sees value in their availability. Communicating the science about the negative health and environmental impacts of plastic bottles to a public grown accustomed to reflexively purchasing and mindlessly discarding them requires incrementalism and patience. As Gostin (2014) wrote about policy directed at reducing the overweight/obesity global crisis, "Politics is the art of the possible, not the ideal." These are grand challenges and wicked problems, not because the evidence to support policy change is lacking, but because policy change is dependent upon drastically modifying value-laden consumer purchasing habits, habits that have been built over time through incessant and effective advertising by bottled water companies, many of which are also sugar, and sugar substitute, sweetened beverage companies.

Shaxson (2009) invoked Kingdon's policy window metaphor as she described the difficulty in approaching such nonlinear, unstructured policy questions: "Science Departments must engage with diverse audiences … in ways tailored for each audience. This means paying greater attention to the changing contexts in which information is received and used, and consequently the mechanisms required to produce and transfer scientific information. For policy audiences in particular, the relevance of the science to the issues of the day, and the crucial importance of timing, underline the need for interactive knowledge brokering approaches that can deliver synergistic combinations of 'science push' and 'policy pull'."

In the plastic bottle example above, proponents of reduced use of plastic bottled water, increased taxes on plastic bottles, or outright bans on their production or use are confronted with the macroeconomics of the manufacturers and distributors and the microeconomics of the end users. When it comes to research, surveillance, and programming to prevent, prepare, mitigate, and respond to infectious disease outbreaks, institutional rigidity, and once again, inertial resistance to policy change, are often encountered.

14.2.3 One Health Research in Emerging Infectious Diseases: Macroeconomic Dilemmas

Even though One Health is about much more than zoonotic diseases, emerging infectious diseases are still a major focus of One Health strategies. Besides the challenges inherent in unstructured, "wicked" problems, we, at least in the USA, place additional hurdles in front of attempts to tackle grand challenges through a One Health motif.

The macroeconomic level is where much of the spending of public tax dollars occurs. The challenges to incorporating the principles of One Health into the allocation of tax dollars may prove to be more entrenched than changing the spending habits of consumers. Implementation of One Health policies and programs requires an interdisciplinary approach to problem solving. Subject matter experts working independently on different aspects of a problem must also work in collaboration with colleagues using a coordinated approach to problem solving. This is in contrast to current funding structures in the USA, in which human health issues are considered in isolation from livestock production, wildlife, or environmental issues, and livestock production issues are considered in isolation from human health, wildlife, and environmental issues (see Chapter 11). Similarly, stakeholders focused on environmental health policy are often at odds with those focused on agricultural production. However, as we have seen in the preceding chapters, many of the current challenges facing policy-makers today occur at the intersection between humans, animals, and the environment. Actions taken on behalf of one sector will impact all three.

How do we get these disparate stakeholder groups to move from working at cross-purposes to working together? How can we enact policies that benefit all of the One Health triad? Reorganization of institutions can be a slow and painful process in which little innovation takes place during the transition period. Rather than attempting to dismantle the silos and institutions that serve different stakeholders, rewarding those who can work effectively between silos and across institutions, will facilitate more rapid progress toward achieving measurable results. One approach that will foster working across subject matter and institutional silos for true interdisciplinary collaboration is for the agencies and institutions that fund research and programmatic activities to evaluate and score proposals though a One Health lens. Whether it is a legislative body considering a new regulation or a review panel evaluating a research or education grant proposal, a One Health approach can be taken in determining which proposals to prioritize for funding.

One method for achieving this is to require that proposal developers conduct a qualitative or quantitative risk assessment of the potential impact of their program or policy on humans, animals, and the environment. This risk assessment should include strategies for mitigation of potential unintended harm to the sectors that are not the focus of the intervention. A second method for facilitating the implementation of programs, research, and policies that are consistent with a One Health perspective is to prioritize funding to those efforts that seek to address more than one component of the triad. Policy-makers, researchers, and program developers should seek to benefit at least two populations: human and animal, animal and environment, or human and environment. Highest priority should be given to policies and activities that seek to enhance the health of all three. In the private sector, the Bill and Melinda Gates Foundation offered grant funding, in 2013, that approached these ideals (Gates Foundation, 2013). But that program, as well as similar programs funded by the federal government, should be the standard rather than the exception.

14.2.4 The Long and Winding Road Forward

In 1971, in support of the second Earth Day in the USA, the cartoonist Walt Kelly invoked the central tenet of environmental stewardship: that we humans are the major cause of environmental degradation. The opossum Pogo, after walking through a forest littered with trash, says to his friend, Porkypine, "We have met the enemy and he is us." A series of fires on the Cuyahoga river, in Cleveland, culminating in the infamous fire of 1969, was just one of many events that led to public outcry loud enough to spawn the modern day movement to clean up our world for present and future generations (Rotman, 2010). In 1978, the appalling health impacts on residents of the Love Canal, NY, housing development, from toxic chemicals leaching into ground, was reported (Beck, 1979). In 1982, the residents of Times Beach, MO, faced a similar fate, that time from dioxin contamination of their land (Hamilton, 2010). In retrospect, many of the chemicals and the levels common in the environment 50 years ago seem shocking now. However, environmental tragedies are not relegated to the past. In 2015, the city of Flint, MI, in a cost-saving move, changed their water supply from Lake Huron to the Flint River, long considered an industrial waterway. Soon after the switch, the city was informed by the US Environmental Protection Agency (EPA) that their water supply had levels of lead that exceeded federal limits by factors of 7 to 20 times (CNN, 2017; EPA, 2017).

Rivers aflame, soil and groundwater contaminated with toxicants, air that you can see – these are all One Health problems. There can be no doubt that we have met and mitigated many threats to ecosystems since that cartoon was first published. Current environmental protections are much stronger, at federal, state, and local levels, than in the past despite recent challenges from the present US administration. And air and water quality in the USA has improved dramatically over the past four decades (Table 14.1). This progress has not been limited to the USA. Over the same time period there have been global efforts to conserve and protect natural resources and more recently to mitigate the impact of climate change. Individual countries, international bodies, and multinational organizations have implemented environmental protection policies and regulations. See Table 14.2 for examples of environmental policies from the European Union, United Nations, and China.

However, the environmental challenges that we face today are perhaps the most daunting and most critical in the history of human civilization. When it comes to climate change, we cannot just blame corporations, many of which are multinational, for One Health problems spawned by extreme weather events, rising sea levels, and elevated temperatures. Corporations that supply the consumption-based economy simply give consumers what they think they want at a price they are willing to pay within the freedom and constraints that our politicians develop for them. We have to look within. We have to take individual responsibility for our environments.

Much of our current extraction-production-distribution-consumption-disposal systems are linear and at odds with the cyclical systems found in nature. Although the dramatic growth in clean energy, especially energy derived from solar technologies that are becoming more cost effective almost monthly, is a step in the right direction, we still have much work to do to account for the true cost of the production, use, and disposal of consumer products, from the smallest trinkets to the largest durables. We cannot separate the business of providing for the wants and needs of a growing population from the social determinants of health and from environmental degradation. Wealth based on the depletion of the very resources that created that wealth is not a sustainable business plan. A focus on infinite growth in the current linear production systems is not possible unless the Earth itself, and its carrying capacity, keeps growing. We need nothing short of a revolution in thinking about an economy based on consumption. The entrepreneur, consultant, and author, Paul Hawken, said it best: "The single greatest flaw of modern accounting is that the cost and losses of destroying the earth are absent from the prices in the marketplace" (Hawken, 2010).

Just as we cannot achieve a sustainable, restorative economy without accounting for the true cost of all of the facets of industrial production, we won't be able to effectively address difficult One Health problems until we account for the true cost of not doing so. A comprehensive, fully integrated, open and effective One Health surveillance system will be expensive, but what will those costs be, in human lives lost, ecosystems diminished, and biodiversity decreased, if we do not do appropriate the necessary funds for such a system? There should be little debate about the contention that the rich countries of the world need to make sure that all member countries of the World Health Organization (WHO) can build the physical and professional infrastructure necessary to rapidly and effectively respond to outbreaks of infectious disease. How many thousands of people have

Table 14.1 Timeline of environmental milestones – USA.

1970	20 million people celebrate the first Earth Day
	President Richard Nixon establishes the US Environmental Protection Agency (EPA) with the mission to protect the environment and public health
	Congress amends the Clean Air Act to set national standards for air quality, auto emission, and anti-pollution
1971	Congress restricts lead-based paint in homes and on cribs and toys
1972	EPA bans DDT, a cancer-causing pesticide, and requires review of all pesticides
	USA and Canada agree to clean up the Great Lakes, which contain 95% of America's fresh water and supply 25 million people with drinking water
	Congress passes the Clean Water Act, limiting raw sewage and other pollutants flowing into lakes, rivers, and streams
1973	EPA begins phasing out lead in gasoline
	EPA issues its first permit limiting a factory's polluted discharges into waterways
1974	Congress passes the Safe Drinking Water Act, allowing EPA to regulate the quality of public drinking water
1975	Congress establishes fuel economy and tail-pipe emission standards for cars, resulting in the introduction of catalytic converters
1976	Congress passes the Resource Conservation Act, regulating hazardous waste from its production to its disposal
	President Gerald Ford signs the Toxic Substances Control Act to reduce environmental and human health risks
	EPA begins phase-out of cancer-causing PCB production and use
1977	President Jimmy Carter signs Clean Air Act amendments to strengthen air quality standards and protect human health
1978	Federal government bans chlorofluorocarbons (CFCs) as propellants in aerosol cans because they destroy the ozone layer
1979	EPA demonstrates scrubber technology for removing air pollution from coal-fired power plants, and the technology becomes widely adopted in the 1980s
	Three Mile Island nuclear power plant accident near Harrisburg, PA, spurs awareness and discussion about nuclear power safety. EPA and other agencies monitor the radioactive fallout
1980	Congress creates Superfund to clean up hazardous waste sites, but polluters are responsible for the most hazardous sites
1981	National Research Council report finds acid rain intensifying in the northeastern USA and Canada
1982	Congress passes laws for safe disposal of nuclear waste
1983	Start of cleanup actions on the Chesapeake Bay to eliminate pollution from sewage treatment plants, urban runoff, and farm waste
	EPA encourages homeowners to test for radon gas, which causes lung cancer
1985	Scientists report that a giant hole in the Earth's ozone layer opens each spring over Antarctica
1986	Congress declares the public has a right to know when toxic chemicals are released into air, land, and water
1987	USA signs the Montreal Protocol, pledging to phase out CFC production
	EPA's "Unfinished Business" report compares relative risk of environmental challenges for the first time
1988	Congress bans ocean dumping of sewage sludge and industrial waste
1989	Exxon Valdez spills 11 million gallons of crude oil into Alaska's Prince William Sound and Exxon is fined $1 billion for the spill

(Continued)

Table 14.1 (Continued)

1990	Congress passes Clean Air Act amendments requiring states to demonstrate progress in air quality improvements
	EPA's Toxic Release Inventory tells which pollutants are being released from specific facilities in communities
	President George Bush signs the Pollution Prevention Act, emphasizing the importance of preventing –not just correcting – environmental damage
	President George Bush signs the National Environmental Education Act, showing the importance of environmental education for scientifically sound, balanced, and responsible decisions
1991	Federal agencies begin using recycled content products
	EPA launches voluntary industry partnership programs for energy efficient lighting and reducing toxic chemical emissions
1992	EPA launches the ENERGY STAR® Program to help consumers identify energy efficient products
1993	EPA reports secondhand smoke contaminates indoor air, posing health risks for nonsmokers
	President Bill Clinton directs the federal government to use its $200 billion annual purchasing power to buy recycled and environmentally preferable products
1994	EPA launches the Brownfields Program to clean up abandoned, contaminated sites to return them to productive use
	EPA issues new standards for chemical plants to reduce toxic air pollution by more than half a million tons each year – the equivalent of taking 38 million vehicles off the road annually
1995	EPA launches an incentive-based acid rain program to reduce sulfur dioxide emissions
	EPA requires municipal incinerators to reduce toxic emission by 90% from 1990 levels
1996	Public drinking supplies are required to inform customers about chemicals and microbes in their water, and funding is made available to upgrade water treatment plants
	EPA requires that home buyers and renters be informed about lead-based paint hazards
	President Bill Clinton signs the Food Quality Protection Act to tighten standards for pesticides used to grow food, including special protections to ensure that foods are safe for children
1997	An Executive Order is issued to protect children from environmental health risks, including childhood asthma and lead poisoning
	EPA issues new air quality standards for smog and soot, an action that improves air quality for 125 million Americans
1998	President Bill Clinton announces the Clean Water Action Plan to continue making waterways safe for fishing and swimming
1999	President Bill Clinton announces new emissions standards requiring cars, sport utility vehicles, minivans, and trucks to be 77–95% cleaner than in 1999
	EPA announces new requirements to improve air quality in national parks and wilderness areas
2000	EPA establishes regulations requiring more than 90% cleaner heavy duty highway diesel engines and fuel
	National Performance Track program is launched to recognize facilities that exceed legal requirements to make measurable environmental progress
2002	President George W. Bush signs the Small Business Liability Relief and Brownfields Revitalization Act to reclaim and restore thousands of abandoned properties
	Clear Skies Initiative and alternative regulations are proposed to keep a "cap and trade" system to reduce SO_2 emissions by 70% and NOx emissions by 65% below current levels
2003	EPA proposes the first ever mercury emissions regulations on power plants
	EPA provides funds for more than 4000 school buses to be retrofitted through the Clean Bus USA program, removing 200 000 pounds of particulate matter from the air over the next 10 years

Table 14.1 (Continued)

2004	New, more protective, 8-hour ozone and fine particulate standards go into effect across the nation
	EPA requires cleaner fuels and engines for off-road diesel machinery such as farm or construction equipment
2005	EPA issues the Clean Air Act Interstate Rule to achieve the largest reduction in air pollution in more than a decade, by permanently capping SO_2 and NOx emissions in the eastern USA
2006	EPA's WaterSense program is created to protect the future water supply with practical ways to use less water
	EPA issues the Ground Water Rule to reduce the risk of contamination in public water systems that use ground water
2007	BP Products North America, Inc. agrees to pay the largest criminal fine to date for air violations, including a $62 million criminal fine plus $400 million on safety upgrades. The penalty was for a 2005 refinery explosion that killed 15 and the 2006 oil spill on the Alaskan tundra, which violated the Clean Air and Water Acts
2008	Stronger lead standards require a tenfold decrease in lead levels
2009	President Barack Obama announces a program that sets the nation's first ever greenhouse gas emission standards for cars
	President Barack Obama signs an Executive Order recognizing the Chesapeake Bay as an important ecosystem and calling the federal government to lead a renewed effort to restore and protect it and its watershed
2010	EPA proposes stricter health standards for smog
	The BP-operated Deepwater Horizon oil rig in the Gulf of Mexico explodes, killing 11 workers and releasing about 4.9 million barrels of crude oil, the largest spill in US history
	President Obama signs an Executive Order forming the Gulf Coast Ecosystem Restoration Task Force, which will coordinate efforts to implement restoration programs and projects in the region
	EPA finalizes a run on the greenhouse gas reporting requirements for facilities that use geological sequestration
	EPA establishes a Chesapeake Bay "pollution diet" to reduce nitrogen, phosphorus, and sediment from the surrounding area to put needed pollution controls in place by 2025
2011	EPA proposes a national standard for mercury pollution from power plants, requiring many to install pollution control technologies to cut emissions
	Next generation of fuel economy labels unveiled
	First national standards for mercury pollution from power plants
2012	EPA updates air pollution standards for oil and natural gas
	EPA proposes first carbon pollution standard for new power plants
	Obama administration finalizes historic 54.5 mpg fuel efficiency standards
	EPA strengthens air standards for fine particles, reducing harmful soot pollution
	New clean air standards for industrial boilers, incinerators, and cement kilns
2013	President Obama announces a climate change strategy focusing on preparing for the effects of climate change, cutting carbon pollution in the USA, and providing international technical assistance
2014	The new "Tier 3" standards, which consider the vehicle and its fuel as an integrated system, set new vehicle emissions standards and lower the sulfur content of gasoline, beginning in 2017
	First guidelines proposed to cut carbon pollution from existing power plants
2016	President Obama signed the Frank R. Lautenberg Chemical Safety for the 21st Century Act, which updates the Toxic Substances Control Act

Adapted from www.epa.gov and http://www.naem.org/?CP_COMP_milestones.

Table 14.2 Summary of international environmental legislation.

Decade	International events	European Union	China
1970s	1972: UN Conference on The Human Environment (Stockholm, Sweden) It was the UN's first major conference on international environmental issues, and marked a turning point in the development of international environmental politics[a]	1973–1976: First Environmental Action Programme (EAP) The first EAP listed 11 Environmental Principles and issued a series of directives focused on air quality, water standards, waste disposal, and noise pollution, many of which were based on existing Dutch and German legislation. This EAP tightly defined pollution standards in areas where the need for action could be readily defended 1977–1981: The Second EAP – focused on international cooperation. Standards on water quality were strengthened and extended. Regulations on dangerous substances were included. For the first time directives covering habitats, endangered bird species, and nature conservation were included in the EAP	1979: First Environmental Protection Law – focused on environmental pollution control due to increasing serious pollution problems
1980s		1982–1986: Third EAP – focused on integrating environmental considerations into other policy areas. It was noted that the new environmental legislation had not been matched with enforcement efforts 1986: The Single European Act – previous regulations of EAPs had been enacted despite the lack of language in the EU treaties giving EU officials the authority to do so. In 1986 environmental matters were formally incorporated into the European Union 1987–1992: The Fourth EAP – a more holistic approach to environmental policy. It created an international task force to investigate the environmental impact of the single market. This report described a "slow but relentless deterioration in Europe's environmental quality" (Bailey, 2017). It concluded that the existing environmental policies had failed to adequately address the environmental problems caused by European Union integration	1983: The Marine Environment Protection Law 1984: Law on Prevention and Control of Water Pollution and Forestry Law 1985: Grassland Law 1986: Fisheries Law, Mineral Resources Law, and Land Administration Law 1987: Law on Prevention and Control of Atmospheric Pollution 1988: Water Law and Law on Protection of Wildlife 1989: Law on Urban and Rural Planning

1990s	1992: UN Conference on Environment and Development – the "Earth Summit" (Rio de Janeiro, Brazil) "Twenty years after the first global environment conference, the UN sought to help Governments rethink economic development and find ways to halt the destruction of irreplaceable natural resources and pollution of the planet"[b] It resulted in two legally binding conventions – the Framework Convention on Climate Change (FCCC) and the Convention on Biological Diversity	1993–2009: Fifth EAP – focused on sustainable development. It concluded that legislation alone is not sufficient to achieve long-term ambitions of sustainable development. More flexible instruments such as environmental taxes and charges, tradable permits, and voluntary agreements are also needed. It identified six issues needing special attention: 1) Sustainable management of natural resources 2) Integrated pollution control and waste prevention 3) Decreased consumption of nonrenewable energy 4) Increased mobility management 5) Urban sustainability 6) Increased public health and safety	1991: Law on Water and Soil Conservation 1993: Surveying and Mapping Law 1996: Law on Prevention and Control of Environmental Pollution by Solid Waste, Electric Power Law, and Law on the Coal Industry 1997: Law on Prevention and Control of Environmental Noise Pollution 1998: Flood Control Law, Law on Energy Conservation, and Law on Protecting Against and Mitigating Earthquake Disasters
2000s	2005: The United Nations Framework Convention on Climate Change (UNFCCC) Kyoto Protocol takes effect – an international agreement that sets internationally binding greenhouse gas emission reduction targets		2000: Meteorology Law 2002: Law on Prevention and Control of Desertification and Law on Administration of the Use of Sea Areas 2003: Law on the Promotion of Cleaner Production, Law on Evaluation of Environmental Effects, and Law on Prevention and Control of Radioactive Pollution 2006 Renewable Energy Law 2009 Law on Promotion of Circular Economy

(Continued)

Table 14.2 (Continued)

Decade	International events	European Union	China

2010s	2016: The UNFCCC Paris Agreement takes effect. It has been described as "the world's first comprehensive climate agreement."[d] It addresses emissions mitigation, adaptation to climate change, and finance	2010–2013: Sixth EAP – "Environment 2010: Our Future, Our Choice" – commends the substantial progress made while also reviewing the ongoing problems and challenges. It continues the focus on sustainable development and the use of flexible policy instruments introduced in the Fifth EAP. It takes a strategic approach to reaching a wider constituency with the participation of all sectors of society. Influenced by the UN Rio Summit in 1992 it sets new priorities:
		
		• Climate Change
		• Nature and Biodiversity
		• Environment and Health
		• Natural Resources and Waste
		
		2014–2020: The Seventh EAP[c] – identifies three key objectives:
		
		• to protect, conserve and enhance the Union's natural capital
		• to turn the Union into a resource-efficient, green, and competitive low-carbon economy
		• to safeguard the Union's citizens from environment-related pressures and risks to health and wellbeing
			2010: Law on the Protection of Offshore Islands
			
			2015: New Environmental Protection Law – described as the most strict environmental legislation in China (Mu et al., 2014).
			
			Three innovations are embodied in this law:
			
			1) Legislative concept:
			  a) This is the fundamental and comprehensive law on the environment in China
			  b) Sustainable Development is a guiding value of the legislation
			  c) Prioritizing Environmental Protection is a basic national policy – requiring that economic development should coordinate with environmental protection
			
			2) Administrative mechanism:
			  a) Multiple governance: government, enterprises, and citizens share the burden of environmental protection
			  b) The public is granted rights of environmental information, knowledge, participation, and supervision
			
			3) Legal approach:
			  The government responsibility for environmental protection is emphasized with periodic supervision and evaluation

a) https://sustainabledevelopment.un.org/milestones/humanenvironment
b) http://www.un.org/geninfo/bp/enviro.html
c) http://ec.europa.eu/environment/action-programme/
d) https://www.cbsnews.com/news/us-china-enter-climate-change-deal/

to die or have their quality of life diminished before we act? The former Swedish Ambassador to the USA and former President of the United Nations General Assembly, Jan Eliasson, commented at a luncheon in Washington DC in 2003: "Without passion, nothing gets done. Without compassion, the wrong things get done" (J. Eliasson, personal communication, 2003).

Even the most ideological reader should be able to put aside his/her prejudices long enough to realize that these humanitarian and environmental justifications for appropriations of substantial sums of money to prevent disease outbreaks and protect the planet are also good business and good policy. In an analysis of the world's response to the Ebola virus disease outbreak in West Africa, Bill Gates issued a global call to action to handle epidemics, centered around a better warning and response system, not only because it is the right thing to do but also because it is essential for our national security. It also makes efficient and therefore, good, business sense (Gates, 2015). It was mentioned earlier in the book that we have allowed, at least in the USA, the framing of environmental protections and the provision of universal health care access as liberal policy proposals that are at odds with a strong economy. Rather than pitting liberal and conservative political ideologies against one another when discussing policy, we need to reframe these prevention-based issues, appropriately, as both: the true conservative approaches that will save money in the long term, while doing the right thing in the short term. Prevention is a fiscally conservative approach that speaks to socially liberal ideals.

Geoffrey Vickers, while serving as Secretary of the Medical Research Council in the UK half a century ago, identified the forces that set the agenda for public health; Vickers noted: "The landmarks of political, economic and social history are the moments when some condition passed from the category of the given into the category of the intolerable. I believe that the history of public health might well be written as a record of successive re-definings of the unacceptable" (Vickers, 1958). Perhaps it is only when we redefine our personal consumption habits, and the short-term profit-seeking by the corporations that we support, as "intolerable" and "unacceptable" that we will be able finally to move the One Health concept from recognition to results.

References

AAAS (American Association for the Advancement of Science) (2017). History. Available at: https://www.aaas.org/about/mission-and-history (accessed August 21, 2017).

Bailey, I. (2017). *New Environmental Policy Instruments in the European Union: Politics, Economics, and the Implementation of the Packaging Waste Directive.* Taylor & Francis.

Beck, E.C. (1979). The Love Canal tragedy. *EPA Journal.* Available at: https://archive.epa.gov/epa/aboutepa/love-canal-tragedy.html (accessed August 14, 2017).

CNN (Cable News Network) (2017). Flint water crisis fast facts. *CNN Library.* Available at: http://www.cnn.com/2016/03/04/us/flint-water-crisis-fast-facts/index.html (accessed August 14, 2017).

EPA (Environmental Protection Agency) (2017). Flint drinking water response. Available at: https://www.epa.gov/flint (accessed August 12, 2017).

Gates, B. (2015). The next epidemic – lessons from Ebola. *N Engl J Med* 372, 1381–1384.

Gates Foundation (2013). The One Health Concept: Bringing Together Human and Animal Health for New Solutions (Round 11). Global Grand Challenges, The Bill and Melinda Gates Foundation. Available at: https://gcgh.grandchallenges.org/challenge/

one-health-concept-bringing-together-human-and-animal-health-new-solutions-round-11 (accessed August 23, 2017).

Geyer, R., Jambeck, J.R., and Law, K.L. (2017). Production, use, and fate of all plastics ever made. *Science Advances* 3(7), e1700782. doi: 10.1126/sciadv.1700782.

Gostin, L. (2014). Limiting what we can eat: A bridge too far? *The Milbank Quarterly* 92(2), 173–176.

Hamilton, J. (2010). A chemical conundrum: how dangerous is dioxin? *Morning Edition*, National Public Radio. Available at: http://www.npr.org/2010/12/28/132368362/a-chemical-conundrum-how-dangerous-is-dioxin (accessed August 10, 2017).

Hawken, P. (2010). *The Ecology of Commerce* (revised edn). New York, NY: Harper Business, HarperCollins.

Kingdon, J.W. (1984). *Agendas, Alternatives, and Public Policies*. Boston: Little, Brown.

Mu, Z., Bu, S., and Xue, B. (2014). Environmental legislation in China: achievements, challenges and trends. *Sustainability* 6(12), 8967–8979.

Nelson, G. (1970). *Face the Nation* [transcript]. CBS NEWS. Available at: http://www.nelsonearthday.net/docs/nelson_157-3_face_the_nation_transcript_19Apr70.pdf (accessed July 13, 2017).

Rotman, M. (2010). Cuyahoga River Fire. Cleveland Historical. Available at: https://clevelandhistorical.org/items/show/63 (accessed August 23, 2017).

Shaxson, L. (2009). Structuring policy problems for plastics, the environment and human health: reflections from the UK. *Philos Trans R Soc Lond B Biol Sci* 364(1526), 2141–2151.

Uchtmann, N., Herrmann, J.A., Hahn, E.C., and Beasley, V.R. (2015). Barriers to, efforts in, and optimization of integrated One Health surveillance: a review and synthesis. *EcoHealth* 12(2) 368–384.

United Nations (2017). World population projected to reach 9.8 billion in 2050, and 11.2 billion in 2100. United Nations Department of Economic and Social Affairs. Available at: https://www.un.org/development/desa/en/news/population/world-population-prospects-2017.html (accessed August 16, 2017).

Vickers, G. (1958). What sets the goals of public health? *Lancet* 271(7021), 599–604.

Index

Note: Page numbers in **bold** indicate tables and those in *italics* indicate figures

Beyond One Health: From Recognition to Results, First Edition.
Edited by John A. Herrmann and Yvette J. Johnson-Walker.
© 2018 John Wiley & Sons, Inc. Published 2018 by John Wiley & Sons, Inc.